Dietary Supplements and Nutraceuticals: A Textbook

Edited by

Mukesh Singh Sikarwar
Amity Institute of Pharmacy
Amity University, Gwalior
Madhya Pradesh
India

Arunachalam Muthuraman
& Sohrab A. Shaikh
Pharmacology, Toxicology and
Basic Health Sciences Unit
Faculty of Pharmacy
AIMST University
Semeling, Bedong, Kedah
Malaysia

Dietary Supplements and Nutraceuticals: A Textbook

Editors: Mukesh Singh Sikarwar, Arunachalam Muthuraman & Sohrab A. Shaikh

ISBN (Online): 979-8-89881-399-4

ISBN (Print): 979-8-89881-400-7

ISBN (Paperback): 979-8-89881-401-4

First published in 2026.

need for a court order if at any point you breach any terms of this License Agreement. In no event will any delay or failure by Bentham Science Publishers in enforcing your compliance with this License Agreement constitute a waiver of any of its rights.

3. You acknowledge that you have read this License Agreement, and agree to be bound by its terms and conditions. To the extent that any other terms and conditions presented on any website of Bentham Science Publishers conflict with, or are inconsistent with, the terms and conditions set out in this License Agreement, you acknowledge that the terms and conditions set out in this License Agreement shall prevail.

Bentham Science Publishers Pte. Ltd.
No. 9 Raffles Place
Office No. 26-01
Singapore 048619
Singapore
Email: subscriptions@benthamscience.net

BENTHAM SCIENCE

CONTENTS

FOREWORD

In today's world, the spectrum of medicine is wide, and innovations are the driving force for the pharmaceutical industry. Nutrition and lifestyle are now equally important as medicine, especially in the case of non-communicable and lifestyle-related diseases. Due to a sedentary lifestyle and its related obesity, chronic conditions like hypertension, cardiovascular disease, and diabetes are on the rise. Nutraceuticals can provide a promising solution to prevent and manage these conditions by combining traditional wisdom with modern science. Nutraceuticals bridge the gap between nutrition and medicine, offering innovative solutions for enhancing well-being.

This book explores the diverse realm of dietary supplements and nutraceuticals, which includes water and fat soluble vitamins, carbohydrates, proteins, micronutrients including zinc, chromium, CoQ10, iodine, selenium, good fat including DHA and EPA, prebiotics, probiotics, various phytochemicals like carotenoids, resveratrol, diallyl sulfides, flavonoids, isoflavones, and rice bran. This book highlights the source, chemistry, applications, and benefits of different nutraceuticals while emphasizing the importance of rigorous standards according to WHO guidelines for assessing the quality of herbal medicines.

Whether you are a healthcare professional, researcher, curious reader, or student, the insights shared by the authors in this book will deepen your understanding of the role of nutraceuticals and dietary supplements in holistic health. May this book inspire you to embrace the potential of nutraceuticals for a healthier future.

SNR. ASSOC. PROF. DR. Sundram M. Karupiah
B.Sc (Hons), MSc (Pharmacy), Ph.D (USM)
AIMST University DU010(K)
Batu 3 1/2, Bukit Air Nasi
Jalan Bedong Semeling, 08100 Bedong
Kedah, Malaysia

Preface

The beginning of an AI and data analytics-driven society is around the corner, and personalized medicine is being revolutionized with innovations. Science-supported health solutions and tailored medicine are on the rise. Before the Human Genome Project, the field of personalized medicine was limited due to the lack of comprehensive genetic information. Changes in gene expressions by environmental factors, including behaviour and food, play key roles in disease development; hence, epigenetics influenced by diet and nutrition shall be considered and addressed in health clinics. Genomic and metabolic profiling can identify individual needs for micronutrient optimization in personalized nutrition. Nutrigenomics is an emerging area that is grounded in molecular biology and studies the interaction of dietary components with the genome; however, in India, Ayurgenomics, originating from the ancient Indian system of medicine Ayurveda, combines the traditional wisdom with genomic insight, recommending key interventions based on diet, lifestyle, and herbal drugs.

Dietary supplements and nutraceuticals play a key role in the management of various diseases. Non-Communicable Diseases (NCDs) are burdened with high oxidative stress due to chronic low-grade inflammation, and such interconnected biological processes are central to the pathogenesis and progression of many NCDs, including cardiovascular diseases, diabetes, cancer, and neurodegenerative disorders. Therapeutic strategies to combat oxidative stress and inflammation include dietary antioxidants and dietary supplements in an anti-inflammatory diet. Micronutrients are the cofactors of enzymes essential for various biochemical pathways. For example, in Cardiovascular Diseases (CVDs), magnesium regulates blood pressure by modulating calcium channels, and selenium is a cofactor for glutathione peroxidase, protecting from oxidative stress and atherosclerosis. Chromium improves insulin action, and zinc supports insulin synthesis in the management of impaired glucose tolerance, insulin resistance, and inflammation. In bone health, calcium and vitamin D are essential for bone mineralization, and magnesium is a cofactor for enzymes regulating bone metabolism.

Vitamin-based nutraceuticals prevent oxidative damage and modulate inflammation, especially in Non-Communicable Diseases (NCDs) and age-related conditions. Vitamins also act as cofactors for enzymes and antioxidants. Short-chain fatty acids produced by gut bacteria play a key role in neuro-immunoendocrine regulation, and these fatty acids can also prevent the growth of pathogenic microorganisms. Modulation of neurochemical pathways through the highly interconnected gut-brain axis has also recently been recognized. Prebiotics may influence the metabolism of minerals by increasing their solubility and absorption. Nutraceuticals for prophylactic and therapeutic purposes are often developed with rigorous clinical research to ensure efficacy and safety in addressing specific health conditions.

Combining dietary supplements through a synergistic approach maximizes their potential to enhance health and manage or prevent diseases. The synergistic approach focuses on bioactive compound interaction to amplify their combined effects rather than individual effects. Ingredients like Shatavari root and ashwagandha are highly regarded in traditional medicine for their adaptogenic properties to help manage stress, reduce hot flashes and night sweats, and maintain hormonal balance. The amino acid L-theanine promotes relaxation, calming, and better sleep, addressing anxiety-driven menopause symptoms. A combination of such products could bring greater relief in menopause symptoms than individual products.

This textbook aims to equip students and researchers with updated information in the field of nutraceuticals. As implied in the title, the dietary supplements, and nutraceuticals, this textbook gives comprehensive knowledge on different dietary supplements and nutraceuticals. This book displays the description of antioxidants, vitamins, macro & micronutrients, essential fatty acids, pre & probiotics, phytochemicals, herbal drugs, and synergistic & clinical nutraceuticals. It focuses on detailed descriptions of selected crude drugs potentially used as dietary supplements and nutraceuticals. This textbook is an easy guide for students and scholars from different domains of health sciences.

As we progress toward precision wellness and the concept of personalized nutrition, this book can be handy in dealing with plant proteins, microalgae-based supplements, probiotics, omega-3, and fermented ingredients to support gut health, cognitive function, and heart health supplements. Challenges such as supply chain transparency, digital health integration, and regulatory compliance will remain areas for further discussion.

Editors would like to extend their heartfelt appreciation to all the authors and contributors who have contributed their time and wisdom in completing this book.

Special thanks to Humaira Hashmi, editorial manager of publications, Bentham Books, for her generous assistance in coordinating throughout the book publication.

Editors are open to suggestions for improvement of this work.

Mukesh Singh Sikarwar
Amity Institute of Pharmacy
Amity University, Gwalior
Madhya Pradesh
India

&

Arunachalam Muthuraman & Sohrab A. Shaikh
Pharmacology, Toxicology and
Basic Health Sciences Unit
Faculty of Pharmacy
AIMST University
Semeling, Bedong, Kedah
Malaysia

Dedication

Thank you to all co-authors for their valuable contributions & support in making this book product for undergraduates & research students, and educators. We are also thankful to Faculty members of Pharmacy, AIMST University, Malaysia, and Amity Institute of Pharmacy, Amity University Madhya Pradesh, Gwalior, Madhya Pradesh, India for their unconditional support. This book is dedicated to Pharmacy students, budding researchers & scientists who are working in this field of research.

List of Contributors

Arunachalam Muthuraman	Pharmacology, Toxicology, and Basic Health Sciences Unit, Faculty of Pharmacy, AIMST University, Bedong 08100, Kedah, Malaysia
Khian Giap Lim	Clinical Pharmacy and Pharmacy Practice Unit, Faculty of Pharmacy, AIMST University, Jalan Bedong-Semeling, Bedong 08100, Kedah, Malaysia
Muthusamy Ramesh	Department of Pharmaceutical Analysis and Quality Assurance, Institute of Pharmaceutical Sciences, Sandip Foundation, Nashik 422213, India
Maulshree Bhandari	Invertis Institute of Pharmacy, Invertis University, Bareilly, Uttar Pradesh, India
Mukesh Singh Sikarwar	Amity Institute of Pharmacy, Amity University, Gwalior, Madhya Pradesh, India
Nallupillai Paramakrishnan	Department of Pharmacognosy, JSS College of Pharmacy, JSS Academy of Higher Education and Research, Mysuru 570015, Karnataka, India
Nazmun Nahar Alam	Faculty of Medicine, AIMST University, Bedong 08100, Kedah, Malaysia
Sumitha Elayaperumal	Department of Biotechnology and Bioinformatics, JSS Academy of Higher Education and Research, Mysore, Karnataka, India
Sohrab A. Shaikh	Pharmacology, Toxicology, and Basic Health Sciences Unit, Faculty of Pharmacy, AIMST University, Bedong 08100, Kedah, Malaysia
Vaibhav Kumar Rathi	Department of Pharmacy, Quantum University, Roorkee (Haridwar), Uttarakhand, India
Yamunna Paramaswaran	Faculty of Pharmacy, AIMST University, Jalan Bedong-Semeling, Bedong 08100, Kedah, Malaysia
Venkata Rathina Kumar Thigarajan	Department of Pharmacognosy, College of Pharmacy, Madurai Medical College, Madurai, 625020, India
Yuvaraj Sivamani	Department of Pharmaceutical Chemistry, Crescent School of Pharmacy, B.S. Abdur Rahman Crescent Institute of Science and Technology, Vandalur, 600048, Chennai, Tamil Nadu, India

CHAPTER 1

Introduction of Dietary Supplements and Nutraceuticals for the Healthcare System

Arunachalam Muthuraman[1,*] and **Sohrab A. Shaikh**[1]

[1] *Pharmacology, Toxicology, and Basic Health Sciences Unit, Faculty of Pharmacy, AIMST University, Bedong 08100, Kedah, Malaysia*

Abstract: Dietary supplements like vitamins, minerals, and herbs, and other products (macronutrients, essential fatty acids, prebiotics, and probiotics) are widely used for various ailments and to improve health status. The evidence of these dietary supplements' action in health benefits is not clear. Hence, the acceptance of these agents as medicine is not recognized in various countries. Moreover, cellular oxidative stress is very common in metabolic and other chronic disorders. However, the common actions of dietary supplements, *i.e.*, free radical scavengers, energy production, and regulation of cellular functions, are well known and reported. Besides, it is identified as safer, has beneficial effects, and has minimal side-effect-causing agents. However, a clear correlation between dietary supplements and nutraceuticals in the clinical Healthcare system. Hence, this book chapter reveals the beneficial effect of dietary supplements in the management of metabolic and inflammatory disorders, along with the correlation of their antioxidant potential.

Keywords: Amino acids, Free radical scavenger, Growth hormone, Non-enzymatic antioxidants, Oil supplements.

INTRODUCTION

Dietary Supplements are essential to maintain the Healthcare system. It is added to conventional food to improve the healthy physiological system [1]. It also reduces the health risks of various diseases. However, the U.S.A. Food and Drug Administration (FDA) is not authorized to review dietary supplement products for safe and effective use in the Healthcare system [2]. Before the intake of dietary supplements, it is necessary to consult healthcare consultants because sometimes dietary supplements can cause potentially unwanted effects [3]. Crucially, a healthy balance between foods and nutrients is needed to consider better health

* **Corresponding author Arunachalam Muthuraman:** Pharmacology, Toxicology, and Basic Health Sciences Unit, Faculty of Pharmacy, AIMST University, Bedong 08100, Kedah, Malaysia; E-mail: muthuraman.a@aimst.edu.my

Mukesh Singh Sikarwar, Arunachalam Muthuraman & Sohrab A. Shaikh (Eds.)

benefits and maintain the healthcare system [4]. Dietary supplements cover minerals, vitamins, herbs, and amino acids, including enzymes [5]. Worldwide, dietary supplements are widely used for ingestible products, and they are distinguishable from conventional foods and drugs. Further, the United States defined that dietary supplements (except tobacco) are products intended to be dietary supplements with one or more of the additional ingredients like minerals, vitamins, herbs, herbal extracts, amino acids, and metabolites [6, 7]. Besides, dietary products like multivitamins, garlic tablets, fish oil capsules, probiotics, natural weight-loss aids, and some kinds of energy drinks are also considered dietary supplements. Further, the dietary supplements are mostly for oral administration [8, 9].

Dietary Supplements

The dietary supplements of marketed products are available in the form of powders, liquids, capsules, tablets, gel caps, and soft gels. Further, dietary supplements should not include chemical compounds like approved drugs or licensed biological products [10]. Mostly, dietary supplements are not intended to be used for the treatment, cure, mitigation, and prevention of any type of disease [7, 11]. In addition, it is not to be viewed as a substitute for conventional medications for any disease. Regulatory bodies outline that dietary supplements are any food products that differ from conventional foods. However, the supplementary products exhibit health benefits and rarely have undesirable side effects [12]. Of course, the side effects are reversible and tolerable [13]. Paradoxically, drugs can cause potential adverse effects, which can be irreversible [14]. Moreover, the dietary supplements must be safe and effective for health and physiological action. Other than in the USA and some other countries, dietary supplements are considered botanical formulations and drugs [15]; and they are proven safe and sold without any prescriptions, like extracts of the Eastern purple coneflower (*Echinacea purpurea*). It is commonly used for the improvement of the healthy immune system [16].

Dietary supplements also provide measurable health benefits. However, clinical usage remains a scientific debate. In conclusion, the general public receives mixed forms of information from the dietary supplement industry and the scientific community of the healthcare system [17]. Significant scientific evidence is still valid for the support, *i.e.*, the role vitamins and minerals play in maintaining a good healthcare system. Moreover, the major questions are the safety and efficacy of vitamins [18]. However, vitamin E and vitamin D are shown to possess remarkable therapeutic actions for the prevention of a variety of chronic diseases [13, 19]. The health claims of botanical dietary supplements remain less convincing. The additional issue of dietary supplement efficacy is the inconsistency and variability of product quality [1]. Furthermore, dietary supplements are often subject to adulteration, and prescribed products may be contaminated with heavy metals and/or pathogenic microbes [20 - 22].

Even though some of the botanical dietary products are strongly considered for the treatment of medicine, such as Saint-John's wort used for depression, anxiety, tiredness, trouble sleeping, and loss of appetite [23, 24]. Hormones like ghrelin are secreted by adipose tissue and influence the hunger and appetite process of the gastrointestinal system [25]. The neuropeptide Y is produced in the brain and used as an appetite stimulant. Besides, melanocyte-stimulating hormones, insulin, and leptin are also used as appetite suppressants by acting on the hypothalamus region of the brain [26, 27]. Some dietary supplements have adequate amounts of essential nutrients and it is important for the improvement of overall health benefits like calcium and vitamin D produce strong bones and reduce bone loss; folic acid decreases the risk of certain birth defects; omega-3 fatty acids of fish oils help to treat the heart disease; and combination of vitamins C and E, zinc, copper, lutein, and zeaxanthin improve the age-related macular degeneration associated vision loss [28, 29]. The class of dietary supplements, examples, and health benefits are tabulated in Table **1**.

Table 1. Class of dietary supplements, examples, and their health benefits.

Class	Example	Health Benefits
Amino acids	Growth hormone and other hormones	Growth activation. Gaining weight [30].
Carbohydrate	Dextrose	Electrolyte balance. Cell growth. Enhance the natural anabolic effect [31].
Food and Foodstuff	Fish oils, carrots, garlic, royal jelly, and yeast (contain minerals and vitamins).	Improves neurovascular health and immune functions [32].
Herbals	Ginseng, Fiber (Contains amino acids, Chicoric acid, and alkylamides) *Allium sativum* (contains Allicin, adenosine *Ginkgo biloba* (contains ginkgolides)	Improves cellular amino acid and protein synthesis. Imuno-stimulants Anti-hypertension. Memory improvements [33].
Minerals	Selenium, multi-mineral.	Enhance the metabolic activity *via* catalytic actions [34].
Multivitamins and Multi-minerals	Vitamin D, calcium.	Improves the visual function. Enhance bone strength [35].

(Table 1) cont.....

Class	Example	Health Benefits
Oil supplements	Cod liver oil, primrose oil (Contains oil base, vitamins, and minerals)	Improves the brain and cardiovascular health [36].
Vitamins	Vitamin C, vitamin B (Essential micronutrients)	Essential micronutrient for cell growth and metabolism [37].

Nutraceuticals

Nutraceutical products are alternatives to biopharmaceutical agents, and they have physiological benefits. The major issues of nutraceutical use are unregulated and exist like dietary supplements and food additives [38, 39]. Nutraceutical products are derived from various food sources, and they have basic nutritional value and provide additional health benefits [40]. These products are known to prevent chronic inflammatory diseases and improve the healthcare system. Nutraceuticals are also called functional foods. It is fortified, enriches the content during processing, and provides limited benefits [38, 41]. However, some additional nutrients, like vitamin D in milk, are also added to nutraceutical products. Generally, nutraceuticals are classified as functional foods, medical foods, designer foods, phytochemicals, and nutritional supplements [42, 43]. Furthermore, these products cover vitamins, diets, herbal products, and genetically engineered foods. It has the potential to produce physiological benefits and prevent disease due to its high concentration of bioactive compounds [44, 45]. Recently, nutraceuticals also covered the daily foods category, *i.e.*, prebiotics, probiotics, processed foods, fortified cereals, and beverages [46]. The definition of nutraceuticals varies from country to country based on their regulation [40]. There is no internationally accepted definition for nutraceutical products [47]. Generally, nutraceuticals are employed in the prevention of cardiovascular disease, diabetes, cancer, and obesity disorders [48].

"Functional foods" is a term used to describe any food or food ingredients that provide basic nutritional value and also offer beneficial effects on disease prevention. Functional foods look like food and it is available as yogurt, snacks, cereal, whole grains, and pasta [49, 50]. The classification of functional foods can be two categories 1) Traditional functional food: It is a nutrient-rich natural food and delivers potential health benefits like omega-3 fatty acids nutrients in salmon food and lycopene nutrients in tomatoes; and 2) Non-traditional functional food: is artificial food. It is prepared by adding additional bioactive components to enhance health and well-being like juice mixed with calcium solution, cereal fortified with irons, and flour mixed with folic acid [51].

These modified functional foods also include recombinant nutraceuticals like yogurt, cheese, bread, and vinegar made with biotechnology techniques [52]. Experimentally, nutraceuticals produce therapeutic effects in diabetes mellitus, obesity, cardiovascular diseases, eye disorders, gastrointestinal disorders, renal disorder, viral infections, Alzheimer's disease, and Parkinson's diseases, including cancer *via* regulation of multiple biological processes like free radical scavenging action, regulates the cell proliferation, improves the healthy gene expression, and maintains the cellular and mitochondrial membrane integrity [53 - 55].

Free Radicals and Associated Clinical Conditions

Free radicals are molecules containing an unpaired electron in their exterior orbit, allowing them to bond with unpaired electrons in other molecules and biological particles, and exhibiting a high level of reactivity [56, 57]. During energetic metabolism, living cells continuously generate free radicals, *i.e.*, Reactive Oxygen Species (ROS). The human body has several inherent ways to counteract oxidative stress, such as producing antioxidants or eating antioxidant-containing foods and supplements. However, when there is an excess of free radicals in the body, oxidative stress occurs. Oxidative stress arises when free radicals outweigh the antioxidative system's ability to neutralize them. Arthritis, arteriosclerosis, cancer, and neurological diseases are now understood to emerge as a result of cumulative tissue damage produced by free radicals [57 - 59].

Clinical Conditions

Disease and oxidative stress-free radicals attack key biological components such as carbohydrates, proteins, lipids, and DNA, all of which are linked to a variety of pathological illnesses, including aging, cancer, cardiovascular disease, diabetes, ischemia, neurological disorders, and other diseases [59, 60]. Table **2** indicates the diseases that are induced due to oxidative stress [61].

Table 2. Oxidative stress-related disorders in humans.

Vital Organs	Clinical Conditions
Lungs	Chronic bronchitis and asthma.
Kidneys	Chronic renal failure and glomerulonephritis.
Brain	Alzheimer's disease, Parkinson's disease, stroke, memory loss, and depression.
Eyes	Cataract.
Heart	Hypertension, arteriosclerosis, ischemia, cardiomyopathy, and heart failure.
Multi-organ	Aging, diabetes, cancer, inflammation, and infection.

Antioxidants

Living organisms have numerous strategies to combat oxidative stress by producing endogenous antioxidants; however, exogenous antioxidants can be obtained through meals [60]. An antioxidant is a substance that binds to free radicals and renders them harmless [62]. Antioxidants are compounds that inhibit oxidation. An antioxidant is currently defined as a substance that can eliminate Reactive Oxygen Species (ROS) and their derivatives (reactive nitrogen species, RNS, or reactive sulfur species, RSS), either directly or indirectly, acting as a defender against oxidative stress or an inhibitor of reactive species production [63]. The primary strategies underpinning antioxidant therapy are agents that boost these defenses. Significant research on antioxidant enzyme stimulation has focused on understanding the regulatory mechanisms and their implications in various diseases [64]. Food and medicinal plants contain a wealth of natural antioxidants. Among these, polyphenols and carotenoids stand out, offering numerous biological advantages such as anti-aging, anti-inflammatory, anticancer, and anti-atherosclerosis properties [65]. Antioxidants obtained from regularly consumed vegetables, cereals, fruits, beverages, and other dietary items, including substances like α-tocopherol (Vitamin E), ascorbic acid (Vitamin C), polyphenols, and carotenoids, have the potential to enhance the body's antioxidative defense mechanisms [66]. The equilibrium of ROS and antioxidants in the body is regulated by the antioxidant systems, *i.e.*, non-enzymatic and enzymatic, which are Glutathione Peroxidase (GPX), Superoxide Dismutase (SOD), Catalase (CAT), lipid-soluble vitamin E, water-soluble vitamin C, and carotenes. Conversely, dietary antioxidants, predominantly sourced from vegetables and fruits, are associated with maintaining a favorable equilibrium between free radicals and antioxidant levels. This equilibrium plays a role in reducing oxidative stress and the associated risks of cardiovascular disease, cancer, and aging [63]. Table **3** indicates the antioxidants classification [59, 67].

Table 3. Antioxidants classification.

<table>
<tr><th colspan="2">Enzymatic Anti-Oxidants</th><th>Non-Enzymatic Anti-Oxidants</th></tr>
<tr><td>Primary enzymes</td><td>Secondary enzymes</td><td rowspan="2">1. Vitamin A, C, E, and K.
2. Polyphenols (Flavonoids, and Phenolic acids).
3. Carotenoids (lycopene, β-carotene, zeaxanthin, and lutein).
4. Antioxidant co-factor (Co-enzyme Q_{10}).
5. Thiol antioxidants.
6. Minerals (Zn, and Se).
7. Melatonin.</td></tr>
<tr><td>1. Superoxide dismutase
2. Catalase
3. Glutathione peroxidase</td><td>1. Glucose 6-phosphate
2. Dehydrogenase glutathione reductase</td></tr>
</table>

Future Directions

Currently, scientists and health professionals agree to use dietary supplements for the improvement of health benefits. However, it should not replace the usage of the drug completely and balance daily meals of food substances [68]. The dietary supplements market is also claimed to improve the health and well-being of the customer. However, the exact benefits are variable from person to person. Crucially, the use of regular drugs and dietary supplements provides physiological or pharmacological effects, and it can cause adverse effects in susceptible individuals [38]. However, more attention is required to the adverse effects and potential interactions to get a better therapeutic outcome [69]. However, self-prescription of dietary supplements should be avoided for patients with old age, pregnant women, young persons, and people living with disabilities [70, 71]. Healthcare practitioners must analyze the patient's history and provide informed guidance regarding the use of dietary supplementation. The overall features of dietary supplements and nutraceuticals have been illustrated in Fig. (**1**).

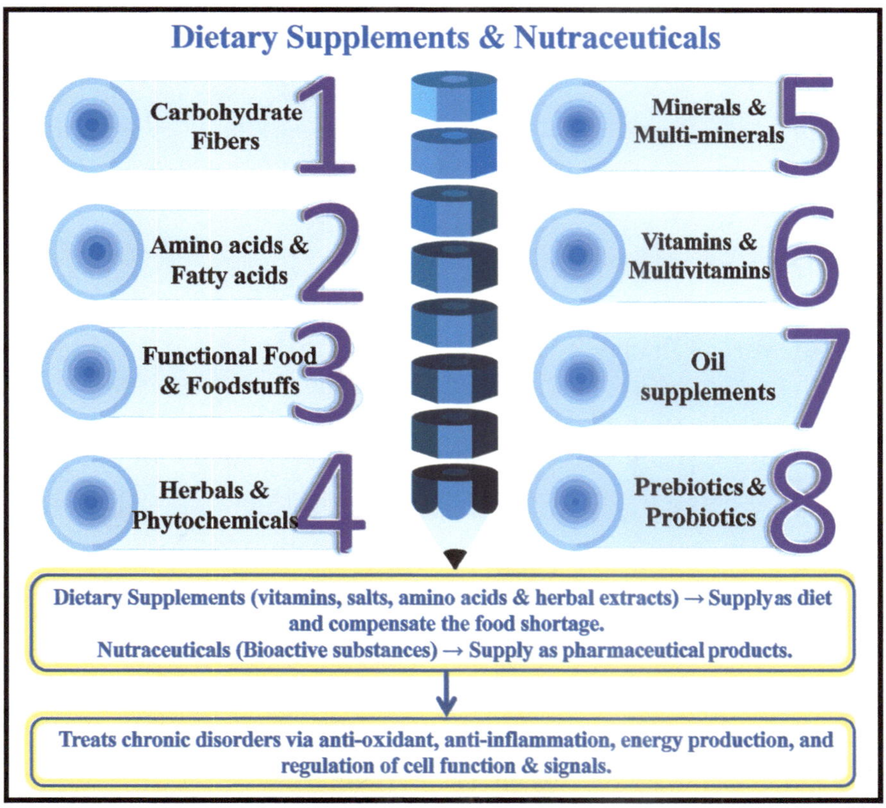

Fig. (1). The overall features of dietary supplements and nutraceuticals.

SUMMARY

Dietary supplements are employed for various health benefits. However, the exact mechanism is not clear, and it is not recognized as a drug in various countries. It is also called nutraceuticals and functional food for the treatment of various disorders. It is employed as a free radical scavenger, for energy production, and as a cellular functional regulator. Cellular oxidative stress is very common in metabolic and various chronic disorders, as it produces safer, beneficial effects and minimal side effects. Hence, dietary supplements are useful for the management of inflammatory disorders due to their antioxidant potential for the reduction of oxidative stress. The various perspectives on nutraceutical effects and their health benefits are discussed in various chapters of this book.

CASE STUDIES AND PRACTICE QUESTIONS

Case 1: *A 62-year-old woman with a previous medical history of significant pre-diabetes, hypertension, hyperlipidemia (HLD), and obesity presented to her primary care physician after a routine six-month follow-up study. She recently became more proactive and had a Myocardial Infarction (MI). In addition to reducing her red meat consumption and walking in the evening, she started taking Red Yeast Rice (RYR) as a dietary supplement. Her clinical report revealed that RYR benefits in lowering cholesterol. She is interested in learning what can lower her risk for future Cardiovascular Disease (CVD), like MI.*

Discussion Questions

a. What is the role of the RYR in the treatment of MI?
b. Explain the mechanism of action of RYR for the treatment of MI.
c. What is the connection of HMG-CoA reductase in the pathogenesis of MI?
d. List the dietary supplements and nutraceuticals' usefulness for this patient.

Case 2: *A 50-year-old male patient has Hashimoto's thyroiditis. His clinical report showed low levels of serum selenium and hypothyroidism.*

Discussion Questions

a. What are the major symptoms reported to selenium deficiency in Hashimoto's thyroiditis?
b. How is selenium important for the functioning of the thyroid gland?
c. What is the connection between selenium deficiency and immune function?
d. Do selenium supplements support thyroid hormone and immune functions?

e. Daily dietary requirement of selenium for healthy thyroid function.

Case 3: *A 40-year-old male patient has fewer incidences of MI. He has taken cod liver oil with regular exercise. The relative risk for total MI incidence was 0.70 (0.44-1.10).*

Discussion Questions

a. What is the major role of cod liver oil for the management of MI?
   a. If cod liver oil can reduce the MI.
b. What are the factors that can cause the pathogenesis of MI?
   a. How can cod liver oil regulate the cardiovascular system?
c. What are the health benefits and mechanisms involved in cardiovascular health?

MCQs Questions

1. Which one of the following trace elements present in tea prevents tooth decay?
   A. Fluoride
   B. Zinc
   C. Copper
   D. Selenium

2. Which one of the following foods is NOT a functional food?
   A. Dietary fiber
   B. Probiotics
   C. Omega-3 polyunsaturated fatty acids
   D. Pills or capsules as part of a daily diet

3. Which one of the following modern methods of extraction of nutraceuticals is based on the acoustic cavitation phenomenon?
   A. Microwave-Assisted Extraction
   B. Ultrasonic-assisted extraction
   C. Enzyme-assisted extraction
   D. Supercritical extraction

4. Which one of the following nutraceuticals has 3-hydroxyphenylpropionic acid as a major dietary metabolite?
   A. Tea extract
   B. Coffee extract
   C. Soybean extract
   D. Grape seed proanthocyanidin extract

5. Which one of the following vitamins is absent in milk?
   A. A
   B. B
   C. C
   D. D

Answers: 1) A; 2) D; 3) B; 4) D; 5) C

REFERENCES

[1] Chen Y, Hamidu S, Yang X, *et al.* Dietary supplements and natural products: an update on their clinical effectiveness and molecular mechanisms of action during accelerated biological aging. Front Genet 2022; 13: 880421.
[http://dx.doi.org/10.3389/fgene.2022.880421] [PMID: 35571015]

[2] Bailey RL. Current regulatory guidelines and resources to support research of dietary supplements in the United States. Crit Rev Food Sci Nutr 2020; 60(2): 298-309.
[http://dx.doi.org/10.1080/10408398.2018.1524364] [PMID: 30421981]

[3] Al-Shatnawi SF, Khasawneh RA, Alhamad H. Healthcare providers' perspectives toward the integration of over the counter supplements during covid-19 pandemic: a cross-sectional study from jordan. Inquiry : a journal of medical care organization, provision and financing 2022; 59: 469580221095825.

[4] Malek L, Umberger WJ, Zhou SJ, Huynh E, Makrides M. Testing the impact of familiarity with health benefits information on dietary supplement choice in pregnancy: an online choice experiment. Nutrients 2022; 14(9): 1707.
[http://dx.doi.org/10.3390/nu14091707] [PMID: 35565674]

[5] Meuffels FM, Isenmann E, Strube M, Lesch A, Oberste M, Brinkmann C. Exercise interventions combined with dietary supplements in type 2 diabetes mellitus patients—a systematic review of relevant health outcomes. Front Nutr 2022; 9: 817724.
[http://dx.doi.org/10.3389/fnut.2022.817724] [PMID: 35356737]

[6] Tan ECK, Eshetie TC, Gray SL, Marcum ZA. Dietary supplement use in middle-aged and older adults. J Nutr Health Aging 2022; 26(2): 133-8.
[http://dx.doi.org/10.1007/s12603-022-1732-9] [PMID: 35166304]

[7] Wierzejska RE. Dietary supplements—for whom? the current state of knowledge about the health effects of selected supplement use. Int J Environ Res Public Health 2021; 18(17): 8897.
[http://dx.doi.org/10.3390/ijerph18178897] [PMID: 34501487]

[8] Pomeroy DE, Tooley KL, Probert B, Wilson A, Kemps E. A systematic review of the effect of dietary supplements on cognitive performance in healthy young adults and military personnel. Nutrients 2020; 12(2): 545.
[http://dx.doi.org/10.3390/nu12020545] [PMID: 32093203]

[9] Brisebois M, Kramer S, Lindsay KG, Wu CT, Kamla J. Dietary practices and supplement use among CrossFit® participants. J Int Soc Sports Nutr 2022; 19(1): 316-35.
[http://dx.doi.org/10.1080/15502783.2022.2086016] [PMID: 35813850]

[10] Hoseini AS, Dehdari T, Solhi M, Janani L, Rahideh ST. Development of an instrument to measure dietary supplement health literacy. Health Lit Res Pract 2022; 6(2): e159-66.
[http://dx.doi.org/10.3928/24748307-20220523-02] [PMID: 35680121]

[11] Crawford C, Avula B, Lindsey AT, *et al.* Analysis of select dietary supplement products marketed to support or boost the immune system. JAMA Netw Open 2022; 5(8): e2226040.
[http://dx.doi.org/10.1001/jamanetworkopen.2022.26040] [PMID: 35947382]

[12] Mah E, Chen O, Liska DJ, Blumberg JB. Dietary supplements for weight management: a narrative review of safety and metabolic health benefits. Nutrients 2022; 14(9): 1787. [http://dx.doi.org/10.3390/nu14091787] [PMID: 35565754]

[13] Mangione CM, Barry MJ, Nicholson WK, *et al.* Vitamin, mineral, and multivitamin supplementation to prevent cardiovascular disease and cancer. JAMA 2022; 327(23): 2326-33. [http://dx.doi.org/10.1001/jama.2022.8970] [PMID: 35727271]

[14] Kozhuharov VR, Ivanov K, Ivanova S. Dietary supplements as source of unintentional doping. BioMed Res Int 2022; 2022(1): 8387271. [http://dx.doi.org/10.1155/2022/8387271] [PMID: 35496041]

[15] Dou J, Weathers P. Specialty molecules from plants and *in vitro* cultures as new drugs: regulatory considerations from flask to patient. Plant Cell Tissue Organ Cult 2022; 149(1-2): 105-11. [http://dx.doi.org/10.1007/s11240-022-02287-4] [PMID: 35345535]

[16] Senica M, Mlinsek G, Veberic R, Mikulic-Petkovsek M. Which plant part of purple coneflower (*Echinacea purpurea* (l.) moench) should be used for tea and which for tincture? J Med Food 2019; 22(1): 102-8. [http://dx.doi.org/10.1089/jmf.2018.0026] [PMID: 30222488]

[17] Lordan R. Dietary supplements and nutraceuticals market growth during the coronavirus pandemic – Implications for consumers and regulatory oversight. PharmaNutrition 2021; 18: 100282. [http://dx.doi.org/10.1016/j.phanu.2021.100282] [PMID: 34513589]

[18] Wang Z, Li WT, Gao Y, *et al.* Analysis of dietary supplement use and influencing factors in the mongolian population. BioMed Res Int 2022; 2022(1): 4064588. [http://dx.doi.org/10.1155/2022/4064588] [PMID: 35360520]

[19] Virtanen JK, Nurmi T, Aro A, *et al.* Vitamin D supplementation and prevention of cardiovascular disease and cancer in the Finnish Vitamin D Trial: a randomized controlled trial. Am J Clin Nutr 2022; 115(5): 1300-10. [http://dx.doi.org/10.1093/ajcn/nqab419] [PMID: 34982819]

[20] Dwyer J, Coates P, Smith M. Dietary supplements: regulatory challenges and research resources. Nutrients 2018; 10(1): 41. [http://dx.doi.org/10.3390/nu10010041] [PMID: 29300341]

[21] Jairoun AA, Shahwan M, Zyoud SH. Heavy metal contamination of dietary supplements products available in the uae markets and the associated risk. Sci Rep 2020; 10(1): 18824. [http://dx.doi.org/10.1038/s41598-020-76000-w] [PMID: 33139833]

[22] Crawford C, Walter AR, Avula B, *et al.* Relative safety and quality of various dietary supplement products U.S. Service Members ask about. Clin Toxicol (Phila) 2022; 60(6): 737-44. [http://dx.doi.org/10.1080/15563650.2022.2036751] [PMID: 35156875]

[23] Khan A, Chauhan K, Ross H, *et al.* A comprehensive review on the use of herbal dietary supplements in the usa, reasons for their use, and review of potential hepatotoxicity. Livers 2022; 2(3): 119-38. [http://dx.doi.org/10.3390/livers2030011]

[24] Klemow KM, Bilbow E, Grasso D, Jones K, McDermott J, Pape E. Medical attributes of St. John's wort (Hypericum perforatum). Oxidative Stress and Disease 2004; 14: 757-80.

[25] Leone A, De Amicis R, Pellizzari M, Bertoli S, Ravella S, Battezzati A. Appetite ratings and ghrelin concentrations in young adults after administration of a balanced meal. Does sex matter? Biol Sex Differ 2022; 13(1): 25. [http://dx.doi.org/10.1186/s13293-022-00434-2] [PMID: 35659737]

[26] Rezitis J, Herzog H, Ip CK. Neuropeptide Y interaction with dopaminergic and serotonergic pathways: interlinked neurocircuits modulating hedonic eating behaviours. Prog Neuropsychopharmacol Biol Psychiatry 2022; 113: 110449. [http://dx.doi.org/10.1016/j.pnpbp.2021.110449] [PMID: 34592387]

[27] Obradovic M, Sudar-Milovanovic E, Soskic S, *et al.* Leptin and obesity: role and clinical implication. Front Endocrinol (Lausanne) 2021; 12: 585887. [http://dx.doi.org/10.3389/fendo.2021.585887] [PMID: 34084149]

[28] Bischoff-Ferrari HA, Freystätter G, Vellas B, *et al.* Effects of vitamin D, omega-3 fatty acids, and a simple home strength exercise program on fall prevention: the DO-HEALTH randomized clinical trial. Am J Clin Nutr 2022; 115(5): 1311-21. [http://dx.doi.org/10.1093/ajcn/nqac022] [PMID: 35136915]

[29] Pellegrini M, Senni C, Bernabei F, *et al.* The role of nutrition and nutritional supplements in ocular surface diseases. Nutrients 2020; 12(4): 952. [http://dx.doi.org/10.3390/nu12040952]

[30] Ranke MB, Wit JM. Growth hormone — past, present and future. Nat Rev Endocrinol 2018; 14(5): 285-300. [http://dx.doi.org/10.1038/nrendo.2018.22] [PMID: 29546874]

[31] Robba C, Rosenstein I, Bilotta F. Fluid and electrolytes management in children undergoing neurosurgery. Fundamentals of Pediatric Neuroanesthesia 2021; 165-77. [http://dx.doi.org/10.1007/978-981-16-3376-8_10]

[32] Gombart AF, Pierre A, Maggini S. A review of micronutrients and the immune system–working in harmony to reduce the risk of infection. Nutrients 2020; 12(1): 236. [http://dx.doi.org/10.3390/nu12010236] [PMID: 31963293]

[33] Abebe W. Review of herbal medications with the potential to cause bleeding: dental implications, and risk prediction and prevention avenues. EPMA J 2019; 10(1): 51-64. [http://dx.doi.org/10.1007/s13167-018-0158-2] [PMID: 30984314]

[34] Kieliszek M, Bano I, Zare H. A comprehensive review on selenium and its effects on human health and distribution in middle eastern countries. Biol Trace Elem Res 2022; 200(3): 971-87. [http://dx.doi.org/10.1007/s12011-021-02716-z] [PMID: 33884538]

[35] Chan H-N, Zhang X-J, Ling X-T, *et al.* Vitamin D and ocular diseases: a systematic review. Vol. 23. Int J Mol Sci 2022.

[36] Al-Okbi SY, Mohammed SE, Al-Siedy ESK, Ali NA. Fish oil and primrose oil suppress the progression of alzheimer's like disease induced by aluminum in rats. J Oleo Sci 2020; 69(7): 771-82. [http://dx.doi.org/10.5650/jos.ess20015] [PMID: 32522946]

[37] Tardy AL, Pouteau E, Marquez D, Yilmaz C, Scholey A. Vitamins and minerals for energy, fatigue and cognition: a narrative review of the biochemical and clinical evidence. Nutrients 2020; 12(1): 228. [http://dx.doi.org/10.3390/nu12010228] [PMID: 31963141]

[38] Chandra S, Saklani S, Kumar P, Kim B, Coutinho HDM. Nutraceuticals: pharmacologically active potent dietary supplements. BioMed Res Int 2022; 2022(1): 2051017. [http://dx.doi.org/10.1155/2022/2051017] [PMID: 35832855]

[39] Das D, Banerjee A, Bhattacharjee A, Mukherjee S, Maji BK. Dietary food additive monosodium glutamate with or without high-lipid diet induces spleen anomaly: A mechanistic approach on rat model. Open Life Sci 2022; 17(1): 22-31. [http://dx.doi.org/10.1515/biol-2022-0004] [PMID: 35128066]

[40] Chopra AS, Lordan R, Horbańczuk OK, *et al.* The current use and evolving landscape of nutraceuticals. Pharmacol Res 2022; 175: 106001. [http://dx.doi.org/10.1016/j.phrs.2021.106001] [PMID: 34826602]

[41] Radziszewska M, Smarkusz-Zarzecka J, Ostrowska L, Pogodziński D. Nutrition and supplementation in ulcerative colitis. Nutrients 2022; 14(12): 2469. [http://dx.doi.org/10.3390/nu14122469] [PMID: 35745199]

[42] Gonçalves AC, Nunes AR, Flores-Félix JD, Alves G, Silva LR. Cherries and blueberries-based

beverages: functional foods with antidiabetic and immune booster properties. Molecules 2022; 27(10): 3294.
[http://dx.doi.org/10.3390/molecules27103294] [PMID: 35630771]

[43] Damián MR, Cortes-Perez NG, Quintana ET, *et al.* Functional foods, nutraceuticals and probiotics: a focus on human health. Microorganisms 2022; 10(5): 1065.
[http://dx.doi.org/10.3390/microorganisms10051065] [PMID: 35630507]

[44] De Conno B, Pesce M, Chiurazzi M, *et al.* Nutraceuticals and diet supplements in crohn's disease: a general overview of the most promising approaches in the clinic. Foods 2022; 11(7): 1044.
[http://dx.doi.org/10.3390/foods11071044] [PMID: 35407131]

[45] Asif M, Mohd I. Prospects of medicinal plants derived nutraceuticals: A re-emerging new era of medicine and health aid. Progress in Chemical and Biochemical Research 2019; 2(4): 150-69.

[46] Küçükgöz K, Trząskowska M. Nondairy probiotic products: functional foods that require more attention. Nutrients 2022; 14(4): 753.
[http://dx.doi.org/10.3390/nu14040753] [PMID: 35215403]

[47] Aronson JK. Defining 'nutraceuticals': neither nutritious nor pharmaceutical. Br J Clin Pharmacol 2017; 83(1): 8-19.
[http://dx.doi.org/10.1111/bcp.12935] [PMID: 26991455]

[48] Casula M, Catapano AL, Magni P. Nutraceuticals for dyslipidaemia and glucometabolic diseases: what the guidelines tell Us (and Do Not Tell, Yet). Nutrients 2022; 14(3): 606.
[http://dx.doi.org/10.3390/nu14030606] [PMID: 35276964]

[49] Baker MT, Lu P, Parrella JA, Leggette HR. Investigating the effect of consumers' knowledge on their acceptance of functional foods: a systematic review and meta-analysis Foods (Basel, Switzerland) 2022; 11(8): 1116.

[50] Poutanen KS, Kårlund AO, Gómez-Gallego C, *et al.* Grains – a major source of sustainable protein for health. Nutr Rev 2022; 80(6): 1648-63.
[http://dx.doi.org/10.1093/nutrit/nuab084] [PMID: 34741520]

[51] Topolska K, Florkiewicz A, Filipiak-Florkiewicz A. Functional food—consumer motivations and expectations. Int J Environ Res Public Health 2021; 18(10): 5327.
[http://dx.doi.org/10.3390/ijerph18105327] [PMID: 34067768]

[52] Zapaśnik A, Sokołowska B, Bryła M. Role of lactic acid bacteria in food preservation and safety Foods (Basel, Switzerland) 2022; 11(9): 1283.
[http://dx.doi.org/10.3390/foods11091283]

[53] Iranshahy M, Javadi B, Sahebkar A. Protective effects of functional foods against Parkinson's disease: A narrative review on pharmacology, phytochemistry, and molecular mechanisms. Phytother Res 2022; 36(5): 1952-89.
[http://dx.doi.org/10.1002/ptr.7425] [PMID: 35244296]

[54] Senesi P, Ferrulli A, Luzi L, Terruzzi I. Diabetes mellitus and cardiovascular diseases: nutraceutical interventions related to caloric restriction. Int J Mol Sci 2021; 22(15): 7772.
[http://dx.doi.org/10.3390/ijms22157772] [PMID: 34360538]

[55] Lewis Luján LM, McCarty MF, Di Nicolantonio JJ, *et al.* Nutraceuticals/drugs promoting mitophagy and mitochondrial biogenesis may combat the mitochondrial dysfunction driving progression of dry age-related macular degeneration. Nutrients 2022; 14(9): 1985.
[http://dx.doi.org/10.3390/nu14091985] [PMID: 35565950]

[56] Di Meo S, Venditti P. Evolution of the knowledge of free radicals and other oxidants. Oxid Med Cell Longev 2020; 2020: 1-32.
[http://dx.doi.org/10.1155/2020/9829176] [PMID: 32411336]

[57] Yaribeygi H, Maleki M, Sathyapalan T, Jamialahmadi T, Sahebkar A. Antioxidative potentials of incretin-based medications: a review of molecular mechanisms. Oxid Med Cell Longev 2021; 2021(1):

9959320.
[http://dx.doi.org/10.1155/2021/9959320] [PMID: 34007411]

[58] Dutta S. Generation and mode of action of free radicals and oxidative stress with special emphasis on health and disease prevention. J Indian Dent Assoc 2021; 42(1): 48-54.

[59] Iannitti T, Iannitti T, Palmieri B. Antioxidant therapy effectiveness: an up to date. Eur Rev Med Pharmacol Sci. 2009 Jul-A.... Eur Rev Med Pharmacol Sci 2009; 13.

[60] Pham-Huy LA, He H, Pham-Huyc C. Free radicals, antioxidants in disease and health. Int J Biomed Sci 2008; 4(2): 89-96.
[http://dx.doi.org/10.59566/IJBS.2008.4089] [PMID: 23675073]

[61] Pham-Huy LA, He H, Pham-Huy C. Free radicals, antioxidants in disease and health. Int J Biomed Sci. 2008; 4(2): 89-96.
[http://dx.doi.org/10.59566/IJBS.2008.4089] [PMID: 23675073] [PMCID: PMC3614697]

[62] Veurink G, Perry G, Singh SK. Role of antioxidants and a nutrient rich diet in Alzheimer's disease. Open Biol 2020; 10(6): 200084.
[http://dx.doi.org/10.1098/rsob.200084] [PMID: 32543351]

[63] Salehi B, Martorell M, Arbiser J, *et al.* Antioxidants: positive or negative actors? Biomolecules 2018; 8(4): 124.
[http://dx.doi.org/10.3390/biom8040124] [PMID: 30366441]

[64] Forman HJ, Zhang H. Targeting oxidative stress in disease: promise and limitations of antioxidant therapy. Nat Rev Drug Discov 2021; 20(9): 689-709.
[http://dx.doi.org/10.1038/s41573-021-00233-1] [PMID: 34194012]

[65] Xu DP, Li Y, Meng X, *et al.* Natural antioxidants in foods and medicinal plants: extraction, assessment and resources. Int J Mol Sci 2017; 18(1): 96.
[http://dx.doi.org/10.3390/ijms18010096] [PMID: 28067795]

[66] Lourenço SC, Moldão-Martins M, Alves VD. Antioxidants of natural plant origins: from sources to food industry applications. Molecules 2019; 24(22): 4132.
[http://dx.doi.org/10.3390/molecules24224132] [PMID: 31731614]

[67] Flora SJS. Structural, chemical and biological aspects of antioxidants for strategies against metal and metalloid exposure. Oxid Med Cell Longev 2009; 2(4): 191-206.
[http://dx.doi.org/10.4161/oxim.2.4.9112] [PMID: 20716905]

[68] Lentjes MAH. The balance between food and dietary supplements in the general population The Proceedings of the Nutrition Society 2019; 78(): 97-109.
[http://dx.doi.org/10.1017/S0029665118002525]

[69] Harnett J, Climstein M, Walsh J, Gifford J. The use of medications and dietary supplements by masters athletes — a review. Curr Nutr Rep 2022; 11(2): 253-62.
[http://dx.doi.org/10.1007/s13668-022-00398-0] [PMID: 35635719]

[70] Jun S, Gahche JJ, Potischman N, *et al.* Dietary supplement use and its micronutrient contribution during pregnancy and lactation in the united states. Obstet Gynecol 2020; 135(3): 623-33.
[http://dx.doi.org/10.1097/AOG.0000000000003657] [PMID: 32028492]

[71] Kominiarek MA, Rajan P. Nutrition recommendations in pregnancy and lactation. Med Clin North Am 2016; 100(6): 1199-215.
[http://dx.doi.org/10.1016/j.mcna.2016.06.004] [PMID: 27745590]

CHAPTER 2

Water-Soluble Vitamins Antioxidant Potential

Sohrab A. Shaikh[1,*]

[1] *Pharmacology, Toxicology, and Basic Health Sciences Unit, Faculty of Pharmacy, AIMST University, Bedong 08100, Kedah, Malaysia*

Abstract: Water-soluble vitamins are essential for the development, growth, and bodily functions. These vitamins are dissolved in water and are not stored in the body; a regular dietary supply is necessary. The key members of this group are vitamin C and the B-complex vitamins. Ascorbic acid (vitamin C) is primarily obtained from fresh fruits and vegetables and acts as a powerful antioxidant, detoxifying free radicals within the body. Thiamin (vitamin B1) plays a crucial role in energy metabolism and exhibits antioxidant activity by inhibiting lipid peroxidation and interacting with free radicals, converting them into less harmful compounds. Riboflavin (vitamin B2), found mainly in milk, is an important yet often overlooked antioxidant that contributes either independently or as part of the glutathione redox cycle, protecting against oxidative damage, particularly during reperfusion. Niacin (vitamin B3), comprising nicotinic acid and nicotinamide, forms the coenzymes Nicotinamide Adenine Dinucleotide (NAD) and Nicotinamide Adenine Dinucleotide Phosphate (NADP), essential for cellular redox processes and energy production. Niacin also functions as an independent antioxidant, enhancing the glutathione cycle and reducing oxidative stress. Coenzyme acid (vitamin B5), as a precursor to coenzyme A (CoA), is vital for metabolic processes involving proteins, lipids, and carbohydrates. Pantothenic acid derivatives panthenol and pantetheine have shown neuroprotective effects by enhancing the glutathione system in preclinical studies, revealing their antioxidant effects. Furthermore, pyridoxine (vitamin B6), biotin (vitamin B7), folic acid (vitamin B9), and cobalamins (vitamin B12) also play significant roles in antioxidant defense, protecting against oxidative stress either by maintaining glutathione levels or reducing reactive oxygen species (ROS) through different pathways. These vitamins collectively contribute to the body's antioxidant mechanisms, highlighting their importance in maintaining overall health and preventing oxidative damage.

Keywords: Antioxidant, B-complex vitamins, Dietary supplements, Oxidative stress, Vitamin C.

* **Corresponding author Sohrab A. Shaikh:** Pharmacology, Toxicology, and Basic Health Sciences Unit, Faculty of Pharmacy, AIMST University, Bedong 08100, Kedah, Malaysia; E-mail: shaikh.sohrab@aimst.edu.my

Mukesh Singh Sikarwar, Arunachalam Muthuraman & Sohrab A. Shaikh (Eds.)

INTRODUCTION

Water-soluble vitamins are a group of vitamins that dissolve in water and are not stored in the body [1], hence need to be supplied through a regular diet for body development, growth, and function [2]. Vitamin C and B complex vitamins are soluble in water [1]. The B vitamins, namely B1, B2, B3, B5, B6, B7, B9, and B12, are recognized, and they are also known as thiamin, riboflavin, niacin, pantothenic acid, pyridoxine, biotin, folate, and cobalamin, respectively. These vitamins are naturally present in the same foods and share the characteristic of being water-soluble. Since the body does not produce B vitamins independently, it is crucial to obtain enough from the diet. Additionally, indirect ingestion through animal sources such as meat, eggs, and dairy is possible. Notably, vitamin B12 is not synthesized by plants but by bacteria, and it is exclusively found in various animal products. The entire spectrum of B vitamins plays essential roles as coenzymes in enzymatic reactions. Some B vitamins have neuro-specific functions and are termed "neurotropic," contributing to both the central and peripheral nervous systems [3]. Moreover, vitamin C is reported to have antioxidant activity by neutralizing free radicals, while B vitamins support antioxidant defenses through their role in metabolic pathways. Regular intake of these vitamins is essential for protecting against oxidative stress, which may help in reducing the risk of various pathological conditions. Hence, the subsequent topics of this chapter provide the information of individual water soluble vitamins along with their antioxidant potential.

VITAMIN C (ASCORBIC ACID)

Ascorbic acid (Fig. **1**), a vital water-soluble vitamin necessary for various bodily functions, is obtained primarily from fresh vegetables and fruits, which serve as key dietary sources [4]. Vitamin C can be obtained from a variety of dietary sources such as asparagus, beet greens, bell peppers, berries, bok choy, broccoli, Brussels sprouts, cabbage, cantaloupe, cauliflower, citrus fruits, collard greens, fennel, grapefruit, green leafy vegetables, kale, kiwifruit, lemons and limes, mustard greens, oranges, papaya, parsley, pineapple, potatoes, raspberries, sea vegetables, spinach, strawberries, sweet potatoes, Swiss chard, tomatoes, and turnip greens [5, 6].

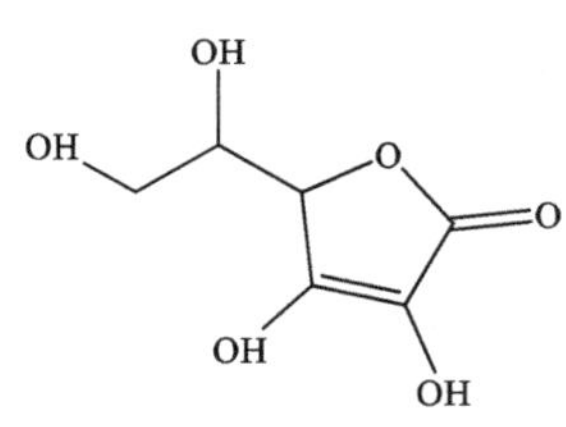

Fig. (1). Chemical structure of ascorbic acid.

The ascorbic acid acts as an antioxidant that detoxifies the free radicals produced within the body [4, 7]. Moreover, recent studies indicate that vitamin C may reduce vulnerability to viral respiratory infections and pneumonia [8]. Biologically, vitamin C plays a role in the metabolic processes of folic acid, tyrosine, and tryptophan. Additionally, it plays a role in synthesizing carnitine and catecholamines. Vitamin C aids in iron absorption and the breakdown of histamine. It also helps form neurotransmitters and is involved in the synthesis and maintenance of collagen. Furthermore, it increases the level of procollagen messenger RNA, acts as a coenzyme, and promotes the growth, development, and maintenance of osteoblasts, delaying the onset of osteoporosis. Vitamin C also protects sperm from oxidative damage, enhances lymphocyte function while reducing bacteriological activity. Additionally, it plays a role in neuronal modulation and the regulation of central nervous system homeostasis.

Additionally, clinical trial findings indicate that increased doses of vitamin C can reduce microvascular complications in type 2 diabetes, lower glycosylated hemoglobin levels, and decrease low-density lipoproteins. This highlights the important role of vitamin C as an adjunct treatment for both type 2 diabetes and atherosclerosis [6, 9, 10]. In another scenario, acute vitamin C deficiency can lead to scurvy [11], hence emphasizing its crucial role in preventing and treating scurvy [5].

Ascorbic Acid Antioxidant Potential

The importance of administering exogenous micronutrients to patients with severe disease to reestablish antioxidant levels has been known for decades [4]. As a potent antioxidant, ascorbic acid functions by contributing electrons to neutralize free radicals. It inhibits the generation of new free radicals through the suppression of the NADPH oxidase pathway. Additionally, it plays a crucial role in the recycling of other antioxidants [12]. This versatile compound is involved in controlling the lipid peroxidation of cellular membranes and nuclear materials within the cell. It mitigates DNA damage by reducing reactive oxygen species and safeguards proteins crucial for DNA repair. Moreover, it acts as a preventive measure against the formation of nitrosamine, a compound that gives rise to reactive nitrogen species. When combined with L-carnitine, it is reported to enhance the antioxidant and anti-inflammatory properties, thereby improving cisplatin-induced nephrotoxicity. High doses of vitamin C have been documented to elevate the production of reactive oxygen species within cells, disrupting the mitochondrial membrane potential. Additionally, at pharmacological doses, vitamin C can generate both ascorbate radicals and hydrogen peroxide. Consequently, the pro-oxidant effects induced by high doses of ascorbic acid have been proposed as a selective mechanism for killing cancer cells. The potential anti-cancer impact may involve the induction of hydrogen peroxide within cells and the depletion of Nicotinamide Adenine Dinucleotide [6].

Ascorbic Acid Supplements

Vitamin C supplements commonly include various formulations such as ascorbic acid, sodium ascorbate, calcium ascorbate, other mineral ascorbates, ascorbic acid paired with bioflavonoids, and combination products featuring calcium ascorbate, dehydroascorbate, calcium threonate, xylonate, and lyxonate [11].

VITAMIN B1 (THIAMIN)

Vitamin B1, also referred to as thiamin (Fig. **2**), is stored briefly in the body and is readily excreted; hence, a diet containing thiamin is required to maintain its proper levels in the blood [13]. Thiamin holds significance as a vital water-soluble vitamin due to its crucial involvement in the process of energy metabolism [14].

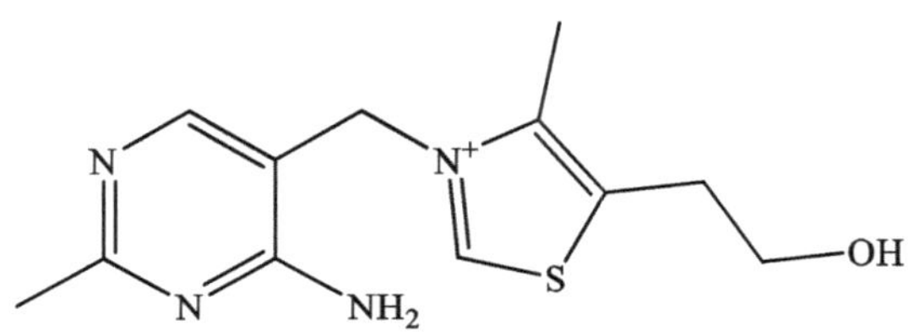

Fig. (2). Chemical structure of thiamin.

Thiamin can be obtained from different dietary sources like meat (beef, pork, poultry, lean meats, tuna), legumes (peas, soybean, navy beans, black beans, lima beans, dried peas, kidney beans, dried beans), whole grains (brown rice, barley, oats), nuts and seeds (sunflower seeds, flax seeds, sesame seeds, peanuts), fortified or enriched grain products (fortified cereals, bread), vegetables (asparagus, brussels sprouts, beet greens, spinach, cabbage, eggplant, romaine lettuce, mushrooms, sweet potato, broccoli, green beans, onions, collard greens), soy products (tofu, soy foods), fruits (pineapple, oranges), processed foods (certain processed foods *e.g.*, fortified cereals) It's important to note that some items, such as fortified cereals, can fall into multiple categories [6, 13, 15, 16].

Thiamin is primarily found in the human body as Thiamin Diphosphate (TDP), also known as Thiamin Pyrophosphate (TPP). This specific form of thiamin serves as a cofactor for many enzymes crucial in the metabolism of proteins, glucose, and lipids [13, 17]. Thiamin contributes to maintaining cellular redox balance and supports mitochondrial oxidative phosphorylation. It is involved in the production of Adenosine Triphosphate (ATP) [15] and contributes to the transmission of nerve impulses and the maintenance of myelin sheaths with an unidentified function [16]. Additionally, it aids in the structural development of brain cells and is involved in alcohol detoxification [6].

In adults, a lack of thiamin can result in encephalopathy, dry beriberi marked by neurological signs and symptoms, or wet beriberi characterized by cardiovascular signs and symptoms [15, 17]. Failure to address or prolonged thiamin deficiency puts individuals at risk of developing advanced-stage symptoms, a condition known as Wernicke-Korsakoff syndrome [13, 16]. Managing thiamin deficiency poses challenges for clinicians, primarily due to its extensive clinical spectrum, referred to as thiamin deficiency disorders, which impact various systems such as metabolic, neurologic, cardiovascular, respiratory, gastrointestinal, and musculoskeletal [14].

Thiamin Antioxidant Potential

The antioxidative properties of thiamin are comparatively limited when compared to vitamin C [18]. Thiamin's reported antioxidant activity involves inhibiting lipid peroxidation in rat liver microsomes and the free radical oxidation of oleic acid *in vitro*. It functions by interacting with free radicals and hydroperoxides, undergoing oxidation to thiochrome and thiamin disulfide [19]. Studies with thiamin pyrophosphate have demonstrated its preventive effect against oxidative stress in the liver induced by cisplatin [20]. Interestingly, a notable finding suggests that a combination of vitamin C and vitamin B1 can mitigate liver cell damage from lead-induced oxidative stress, with the antioxidant effects dependent on their concentrations [21]. Additional research indicates that thiamin and TDP exert significant suppressive effects on superoxide generation in hypoxanthine and xanthine oxidase systems [22]. Furthermore, thiamin has displayed antioxidant potential in various pro-oxidant conditions [23].

Thiamin Supplements

Many dietary supplements can fulfill the thiamin requirement; however, it is also supplied in the form of multivitamin/multimineral supplements. Thiamin can be found in supplements that contain B-complex vitamins (including thiamin) or in those specifically targeting thiamin. Commonly used forms of thiamin in supplements include thiamin mononitrate and thiamin hydrochloride, which are valued for their stability and ability to dissolve in water. Some dietary supplements also incorporate benfotiamine, a synthetic derivative of thiamin [24].

VITAMIN B2 (RIBOFLAVIN)

Riboflavin (Fig. **3**), also known as vitamin B2, is a vital water-soluble vitamin primarily obtained from milk. It exists in two coenzyme forms: Flavin

Mononucleotide (FMN) and Flavin Adenine Dinucleotide (FAD), both crucial for supporting enzymatic functions [25]. Unlike cooking, which does not affect riboflavin levels, exposure to light can cause its degradation [26].

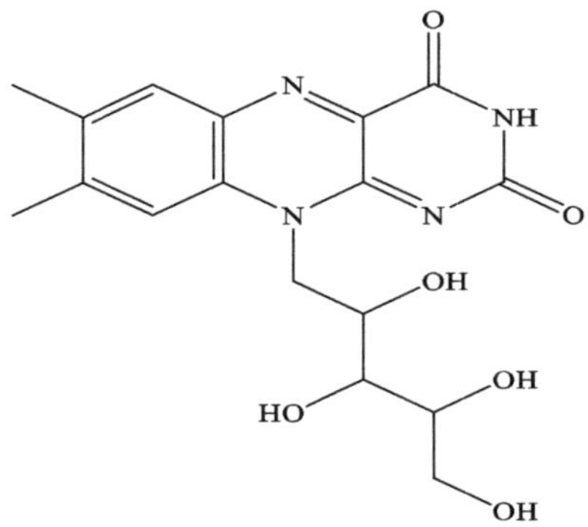

Fig. (3). Chemical structure of riboflavin.

Riboflavin is found in many foods and natural sources like meat and dairy products (milk, organ meats (especially calf liver), cheese, yogurt, turkey, sardines, tuna), eggs, seafood (salmon), nuts (almonds), fruits, vegetables (dark green leafy vegetables, spinach, beet greens, asparagus, collard greens, broccoli, swiss chard, green beans, mushrooms, turnip greens, kale, mustard greens, soybeans, green peas, sweet potato, carrots, cabbage) grains and legumes (wild rice, yeast, beer), and nutritional supplements (synthetic riboflavin rather than deriving it directly from food sources) cabbage are all good sources of vitamin B2 [6, 25, 26].

FMN and FAD both serve important roles as cofactors in energy metabolism and are indispensable for coenzyme function in various oxidation and reduction processes across all aerobic life forms [26]. Vitamin B2 has the vital function of regenerating glutathione, the body's primary antioxidant that defends against free radicals. A deficiency in Vitamin B2 heightens the risk of anemia due to the essential role of iron in red blood cell production [6]. Riboflavin, with its limited absorption in humans, exhibits poor retention in vertebrates. To prevent ariboflavinosis, characterized by cheilitis, a sore tongue, and a scaly rash on the scrotum or vulva, it is essential to orally consume riboflavin through a nutritious diet [26]. Additionally, a deficiency in riboflavin may elevate the risk of certain cancers [25].

Riboflavin has found application in dietary supplements and the management of inflammatory conditions like cataracts, cheilitis, glossitis, migraine headaches, and sepsis. Biotechnological methods are utilized for incorporating riboflavin into fermented functional meals. Research is underway on the use of lactic acid bacteria in the production of vitamin-enriched foods through food fermentation [26].

Riboflavin Antioxidant Potential

Riboflavin, an often-overlooked antioxidant nutrient, possesses the potential for antioxidant effects either independently or as part of the glutathione redox cycle. This vitamin plays a significant role in shielding the body from oxidative stress, particularly in countering lipid peroxidation and oxidative damage during reperfusion [25, 27]. Riboflavin serves as a coenzyme for redox enzymes in the forms of FAD and FMN, contributing to its antioxidant function. The FAD coenzyme is critical for the function of glutathione reductase, which is essential for converting oxidized glutathione to its reduced form. Reduced glutathione acts as an antioxidant within cells, neutralizing reactive oxygen species generated during oxidation and playing a crucial role in deactivating peroxides, especially hydroperoxides [6]. Additionally, riboflavin exhibits both antioxidant and anti-inflammasome functions, contributing to the modulation of the inflammatory response [28 - 30].

Riboflavin Supplements

Riboflavin is present in numerous dietary supplements. Multivitamin/multimineral supplements that include riboflavin usually provide a dosage of 1.3 mg. Additionally, there are riboflavin-only supplements and B-complex vitamins (which incorporate riboflavin) available. While the majority of supplements contain riboflavin in its free form, certain products include riboflavin 5'-phosphate [31].

VITAMIN B3 (NIACIN)

Niacin, also known as “vitamin B3” or “vitamin PP,” comprises two vitamers: nicotinic acid (Fig. **4A**) and nicotinamide (Fig. **4B**). These substances combine to form the coenzymes Nicotinamide Adenine Dinucleotide (NAD) and Nicotinamide Adenine Dinucleotide Phosphate (NADP) [6, 32, 33]. Dietary sources of vitamin B3 are found in vegetables (mushrooms, cauliflower, sweet potato, broccoli, beet greens, asparagus, turnip greens, bell peppers, cucumber, celery, avocado, potatoes, papaya, winter squash), legumes (lentils, dried peas), meat (chicken, turkey, beef, red meat, poultry, fish, shrimps), dairy (yogurt, cow milk), grains (rye, wheat, corn, whole-grain cereals, bran), protein sources (eggs, salmon), and other sources like yeast, peanuts and seeds [6, 33, 34]. It's worth noting that some items could fit into multiple categories, as they may provide various nutrients from different sources. For example, yogurt provides protein and dairy, and eggs provide protein and are categorized as poultry. NAD(P) serves as a vitamin in meat and fish, with unprocessed meals containing higher concentrations compared to processed foods, where enzymatic hydrolysis during preparation may decrease levels. In mature cereal grains, particularly corn, niacin is primarily in the form of niacin-glycoside and, to a lesser degree, as peptide-bound niacin, collectively termed "niacinogens" [35].

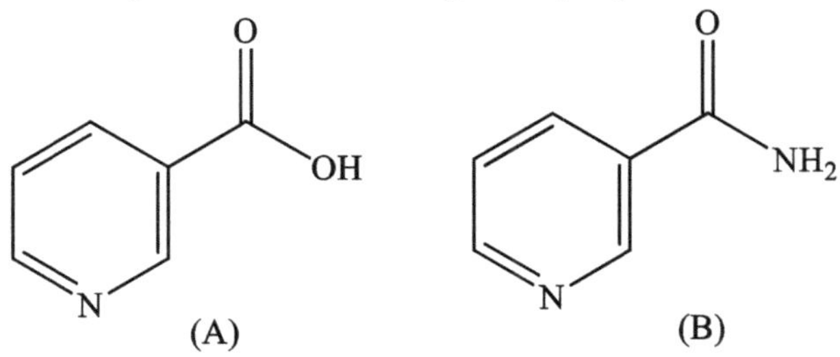

Fig. (4). Chemical structure of nicotinic acid (**A**) and nicotinamide (**B**).

NAD and NADP serve as vital cofactors in numerous cellular redox processes, playing a crucial role in sustaining cellular metabolism and respiration. These coenzymes are indispensable for oxidative reactions essential in energy production. Additionally, a diverse array of ADP-ribosylation enzymes utilizes NAD as a cosubstrate, showcasing various activities [36]. Beyond their involvement in redox processes, both NAD and NADP function as substrates for enzymes participating in non-redox signaling pathways. These pathways, in turn, regulate crucial biological functions such as cell cycle progression, DNA repair, gene expression, and cell death [32]. Notably, niacin, a pharmacotherapeutic drug since 1955, stands as the oldest pleiotropic hypolipidemic medication. Niacin is essential for the proper functioning of the central nervous system and neuronal growth, impacting both neuroprotection and neuronal death [32, 37]. Furthermore, it is worth highlighting that NAD, NADP, and niacin-containing enzymes also serve as antioxidants, contributing to cellular protection [6].

Pellagra arises from a deficiency in vitamin B3. The standard treatment for pellagra involves the administration of niacin until the symptoms resolve, particularly for alleviating skin issues [33]. According to guidelines from the World Health Organization, pellagra should be treated with a daily intake of 300 mg of nicotinamide, distributed in divided doses over a period of 3-4 weeks. Additionally, the recommendation suggests using a B-complex supplement or a yeast product to address possible deficiencies in other B vitamins that may be linked to pellagra [34].

Niacin Antioxidant Potential

Niacin is an often-overlooked antioxidant vitamin that can act independently as an antioxidant and also as a component of the glutathione redox cycle. Nicotinamide demonstrates strong antioxidant properties, as evidenced by both *in vitro* and *in vivo* studies. Its protective effects against oxidative stress include maintaining the glutathione redox cycle, lowering the NADPH/total NADP+ ratio, and boosting NAD+ levels [38 - 41]. Additionally, niacin is recognized for enhancing lipid metabolism and delivering antioxidant and anti-inflammatory effects. Consequently, supplementing with niacin may alleviate oxidative stress, inflammation, and tissue damage [6, 42, 43].

Niacin Supplements

Niacin is available in multivitamin-mineral supplements, supplements that include various other B-complex vitamins, and those specifically focused on niacin. The two main forms of niacin typically found in these supplements are nicotinic acid and nicotinamide [44].

VITAMIN B5 (PANTOTHENIC ACID)

Pantothenic acid (Fig. **5**) plays an essential role as a precursor to coenzyme A (CoA), a vital component in various metabolic processes involving proteins, lipids, and carbohydrates. Its presence in the form of CoA and as part of acyl carrier protein contributes to diverse metabolic activities. While pantothenic acid deficiency is rare in humans due to its abundance in animal and plant sources [45 - 47], it can manifest in individuals experiencing severe malnutrition [48]. Studies have demonstrated a significant reduction in pantothenic acid levels in multiple brain regions associated with Alzheimer's disease and Huntington's disease [49].

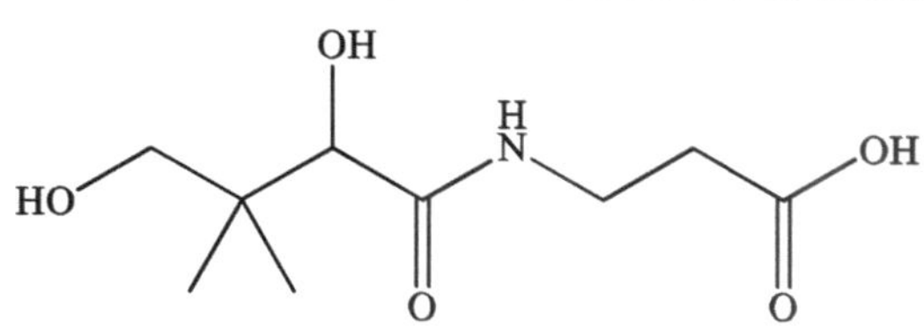

Fig. (5). Chemical structure of pantothenic acid.

Pantothenic acid is present in different quantities in nearly all foods derived from plants and animals. Some of the most nutrient-rich dietary sources come from animal sources (chicken, beef, organ meats (*e.g.*, liver, kidney, heart), fish (*e.g.*, salmon, shrimps) and turkey), dairy products (eggs, cow's milk, yogurt), vegetables (cauliflower, sweet potato, potatoes, broccoli, beet greens, asparagus, turnip greens, bell peppers, cucumber, celery, avocado, mustard greens, tomatoes,

Romaine lettuce, winter squash, sea vegetables), legumes (lentils, dried peas), whole grains (rye, wheat, corn), fruits (papaya). Pantothenic acid is incorporated into several food products, including certain breakfast cereals and beverages like energy drinks. Edible tissues from both animals and plants naturally contain high levels of pantothenic acid. However, the process of food manufacturing can lead to notable reductions in the content of this compound [6, 48, 50].

Vitamin B5 Antioxidant Potential

Preclinical investigations of pantothenic acid derivatives in a Parkinson's disease model reveal that panthenol and pantethine have neuroprotective action by increasing the glutathione system's reduction potential, therefore reducing the consequences of oxidative stress [51]. Additionally, investigations reveal that pantothenic acid therapy significantly diminishes oxidative stress and improves brain damage in rats exposed to gamma irradiation [6]. Consequently, these studies suggest the antioxidant capabilities of vitamin B5.

Vitamin B5 Supplements

Pantothenic acid is available in dietary supplements either by itself or as part of multivitamin/multimineral combinations that include other B-complex vitamins. Some supplements also contain pantethine (a dimeric form of pantetheine) or, more frequently, calcium pantothenate [50].

VITAMIN B6 (PYRIDOXINE, PYRIDOXAL, PYRIDOXAMINE)

Vitamin B6 encompasses pyridoxine (Fig. **6A**), pyridoxal (Fig. **6B**), pyridoxamine (Fig. **6C**), and their respective 5′-phosphate forms [52, 53]. Vitamin B-6, a crucial water-soluble vitamin, is found in a diverse range of foods such as meat (tuna, turkey, beef, chicken, salmon, shrimps), legumes (lentils, pinto beans, green peas, lima beans), seeds (sunflower seeds), cereals, vegetables (spinach, cabbage, bell peppers, turnip greens, garlic, cauliflower, sweet potato, winter squash, broccoli, brussels sprouts, collard greens, beet greens, kale, carrots, swiss chard, asparagus, mustard greens, tomatoes, leeks, summer squash, chili peppers, onions), and fruits (bananas, pineapple, avocado) [6, 54].

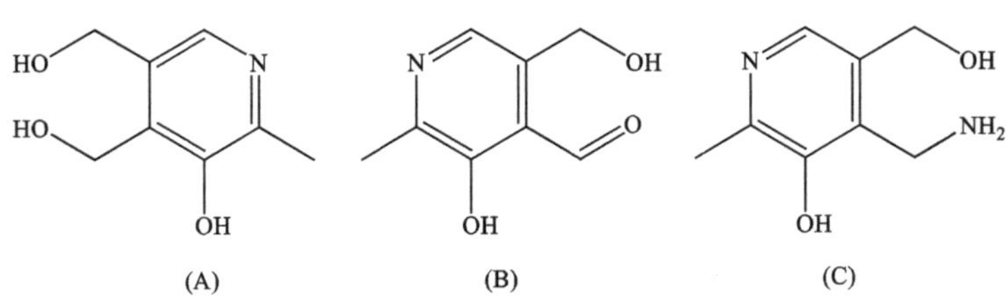

Fig. (6). Chemical structure of pyridoxine (**A**), pyridoxal (**B**), and pyridoxamine (**C**).

Over 140 coenzymatic actions have been linked to vitamin B6 (pyridoxine). Although it has many other functions, it is best recognized for its role in the production of neurotransmitters such as dopamine from levodopa (L-DOPA), gamma-aminobutyric acid (GABA) from glutamate, and serotonin from 5-hydroxytryptophan (5HTP). Pyridoxine impacts the adrenergic, serotonergic, and glutamatergic systems as a result of its activity for the aforementioned neurotransmitters [3, 55]. The use of pyridoxamine dihydrochloride as a dietary supplement has demonstrated its ability to inhibit the formation of Advanced Glycation End (AGE) products resulting from glycated proteins, which has attracted the interest of diabetologists and others researching diabetic complications [53]. Interestingly, a recent research study indicates that pyridoxine supplementation may have a positive impact on reducing symptoms associated with COVID-19. This is attributed to improved immune responses, decreased levels of pro-inflammatory cytokines, support for endothelial integrity, and a reduction in hypercoagulability [56].

Signs of a deficiency in vitamin B6 include a swollen tongue, itchy rashes, cracks at the corners of the mouth, anemia, and scaly skin on the lips. Depression, confusion, and a weakened immune system (innate/adaptive immunity) are further signs of severely low vitamin B6 levels. Infants who are deficient in vitamin B6 might display irritability, heightened sensitivity to hearing, or may even encounter seizures [56, 57]. High and continuous alcohol consumption, as well as some antiepileptic medicines and severe renal disorders, might induce deficiencies. In addition, several malabsorption syndromes, like Crohn's disease, ulcerative colitis, or celiac disease, can induce vitamin B6 insufficiency, and certain hereditary abnormalities, such as homocystinuria, can cause vitamin B6 deficiency. Moreover, Vitamin B6 insufficiency can occur in the majority of people with chronic renal failure and patients undergoing various forms of renal replacement treatment for a variety of reasons [56, 58]. Vitamin B6 is therefore recommended in cases of insufficiency; nevertheless, insufficient vitamin B6 intake is an uncommon cause of deficiency [55].

Vitamin B6 Antioxidant Potential

A lack of vitamin B6 is associated with atherogenesis, affecting the production of long-chain polyunsaturated fatty acids, promoting lipid peroxidation, and affecting the body's antioxidant defenses [6]. Consequently, vitamin B6 appears to play a crucial role in the antioxidant mechanism [59]. Due to the presence of both hydroxyl (–OH) and amine (–NH2) groups on a pyridine ring in its molecules, vitamin B6 can directly interact with peroxy radicals, effectively scavenging radicals and preventing lipid peroxidation. The physiological coenzyme form of vitamin B6, plasma pyridoxal 5′-phosphate (PLP), plays a crucial role in the transsulfuration pathway, converting homocysteine to cysteine and contributing to the indirect antioxidative effect of vitamin B6. Inadequate plasma PLP levels may lead to homocysteine accumulation, restricting cysteine synthesis. The oxidation of homocysteine can generate oxygen-free radicals, increasing oxidative stress and reducing DNA methylation in vital tissues [60]. Additionally, vitamin B6's antioxidant and radical scavenging activities have been extensively explored in the literature, such as its role in reducing oxidative stress markers related to homocysteinemia or preventing the production of reactive oxygen species and lipid peroxidation in cellular models [61 - 63]. Moreover, following polymicrobial sepsis, vitamin B6 has demonstrated anti-inflammatory and antioxidant effects in peripheral organs, contributing to its role in stress responses [64, 65].

Vitamin B6 Supplements

Pyridoxine is a prevalent form of Vitamin B6 in dietary supplements, commonly present in most multivitamin-mineral supplements. Some dietary supplements may exclusively contain vitamin B6 or combine it with other B vitamins [66].

VITAMIN B7 (BIOTIN)

Biotin, a vitamin soluble in water, functions as a cofactor in carboxylation reactions. Within humans, there are five biotin-dependent carboxylases: propionyl-CoA carboxylase, methylcrotonyl-CoA carboxylase, pyruvate carboxylase, and two forms of acetyl-CoA carboxylase. Biotin plays a crucial role in maintaining metabolic balance as these enzymes catalyze essential reactions in gluconeogenesis, fatty acid metabolism, and amino acid catabolism [67]. Additionally, biotin has been noted for its impact on chromatin structure and its involvement in gene regulation [68]. The chemical structure of biotin is illustrated in Fig. (7).

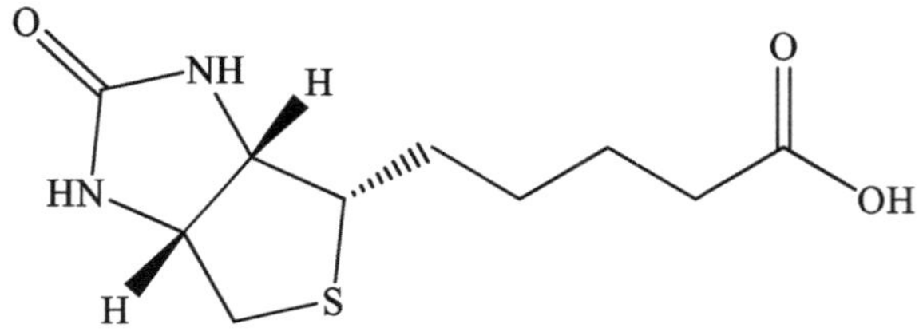

Fig. (7). Chemical structure of biotin.

The good sources of biotin are found in animal meat (liver, salmon), egg yolk, cereals (wheat, oats), rice, dairy products (yogurt, cow's milk), fruits (banana, raspberries, strawberries, watermelon, grapefruit), vegetables (spinach, mushrooms, tomatoes, onions, carrots, romaine lettuce, cauliflower, sweet potato, peanuts, walnuts, cucumber) [6]. Moreover, biotin can also be produced by intestinal microbes [69]. Biotin affects the expression of genes and exerts various effects on systemic functions beyond its role as a carboxylase prosthetic group. This vitamin plays a regulatory role in essential genes that control intermediary metabolism: Biotin acts as a stimulator of genes that promote hypoglycemia [70]. In addition, biotin plays a crucial role in fat metabolism. A deficiency in biotin can lead to skin rashes and is necessary for the deposition of fat in the skin. Furthermore, increased biotin intake in the meals of lactating women may help newborns with cradle cap symptoms [6].

Biotin deficiency causes a variety of symptoms, the most common of which are neurological and cutaneous problems [69]. The term "Biotin deficiency facies" pertains to the distinctive facial rash and atypical distribution of facial fat observed in individuals lacking sufficient biotin [71]. Biotin's precise indications have only been confirmed in a few studies. Biotinidase deficiency is a rare but well-known condition. In children, biotinidase deficiency can cause conjunctivitis, ataxia, seizures, skin infections, and developmental delays. Those with pathologic brittle hair syndrome or uncombable hair syndrome may benefit from biotin. Otherwise, supplementing indications are unnecessary in healthy people. Biotin may help with hair and nail development, but there isn't much proof to back it up [72].

Vitamin B7 Antioxidant Potential

Biotin is reported to have antioxidant activities by decreasing ROS overproduction, protein and lipid oxidation products [73]. In preclinical trials, the administration of 6 mg of biotin demonstrated a significant decrease in oxidative stress within the rat hippocampus. This was supported by reduced levels of 4-hydroxynonenal, total nitrate/nitrite, and xanthine oxidase, together with elevated glutathione levels and increased activities of superoxide dismutase and catalase. Biotin also exhibited the ability to lower pro-inflammatory cytokines, serum S100 protein, and neuron-specific enolase levels [74]. Furthermore, high-dose biotin studies indicated the restoration of redox balance, energy, and lipid homeostasis, as well as improvement in axonal health in an adrenoleukodystrophy model [75]. These findings strongly suggest that biotin plays a role as an effective antioxidant.

VITAMIN B9 (FOLATE)

Folate, previously known as "folacin" or sometimes "vitamin B9," is a water-soluble vitamin belonging to the B complex. It covers naturally occurring food folates and includes folic acid (Fig. **8**), which is present in dietary supplements and fortified foods [76]. Vitamin B9 is vital, as it plays a crucial role in promoting human brain health, supporting cardiovascular function, and maintaining the nervous system [6]. Additionally, it plays a vital role in the biosynthesis of Deoxyribonucleic Acid (DNA) [77].

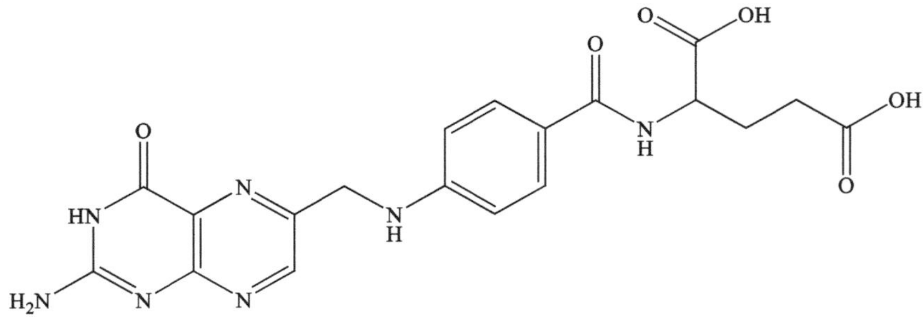

Fig. (8). Chemical structure of folic acid.

Folate is found naturally in various foods and must be consumed regularly because humans and other animals are unable to synthesize it. Sources of folate in the diet include leafy green vegetables (spinach, broccoli, asparagus, turnip greens, romaine lettuce, bok choy, cauliflower, parsley, brussels sprouts) [6], meats (liver), eggs and dairy products (eggs, milk) [77], legumes and beans (lentils, pinto beans, garbanzo beans (chickpeas), black beans, navy beans, kidney beans), papaya, nuts, seafood, poultry, grains and fruits and fruit juices. The foods with the highest levels of folate are spinach, liver, asparagus, and brussels sprouts [76].

Folates play a crucial role in regulating homocysteine levels, influencing factors that contribute to cardiovascular disease risk. Elevated homocysteine levels signify an increased susceptibility to cardiovascular disease. Folate stands as a vital nutrient essential for maintaining heart health, as it is needed for the production of red blood cells [6]. Folate acts as a coenzyme or cosubstrate in single-carbon transfers necessary for synthesizing nucleic acids (DNA and RNA) and metabolizing amino acids. Normal cell division relies on folate, particularly in the methylation of deoxyuridylate to thymidylate during DNA synthesis. Disruptions in this process can lead to megaloblastic anemia, a common symptom of folate deficiency [76, 77]. In the formation of the central nervous system, folate emerges as a crucial element. To lessen the risk of neural tube abnormalities (NTDs), such as spina bifida, in the developing baby, pregnant women should take folic acid supplements [77].

Vitamin B9 Antioxidant Potential

The reduced forms of folic acid have been observed to exhibit antioxidant properties comparable to vitamins C and E. Tetrahydrofolate is particularly effective in protecting against lipid peroxidation, while dihydrofolate shows significant effectiveness against ABTS+ cations. Numerous studies have indicated that folate contributes to the prevention or improvement of hematological disease, cancer, neurological issues, and neural tube defects. The antioxidant ability of folates has been postulated as a reason for its preventive role in various disorders [6].

Vitamin B9 Supplements

Folic acid is present in multivitamins, prenatal vitamins, supplements containing other B-complex vitamins, and separate folic acid supplements. Additionally, there are dietary supplements containing 5-methyl-THF, also known as methyl folate, which is a reduced form of folate. In certain cases, individuals may find supplementation with 5-methyl-THF more advantageous than with folic acid [78].

VITAMIN B12 (CYANOCOBALAMIN, HYDROXOCOBALAMIN, METHYLCOBALAMIN)

Substances exhibiting vitamin B12 activity are denoted as "cobalamins" due to the presence of the element cobalt in vitamin B12 [79]. Cobalamin is a cofactor that works by transferring one-carbon through methylation and chemical rearrangement. These processes are carried out in the amino acid, fatty acid, and nucleic acid metabolic pathways [80]. Being water-soluble, cobalamin is crucial for human well-being [81].

Vitamin B12 is normally obtained from animal sources. Unlike other B vitamins, plant-based foods generally lack vitamin B12, with the exception of rare algae. Commonly consumed plant foods only contain vitamin B12 if they have undergone bacterial processes generating the vitamin, been contaminated with substances like soil or insects that contain B12, or have been fortified with B12. Shellfish, organ meats like liver, certain game meats, and a few types of fish, which are not commonly included in most people's diets, are the richest sources of vitamin B12 [82, 83]. Cow's milk, yogurt, cheese, eggs, chicken, turkey, cattle, lamb, mushrooms, breakfast cereals, cod, tuna, salmon, sardines, shrimp, and scallops are all good sources of Vitamin B12 [6].

Vitamin B12 is crucial for red blood cell formation, nervous system health, myelin synthesis, cellular growth support, and DNA synthesis. The active forms of vitamin B12 include hydroxo-, adenosyl-, and methyl-cobalamin. Inadequate levels of vitamin B12 can elevate methylmalonic acid and homocysteine, leading to heightened inflammation, reactive oxygen species, and oxidative stress [84, 85]. Even with a well-balanced diet that supplies adequate cobalamin, certain diseases can cause a deficiency in this vitamin [81].

Reversible megaloblastic anaemia, demyelinating illness, or both are symptoms of vitamin B12 insufficiency. Its absence has been linked to a variety of neuropsychiatric diseases. In addition, the role of vitamin B12 deficiency in hyperhomocysteinemia and atherosclerosis promotion is being investigated [86, 87].

Vitamin B12 Antioxidant Potential

A subclinical deficiency in vitamin B12 results in the production of reactive oxygen species, impacting vitamin B12 intake. Oxidative stress can cause the formation of advanced glycation end products, further hindering B12 intake. Some researchers suggest that vitamin B12 may directly scavenge superoxide radicals. Vitamin B12's antioxidant properties are linked to its ability to maintain glutathione levels. It can protect against oxidative stress by altering the activity of nuclear factor-K. Additionally, it facilitates the conversion of homocysteine into methionine; hence, a deficiency in vitamin B12 leads to elevated homocysteine levels. Through its involvement in homocysteine metabolism, vitamin B12 indirectly provides protection against oxidative stress [6]. Vitamin B12 modulates the production of cytokines and growth factors, shielding the body from oxidative stress triggered by immune responses [85]. Consequently, vitamin B12 plays a crucial role in the cycle of oxidative stress. External antioxidant treatments, especially vitamins such as "vitamin B12," are employed to diminish oxidative stress and reestablish equilibrium between antioxidants and oxidants [88].

Vitamin B12 Supplements

Various options exist for vitamin B12 supplementation, including multivitamin/mineral supplements, B-complex vitamin supplements, and standalone vitamin B12 supplements. Cyanocobalamin is the most common form of vitamin B12 in dietary supplements. Other forms include adenosylcobalamin, methylcobalamin, and hydroxycobalamin. Vitamin B12 is also available in sublingual tablets or lozenges, besides traditional oral supplements [89].

SUMMARY

Water-soluble vitamins are essential for several bodily functions, including energy metabolism, DNA synthesis, immune support, and nerve function. These water-soluble vitamins are not stored in the body and must be obtained from diverse sources like vegetables, fruits, lean proteins, and whole grains. Their antioxidant activity helps protect cells from oxidative stress, thereby reducing the risk of developing various chronic pathological conditions like cardiovascular disease, cancer, and neurodegenerative disorders. Furthermore, ensuring enough consumption is very important for groups at higher risk of deficiency, such as pregnant women, older adults, and those with certain health conditions. Identifying the different roles and health benefits of water-soluble vitamins highlights the significance of a balanced diet in maintaining overall health and well-being. Continuing research on water-soluble vitamins discloses new understandings into their therapeutic potential, emphasizing their critical role in nutraceuticals.

CASE STUDIES AND PRACTICE QUESTIONS

Case 1: *A 45-year-old male presents with symptoms of fatigue, bleeding gums, joint pain, and slow wound healing associated with scurvy. His diet consists mainly of preserved meat and biscuits, lacking fresh fruits and vegetables.*

Discussion Questions

a. What vitamin deficiency is most likely causing his symptoms?
b. Explain the biochemical role of the vitamin that is deficient in this case, in collagen synthesis.
c. How does the vitamin that is deficient in this case function as an antioxidant?
d. List dietary sources of the vitamin that is deficient in this patient.

Case 2: *A 28-year-old pregnant woman did not take any prenatal supplements during the first trimester of her pregnancy. An ultrasound examination reveals signs of neural tube defects in the fetus.*

Discussion Questions

a. Which vitamin is most likely deficient in this case, and why is it important for fetal development?
b. What dietary sources of the deficient vitamin can help manage or prevent this patient's condition?
c. List the different forms or types of supplements available for the deficient vitamin in this case.

Case 3: *A 42-year-old male patient complains of fatigue, low mood, cracked lips, and frequent infections. On examination, he has a swollen tongue, scaly lips, and a mild rash on his hands; laboratory results show mild anemia and elevated homocysteine.*

Discussion Questions

a. What is the most likely vitamin deficiency in this patient?
b. What does the presence of elevated homocysteine suggest about the patient's metabolic status in this case?
c. How does the vitamin that is deficient in this patient contribute to the body's antioxidant defense system?
d. List two food sources that could help improve this patient's condition.

REFERENCES

[1] Lykstad J, Sharma S. Biochemistry, water soluble vitamins. StatPearls. Treasure Island, FL: StatPearls Publishing 2022. Internet Available from: http://www.ncbi.nlm.nih.gov/books/NBK538510/

[2] Yaman M, Çatak J, Uğur H, *et al.* The bioaccessibility of water-soluble vitamins: A review. Trends Food Sci Technol 2021; 109: 552-63.
[http://dx.doi.org/10.1016/j.tifs.2021.01.056]

[3] Calderón-Ospina CA, Nava-Mesa MO. B Vitamins in the nervous system: Current knowledge of the biochemical modes of action and synergies of thiamine, pyridoxine, and cobalamin. CNS Neurosci Ther 2020; 26(1): 5-13.
[http://dx.doi.org/10.1111/cns.13207] [PMID: 31490017]

[4] Berretta M, Quagliariello V, Maurea N, *et al.* Multiple effects of ascorbic acid against chronic diseases: updated evidence from preclinical and clinical studies. Antioxidants 2020; 9(12): 1182.
[http://dx.doi.org/10.3390/antiox9121182] [PMID: 33256059]

[5] Abdullah M, Jamil RT, Attia FN. Vitamin C (Ascorbic Acid). StatPearls. Treasure Island, FL: StatPearls Publishing 2022. Internet Available from: http://www.ncbi.nlm.nih.gov/books/NBK499877/

[6] Sinbad OO, Folorunsho AA, Olabisi OL, Ayoola OA, Temitope EJ. Vitamins as antioxidants. Journal of Food Science and Nutrition Research 2019; 2(3): 214-35.

[7] Smirnoff N. Ascorbic acid metabolism and functions: A comparison of plants and mammals. Free Radic Biol Med 2018; 122: 116-29.
[http://dx.doi.org/10.1016/j.freeradbiomed.2018.03.033] [PMID: 29567393]

[8] Bauer SR, Kapoor A, Rath M, Thomas SA. What is the role of supplementation with ascorbic acid, zinc, vitamin D, or N-acetylcysteine for prevention or treatment of COVID-19? CCJM [Internet]. 2020 Jun 8 [cited 2022 Feb 14]; Available from: https://www.ccjm.org/content/early/2020/06/08/ccjm.87a.ccc046

[9] Moretti M, Rodrigues ALS. Functional role of ascorbic acid in the central nervous system: a focus on neurogenic and synaptogenic processes. Nutr Neurosci 2021; 0(0): 1-11.
[PMID: 34493165]

[10] Santosh H, David C. Role of ascorbic acid in diabetes mellitus: A comprehensive review. Journal of Medicine, Radiology. Pathology and Surgery 2017; 4: 1-3.

[11] Office of Dietary Supplements - Vitamin C [Internet]. [cited 2022 Apr 9]. Available from: https://ods.od.nih.gov/factsheets/VitaminC-HealthProfessional/

[12] Moskowitz A, Andersen LW, Huang DT, *et al.* Ascorbic acid, corticosteroids, and thiamine in sepsis: a review of the biologic rationale and the present state of clinical evaluation. Crit Care 2018; 22(1): 283.
[http://dx.doi.org/10.1186/s13054-018-2217-4] [PMID: 30373647]

[13] Martel JL, Kerndt CC, Doshi H, Franklin DS. Vitamin B1 (Thiamine). StatPearls. Treasure Island, FL: StatPearls Publishing 2022. Internet Available from: http://www.ncbi.nlm.nih.gov/books/NBK482360/

[14] Smith TJ, Johnson CR, Koshy R, *et al.* Thiamine deficiency disorders: a clinical perspective. Ann N Y Acad Sci 2021; 1498(1): 9-28.
[http://dx.doi.org/10.1111/nyas.14536] [PMID: 33305487]

[15] Belsky JB, Wira CR, Jacob V, Sather JE, Lee PJ. A review of micronutrients in sepsis: the role of thiamine, L -carnitine, vitamin C, selenium and vitamin D. Nutr Res Rev 2018; 31(2): 281-90.
[http://dx.doi.org/10.1017/S0954422418000124] [PMID: 29984680]

[16] Wiley KD, Gupta M. Vitamin B1 thiamine deficiency. StatPearls. Treasure Island, FL: StatPearls Publishing 2022. Internet Available from: http://www.ncbi.nlm.nih.gov/books/NBK537204/

[17] Polegato BF, Pereira AG, Azevedo PS, *et al.* Role of thiamin in health and disease. Nutr Clin Pract 2019; 34(4): 558-64.

[http://dx.doi.org/10.1002/ncp.10234] [PMID: 30644592]

[18] Piechocka J, Szymandera-Buszka K, Kobus-Cisowska J, Gramza-Michałowska A, Jędrusek-Golińska A. The effect of thiamine concentration on the antioxidative activity indices in tea extracts. Antioxidants 2019; 8(11): 555. [http://dx.doi.org/10.3390/antiox8110555] [PMID: 31731638]

[19] Lukienko PI, Mel'nichenko NG, Zverinskii IV, Zabrodskaya SV. Antioxidant properties of thiamine. Bull Exp Biol Med 2000; 130(9): 874-6. [http://dx.doi.org/10.1023/A:1015318413076] [PMID: 11177269]

[20] Turan MI, Siltelioglu Turan I, Mammadov R, Altınkaynak K, Kisaoglu A. The effect of thiamine and thiamine pyrophosphate on oxidative liver damage induced in rats with cisplatin. BioMed Res Int 2013; 2013: 1-6. [http://dx.doi.org/10.1155/2013/783809] [PMID: 23841092]

[21] Wang C, Liang J, Zhang C, Bi Y, Shi X, Shi Q. Effect of ascorbic acid and thiamine supplementation at different concentrations on lead toxicity in liver. Ann Occup Hyg 2007; 51(6): 563-9. [PMID: 17878260]

[22] Okai Y, Higashi-Okai K, F Sato E, Konaka R, Inoue M. Potent radical-scavenging activities of thiamin and thiamin diphosphate. J Clin Biochem Nutr 2007; 40(1): 42-8. [http://dx.doi.org/10.3164/jcbn.40.42] [PMID: 18437212]

[23] Gonçalves Á de C, Soldi LR, Portari GV. Thiamine, oxidative stress, and ethanol. In: Patel VB, Ed. Molecular Nutrition. Academic Press 2020; pp. 207-23. [Internet] Available from: https://www.sciencedirect.com/science/article/pii/B978012 811907500018X [http://dx.doi.org/10.1016/B978-0-12-811907-5.00018-X]

[24] Office of Dietary Supplements - Thiamin [Internet]. [cited 2022 Apr 9]. Available from: https://ods.od.nih.gov/factsheets/Thiamin-HealthProfessional/

[25] Saedisomeolia A, Ashoori M. Chapter Two - Riboflavin in Human Health: A Review of Current Evidences. In: Eskin NAM, editor. Advances in Food and Nutrition Research [Internet]. Academic Press; 2018 [cited 2022 Feb 15]. p. 57–81. (New Research and Developments of Water-Soluble Vitamins; vol. 83). Available from: https://www.sciencedirect.com/science/article/pii/S1043452617300384

[26] Suwannasom N, Kao I, Pruß A, Georgieva R, Bäumler H. Riboflavin: The health benefits of a forgotten natural vitamin. Int J Mol Sci 2020; 21(3): 950. [http://dx.doi.org/10.3390/ijms21030950] [PMID: 32023913]

[27] Ashoori M, Saedisomeolia A. Riboflavin (vitamin B_2) and oxidative stress: a review. Br J Nutr 2014; 111(11): 1985-91. [http://dx.doi.org/10.1017/S0007114514000178] [PMID: 24650639]

[28] Ahn H, Lee GS. Riboflavin, vitamin B2, attenuates NLRP3, NLRC4, AIM2, and non-canonical inflammasomes by the inhibition of caspase-1 activity. Sci Rep 2020; 10(1): 19091. [http://dx.doi.org/10.1038/s41598-020-76251-7] [PMID: 33154451]

[29] M MH. Riboflavin antioxidant scavenging activity in the presence of sunlight 2020; 17(165): 15-24.

[30] Hoffman MD, Valentino TR, Stuempfle KJ, Hassid BV. A placebo-controlled trial of riboflavin for enhancement of ultramarathon recovery. Sports Med Open 2017; 3(1): 14. [http://dx.doi.org/10.1186/s40798-017-0081-4] [PMID: 28349501]

[31] Office of Dietary Supplements - Riboflavin [Internet]. [cited 2022 Apr 9]. Available from: https://ods.od.nih.gov/factsheets/Riboflavin-HealthProfessional/

[32] Niacin. In: LiverTox: Clinical and research information on drug-induced liver injury [internet]. bethesda (md): national institute of diabetes and digestive and kidney diseases; 2012 [cited 2022 Feb 17]. Available from: http://www.ncbi.nlm.nih.gov/books/NBK548176/

[33] Peechakara BV, Gupta M. Vitamin B3. StatPearls. Treasure Island, FL: StatPearls Publishing 2022. Internet Available from: http://www.ncbi.nlm.nih.gov/books/NBK526107/

[34] Office of Dietary Supplements - Niacin [Internet]. [cited 2022 Mar 27]. Available from: https://ods.od.nih.gov/factsheets/Niacin-HealthProfessional/

[35] Gasperi V, Sibilano M, Savini I, Catani MV. Niacin in the central nervous system: an update of biological aspects and clinical applications. Int J Mol Sci 2019; 20(4): 974. [http://dx.doi.org/10.3390/ijms20040974] [PMID: 30813414]

[36] Kirkland JB, Meyer-Ficca ML. Chapter Three - Niacin. In: Eskin NAM, editor. Advances in Food and Nutrition Research [Internet]. Academic Press; 2018 [cited 2022 Feb 17]. p. 83–149. (New Research and Developments of Water-Soluble Vitamins; vol. 83). Available from: https://www.sciencedirect.com/science/article/pii/ S1043452617300396

[37] Djadjo S, Bajaj T. Niacin. StatPearls. Treasure Island, FL: StatPearls Publishing 2022. Internet Available from: http://www.ncbi.nlm.nih.gov/books/NBK541036/

[38] Ilkhani F. Niacin and oxidative stress: a mini-review. J Nutri Med Diet Care [Internet] 2016; 2(1) Available from: https://clinmedjournals.org/articles/jnmdc/journal-of-nutritional-medicine-and-diet-care-jnmdc-2-014.php?jid=jnmdc

[39] Keskin A, Büyüköztürk Karul A. The effect of niacin and melatonin supplementation on the antioxidant system and lipid peroxidation in exercised rats. Meandros 2022; 23(1): 60-6.

[40] Luo D, Peng Z, Yang L, *et al.* Niacin protects against butyrate-induced apoptosis in rumen epithelial cells. Oxid Med Cell Longev 2019; 2019: 1-8. [http://dx.doi.org/10.1155/2019/2179738] [PMID: 31737165]

[41] Silva de Paula E, Carneiro MFH, Grotto D, Hernandes LC, Antunes LMG, Barbosa F Jr. Protective effects of niacin against methylmercury-induced genotoxicity and alterations in antioxidant status in rats. J Toxicol Environ Health A 2016; 79(4): 174-83. [http://dx.doi.org/10.1080/15287394.2015.1137264] [PMID: 26914397]

[42] Cho K, Kim H, Rodriguez-Iturbe B, Vaziri ND. Niacin ameliorates oxidative stress, inflammation, proteinuria, and hypertension in rats with chronic renal failure. Am J Physiol Renal Physiol 2009; 297(1): F106-13. [http://dx.doi.org/10.1152/ajprenal.00126.2009] [PMID: 19420110]

[43] Hamoud S, Hayek T, Hassan A, *et al.* Niacin administration significantly reduces oxidative stress in patients with hypercholesterolemia and low levels of high-density lipoprotein cholesterol. Am J Med Sci 2013; 345(3): 195-9. [http://dx.doi.org/10.1097/MAJ.0b013e3182548c28] [PMID: 22990043]

[44] Office of Dietary Supplements - Niacin [Internet]. [cited 2022 Apr 10]. Available from: https://ods.od.nih.gov/factsheets/Niacin-HealthProfessional/

[45] Gheita AA, Gheita TA, Kenawy SA. The potential role of B5: A stitch in time and switch in cytokine. Phytother Res 2020; 34(2): 306-14. [http://dx.doi.org/10.1002/ptr.6537] [PMID: 31691401]

[46] Miller JW, Rucker RB. Chapter 16 - Pantothenic acid. In: Marriott BP, Birt DF, Stallings VA, Yates AA, editors. Present knowledge in nutrition (eleventh edition) [internet]. academic press; 2020 [cited 2022 Mar 16]. p. 273–87. Available from: https://www.sciencedirect.com/science/article/pii/ B978032366 1621000160

[47] Peterson CT, Rodionov DA, Osterman AL, Peterson SN. B vitamins and their role in immune regulation and cancer. Nutrients 2020; 12(11): 3380. [http://dx.doi.org/10.3390/nu12113380] [PMID: 33158037]

[48] Sanvictores T, Chauhan S. Vitamin B5 (Pantothenic Acid). StatPearls. Treasure Island, FL: StatPearls Publishing 2022. Internet Available from: http://www.ncbi.nlm.nih.gov/books/NBK563233/

[49] Scholefield M, Church SJ, Xu J, *et al.* Substantively lowered levels of pantothenic acid (vitamin b5) in several regions of the human brain in parkinson's disease dementia. Metabolites 2021; 11(9): 569. [http://dx.doi.org/10.3390/metabo11090569] [PMID: 34564384]

[50] Office of Dietary Supplements - Pantothenic Acid [Internet]. [cited 2022 Mar 16]. Available from: https://ods.od.nih.gov/factsheets/PantothenicAcid-HealthProfessional/

[51] Semenovich DS, Lukienko EP, Kanunnikova NP. Modulating oxidative stress indices and thiol-disulfide balance in the brain structures by pantothenic acid derivatives in an experimental model of parkinson's disease. Neurochem J 2021; 15(1): 24-9. [http://dx.doi.org/10.1134/S1819712421010128]

[52] Bonetti F, Brombo G, Zuliani G. Chapter 15 - The role of b group vitamins and choline in cognition and brain aging. In: Watson RR, editor. Nutrition and functional foods for healthy aging [internet]. Academic Press; 2017 [cited 2022 Mar 11]. p. 139–58. Available from: https://www.sciencedirect.com/science/article/pii/ B9780128053768000150

[53] Telen MJ. Pyridoxamine: another vitamin for sickle cell disease? Haematologica 2020; 105(10): 2348-50. [http://dx.doi.org/10.3324/haematol.2020.257998] [PMID: 33054072]

[54] Hadtstein F, Vrolijk M. Vitamin b-6-induced neuropathy: exploring the mechanisms of pyridoxine toxicity. Adv Nutr 2021; 12(5): 1911-29. [http://dx.doi.org/10.1093/advances/nmab033] [PMID: 33912895]

[55] Abosamak NR, Gupta V. Vitamin B6 (Pyridoxine). StatPearls. Treasure Island, FL: StatPearls Publishing 2022. Internet Available from: http://www.ncbi.nlm.nih.gov/books/NBK557436/

[56] Kumar P, Kumar M, Bedi O, *et al.* Role of vitamins and minerals as immunity boosters in COVID-19. Inflammopharmacology 2021; 29(4): 1001-16. [http://dx.doi.org/10.1007/s10787-021-00826-7] [PMID: 34110533]

[57] Available from: https://ods.od.nih.gov/factsheets/VitaminB6-HealthProfessional/

[58] Parra M, Stahl S, Hellmann H. Vitamin B6 and its role in cell metabolism and physiology. Cells 2018; 7(7): 84. [http://dx.doi.org/10.3390/cells7070084] [PMID: 30037155]

[59] Hsu CC, Cheng CH, Hsu CL, Lee WJ, Huang SC, Huang YC. Role of vitamin B6 status on antioxidant defenses, glutathione, and related enzyme activities in mice with homocysteine-induced oxidative stress. Food Nutr Res 2015; 59(1): 25702. [http://dx.doi.org/10.3402/fnr.v59.25702] [PMID: 25933612]

[60] Cheng SB, Lin PT, Liu HT, Peng YS, Huang SC, Huang YC. Vitamin B-6 supplementation could mediate antioxidant capacity by reducing plasma homocysteine concentration in patients with hepatocellular carcinoma after tumor resection. BioMed Res Int 2016; 2016: 1-7. [http://dx.doi.org/10.1155/2016/7658981] [PMID: 27051670]

[61] Choi EY, Cho YO. Effect of vitamin B6 deficiency on antioxidative status in rats with exercise-induced oxidative stress. Nutr Res Pract 2009; 3(3): 208-11. [http://dx.doi.org/10.4162/nrp.2009.3.3.208] [PMID: 20090886]

[62] Mahfouz MM, Zhou SQ, Kummerow FA. Vitamin B6 compounds are capable of reducing the superoxide radical and lipid peroxide levels induced by H_2O_2 in vascular endothelial cells in culture. Int J Vitam Nutr Res 2009; 79(4): 218-29. [http://dx.doi.org/10.1024/0300-9831.79.4.218] [PMID: 20209473]

[63] Tunali S. The effects of vitamin B6 on lens antioxidant system in valproic acid-administered rats. Hum Exp Toxicol 2014; 33(6): 623-8. [http://dx.doi.org/10.1177/0960327113506233] [PMID: 24107455]

[64] Giustina AD, Danielski LG, Novochadlo MM, *et al.* Vitamin B6 reduces oxidative stress in lungs and

liver in experimental sepsis 2019. Available from: http://www.scielo.br/j/aabc/a/DYfxS4593bPWprBFDm3cGhh/?lang=en [http://dx.doi.org/10.1590/0001-3765201920190434]

[65] Samsatly J, Bayen S, Jabaji SH. Vitamin B6 is under a tight balance during disease development by *Rhizoctonia solani* on different cultivars of potato and on *Arabidopsis thaliana* mutants. Front Plant Sci 2020; 11: 875. Available from: https://www.frontiersin.org/article/10.3389/fpls.2020.00875 [http://dx.doi.org/10.3389/fpls.2020.00875] [PMID: 32670323]

[66] Office of Dietary Supplements - Vitamin B6 [Internet]. [cited 2022 Apr 10]. Available from: https://ods.od.nih.gov/factsheets/VitaminB6-Consumer/

[67] Pacheco-Alvarez D, Solórzano-Vargas RS, Del Río AL. Biotin in metabolism and its relationship to human disease. Arch Med Res 2002; 33(5): 439-47. [http://dx.doi.org/10.1016/S0188-4409(02)00399-5] [PMID: 12459313]

[68] Zempleni J, Wijeratne SSK, Hassan YI. Biotin. Biofactors 2009; 35(1): 36-46. [http://dx.doi.org/10.1002/biof.8] [PMID: 19319844]

[69] Saleem F, Soos MP. Biotin deficiency. StatPearls. Treasure Island, FL: StatPearls Publishing 2022. Internet Available from: http://www.ncbi.nlm.nih.gov/books/NBK547751/

[70] Fernandez-Mejia C. Pharmacological effects of biotin. J Nutr Biochem 2005; 16(7): 424-7. [http://dx.doi.org/10.1016/j.jnutbio.2005.03.018] [PMID: 15992683]

[71] Office of Dietary Supplements - Biotin [Internet]. [cited 2022 Apr 10]. Available from: https://ods.od.nih.gov/factsheets/Biotin-HealthProfessional/

[72] Bistas KG, Tadi P. Biotin. StatPearls. Treasure Island, FL: StatPearls Publishing 2022. Internet Available from: http://www.ncbi.nlm.nih.gov/books/NBK554493/

[73] Sghaier R, Zarrouk A, Nury T, *et al.* Biotin attenuation of oxidative stress, mitochondrial dysfunction, lipid metabolism alteration and 7β-hydroxycholesterol-induced cell death in 158N murine oligodendrocytes. Free Radic Res 2019; 53(5): 535-61. [http://dx.doi.org/10.1080/10715762.2019.1612891] [PMID: 31039616]

[74] Abdel-Magied N, Shedid SM, Ahmed AG. Mitigating effect of biotin against irradiation-induced cerebral cortical and hippocampal damage in the rat brain tissue. Environ Sci Pollut Res Int 2019; 26(13): 13441-52. [http://dx.doi.org/10.1007/s11356-019-04806-x] [PMID: 30911963]

[75] Fourcade S, Goicoechea L, Parameswaran J, *et al.* High-dose biotin restores redox balance, energy and lipid homeostasis, and axonal health in a model of adrenoleukodystrophy. Brain Pathol 2020; 30(5): 945-63. [http://dx.doi.org/10.1111/bpa.12869] [PMID: 32511826]

[76] Office of Dietary Supplements - Folate [Internet]. [cited 2022 Apr 9]. Available from: https://ods.od.nih.gov/factsheets/Folate-HealthProfessional/

[77] Merrell BJ, McMurry JP. Folic acid. StatPearls. Treasure Island, FL: StatPearls Publishing 2022. Internet Available from: http://www.ncbi.nlm.nih.gov/books/NBK554487/

[78] Office of Dietary Supplements - Folate [Internet]. [cited 2022 Apr 23]. Available from: https://ods.od.nih.gov/factsheets/Folate-HealthProfessional/

[79] Office of Dietary Supplements - Vitamin B12 [Internet]. [cited 2022 Apr 10]. Available from: https://ods.od.nih.gov/factsheets/VitaminB12-HealthProfessional/

[80] Rizzo G, Laganà A, Rapisarda A, *et al.* Vitamin B12 among vegetarians: status, assessment and supplementation. Nutrients 2016; 8(12): 767. [http://dx.doi.org/10.3390/nu8120767] [PMID: 27916823]

[81] Rizzo G, Laganà AS. A review of vitamin B12. In: Patel VB, Ed. Molecular Nutrition. Academic Press 2020; pp. 105-29. [Internet] Available from: https://www.sciencedirect.com/science/article/

pii/B9780128119075000051
[http://dx.doi.org/10.1016/B978-0-12-811907-5.00005-1]

[82] Institute of Medicine (US) Standing Committee on the Scientific Evaluation of Dietary Reference Intakes and its Panel on Folate, Other B Vitamins, and Choline. Dietary Reference Intakes for Thiamin, Riboflavin, Niacin, Vitamin B6, Folate, Vitamin B12, Pantothenic Acid, Biotin, and Choline [Internet]. Washington (DC): National Academies Press (US); 1998 [cited 2022 Mar 13]. (The National Academies Collection: Reports funded by National Institutes of Health). Available from: http://www.ncbi.nlm.nih.gov/books/NBK114310/

[83] Watanabe F. Vitamin B12 sources and bioavailability. Exp Biol Med (Maywood) 2007; 232(10): 1266-74.
[http://dx.doi.org/10.3181/0703-MR-67] [PMID: 17959839]

[84] Shakoor H, Feehan J, Mikkelsen K, *et al.* Be well: A potential role for vitamin B in COVID-19. Maturitas 2021; 144: 108-11.
[http://dx.doi.org/10.1016/j.maturitas.2020.08.007] [PMID: 32829981]

[85] van de Lagemaat EE, de Groot LCPGM, van den Heuvel EGHM. Vitamin B_{12} in relation to oxidative stress: a systematic review. Nutrients 2019; 11(2): 482.
[http://dx.doi.org/10.3390/nu11020482] [PMID: 30823595]

[86] Oh R, Brown DL. Vitamin B12 deficiency. Am Fam Physician 2003; 67(5): 979-86.
[PMID: 12643357]

[87] Stabler SP. Vitamin B_{12} deficiency. N Engl J Med 2013; 368(2): 149-60.
[http://dx.doi.org/10.1056/NEJMcp1113996] [PMID: 23301732]

[88] Abdelfattah E. Effect of different concentration and application time of vitamin B12 on antioxidant response of Physiophora alceae. African Journal of Biological Sciences 2021; 0(0): 189-203.
[http://dx.doi.org/10.21608/ajbs.2021.88898.1021]

[89] Office of Dietary Supplements - Vitamin B12 [Internet]. [cited 2022 Apr 10]. Available from: https://ods.od.nih.gov/factsheets/VitaminB12-HealthProfessional/

CHAPTER 3

Fat-Soluble Vitamins Antioxidant Potential

Sohrab A. Shaikh[1,*]

[1] *Pharmacology, Toxicology, and Basic Health Sciences Unit, Faculty of Pharmacy, AIMST University, Bedong 08100, Kedah, Malaysia*

Abstract: The fat-soluble vitamins A, D, E, and K play important roles in maintaining overall health. These vitamins are stored in the body for future use and are mostly found in fruits, vegetables, nuts, and animal products. Vitamin A is essential for various physiological functions, including vision, epithelial integrity, red blood cell synthesis, growth, development, immune response, and reproduction. Moreover, vitamin A, along with carotenoids, can engage in electron transfer and quench singlet oxygen, suggesting their potential role in a biological antioxidant network. Furthermore, another fat-soluble vitamin, vitamin D, known as the "sunshine vitamin" due to its production in the skin upon sunlight exposure, is vital for musculoskeletal health and maintaining serum calcium levels. Additionally, vitamin D is reported to reduce the generation of Reactive Oxygen Species (ROS) through NADPH oxidase and enhance the antioxidant defenses by increasing the activity of enzymes like superoxide dismutase. Another vitamin in this group is Vitamin E, a potent fat-soluble antioxidant, which comprises eight isomers: four tocopherols and four tocotrienols. Each isoform has distinct biological effects and acts as a powerful scavenger of free radicals, contributing to the body's antioxidant defense. Vitamin K is another fat-soluble vitamin obtained from certain foods and dietary supplements, and is integral to the body's coagulation pathways. Additionally, vitamin K plays a role in preventing oxidative damage by inhibiting the activation of 12-lipoxygenase, an enzyme involved in arachidonic acid metabolism, thereby reducing ROS production. Collectively, these fat-soluble vitamins contribute to antioxidant defense and overall health, supporting various physiological functions and protecting against oxidative stress.

Keywords: Antioxidants, Dietary supplements, Oxidative stress, Vitamin A, Vitamin D, Vitamin E, Vitamin K.

INTRODUCTION

The fat-soluble vitamins A, D, E, and K possess unique properties that enhance overall health. These vitamins are commonly found in fruits, vegetables, nuts, and

* **Corresponding author Sohrab A. Shaikh:** Pharmacology, Toxicology, and Basic Health Sciences Unit, Faculty of Pharmacy, AIMST University, Bedong 08100, Kedah, Malaysia; E-mail: shaikh.sohrab@aimst.edu.my

Mukesh Singh Sikarwar, Arunachalam Muthuraman & Sohrab A. Shaikh (Eds.)

animal products. After being consumed and metabolized, they are stored in the body for later use [1]. The main fat-soluble microconstituents in the human diet consist of carotenoids and phytosterols [2]. Fat-soluble vitamins are essential for various physiological functions, including supporting vision, maintaining bone health, enhancing immune function, and aiding in blood coagulation [3]. Vitamin A aids in vision, while vitamin D assists in regulating calcium and phosphate balance, vitamin E helps with antioxidant activity, and vitamin K helps with blood coagulation. Although vitamin D was once regarded as merely a vitamin, it is now also recognized to be a prohormone [4]. In the past two decades, a lack of these vitamins has been associated with elevated risks of cancer, type 2 diabetes, and various issues with the immune system [5].

VITAMIN A

Vitamin A is made up of fat-soluble retinoids such as retinal (Fig. **1A**), retinol (Fig. **1B**), and retinyl esters [6]. Vitamin A is a necessary vitamin for the body's healthy functioning, including the visual system, epithelial integrity, red cell synthesis, growth and development, immunological and reproductive function, and so on. However, because the human body does not synthesize this vitamin, appropriate daily consumption is required to avoid micronutrient deficit and impairment of the body's proper functioning [7].

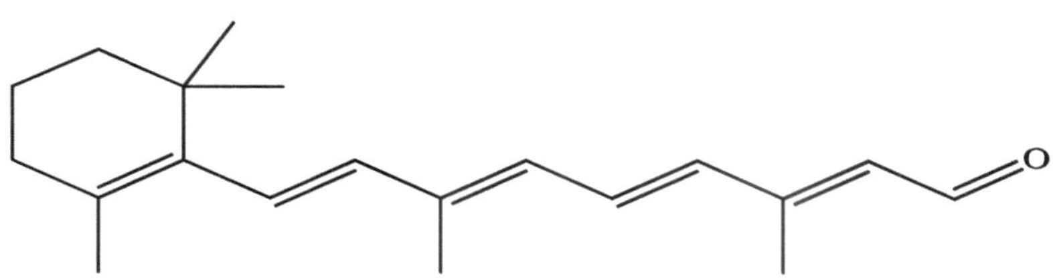

(A)

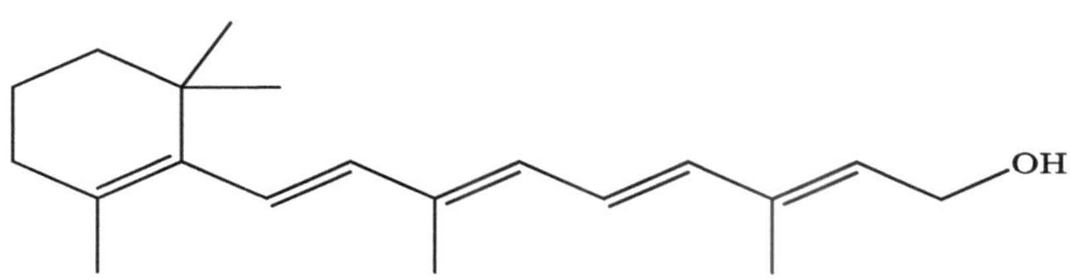

(B)

Fig. (1). Chemical structure of retinal (**A**) and retinol (**B**).

Dietary sources provide vitamin A in two forms. Preformed vitamin A, found as retinol and retinyl ester, can be obtained from foods like meat, whole milk, yogurt, cheese, margarine, butter, eggs, chicken, chicken liver, processed meats, pizza, and fish oils. Provitamin A, or beta-carotene, is found in colorful fruits and vegetables such as carrots, pumpkins, papayas, sweet potatoes, and red palm oil. Both forms of ingested vitamin A must be converted into retinal and retinoic acid after absorption to support biological functions [8 - 10]. A deficiency in vitamin A leads to the replacement of normal epithelial tissue with stratified, keratinizing epithelium in the eyes, periocular glands, respiratory system, digestive tract, and genitourinary tract. Vitamin A is required for gene regulation because of its role in cell morphogenesis, differentiation, and proliferation [8]. Vitamin A is essential for regenerating visual pigments, maintaining the integrity of mucosal membranes, and supporting the immune system. A deficiency in vitamin A can hinder the regeneration of visual pigment in retinal rods, leading to night blindness. If untreated, this deficiency can cause the deterioration of rods, resulting in xerophthalmia and potentially leading to blindness. Additionally, deficiencies may manifest as xerosis and breakdown of mucosal membranes in the intestines and lungs, along with compromised immune function, leading to frequent infections [9, 11].

Vitamin A supplements are used to treat xerophthalmia, severe malnutrition, measles, and to prevent deficiency among pregnant women living in regions where vitamin A deficiency is prevalent. Notably, the treatment of xerophthalmia holds significance as it stands out among vitamin-deficient illnesses that have escalated to epidemic levels. Administering vitamin A supplements has proven efficacy in addressing xerophthalmia, effectively averting night blindness, a significant issue in developing nations [8].

Vitamin A Antioxidant Potential

Vitamin A and carotenoids can receive and transfer electrons under certain conditions, and carotenoids can also quench singlet oxygen. As a result, both sets of chemicals have the potential to be part of a biological antioxidant network [12]. Although vitamin A is not widely recognized as an antioxidant, some research suggests it may have an indirect antioxidant role. Studies have shown that all-trans retinoic acid can inhibit thioredoxin-interacting protein, which reduces the activation of hepatic stellate cells (linked to liver cancer) and lowers oxidative stress. Additionally, retinoic acid, a metabolite of vitamin A, has been found to increase the expression of antioxidant genes in mature buffalo oocytes *in vitro*. Furthermore, in both normal and varicocele sperm, all-trans retinoic acid has been shown to enhance superoxide dismutase and glutathione transferase activity, while decreasing levels of malondialdehyde and reactive oxygen species. These findings suggest that retinol may boost the activity of antioxidant enzymes. As a result, growing evidence indicates that vitamin A might help protect the body from oxidative stress [13]. In addition to providing a metabolic source of retinol, beta-carotene and other dietary carotenoids act as antioxidants, reducing the quantities of free radicals that cause DNA damage and so preventing carcinogenesis [14]. Vitamin A, carotenoids, and provitamin A carotenoids have also been found to be efficient antioxidants in the prevention of heart disease [15].

Vitamin A Supplementation

Vitamin A is available in several forms, including retinyl palmitate, retinyl acetate, provitamin A beta-carotene, or a combination of these, in both individual supplements and most multivitamins [16].

VITAMIN D

Vitamin D is often called the "sunshine vitamin" because it is produced in the skin when exposed to sunlight [17]. Vitamin D, also called "calciferol," is biologically inactive and needs to undergo two hydroxylation processes in the body to become active. It can be obtained from sunlight, diet, and supplements. The first hydroxylation, occurring in the liver, converts vitamin D into "calcidiol," while the second hydroxylation, which mainly happens in the kidneys, produces the physiologically active form known as "calcitriol" [18]. The term "Vitamin D" refers to both vitamin D2 and vitamin D3, also known as ergocalciferol (Fig. **2A**) and cholecalciferol (Fig. **2B**). Vitamin D2 is formed in plants when ergosterol is exposed to ultraviolet B (UVB) radiation, whereas vitamin D3 is generated in the skin of humans and animals when exposed to UVB radiation [19]. Vitamin D is necessary for musculoskeletal health to keep serum calcium concentrations within the normal physiologic range [17].

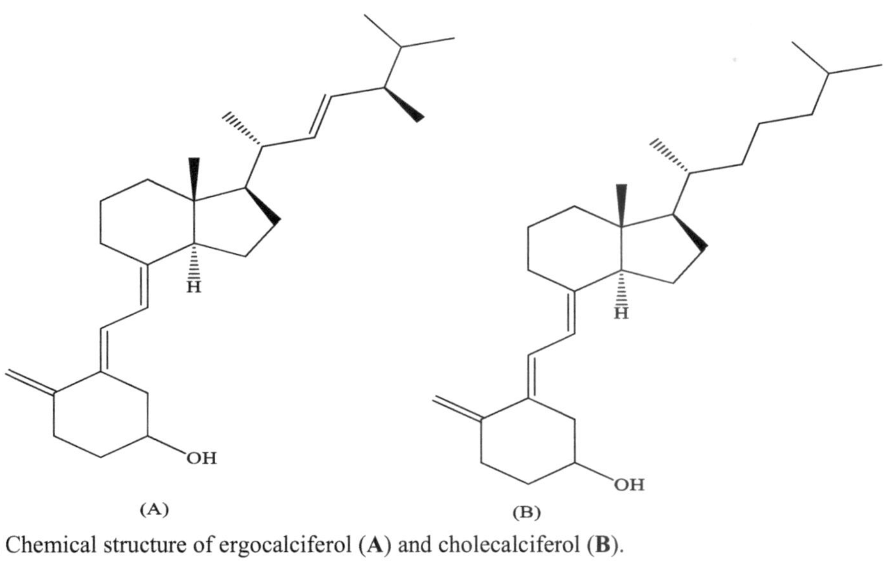

(A) (B)

Fig. (2). Chemical structure of ergocalciferol (**A**) and cholecalciferol (**B**).

Vitamin D is primarily obtained from three sources: sunlight, dietary intake, and supplementation [20]. Exposure of human skin to direct sunlight, which includes UVB radiation within the wavelength range of 290–315 nm, leads to the synthesis of vitamin D [19]. Vitamin D can be sourced from various foods, such as fatty fish like salmon, sardines, tuna, cod liver oil, swordfish, portabella mushrooms, egg yolks, and fortified foods like breakfast cereal, milk, infant formula, cheese, and orange juice [21]. Fortified foods, including milk (from cows or plant-based sources), margarine, butter, and breakfast cereals enriched with either ergocalciferol or cholecalciferol, are major sources of dietary vitamin D in many countries. The option of adding vitamin D to meals appears to be beneficial, however, its uptake is highly variable. As a result, its role in alleviating vitamin D insufficiency is unknown [22, 23]. Moreover, chocolate and cocoa are also identified as dietary sources of vitamin D [24].

The critical role of vitamin D in supporting skeletal growth and maintenance is well-known, and recent studies have highlighted its positive impact on non-skeletal health aspects such as cardiovascular health, immune function, and cancer. The main biological function of active vitamin D is to maintain the balance of calcium and phosphorus in the blood, which is vital for bone mineralization and neuromuscular function. The finding that the vitamin D receptor is present in nearly every cell of the human body has led to the realization that vitamin D may be involved in many more functions than previously known [19, 21]. The hormone-like activity of vitamin D has been demonstrated in various metabolic, enzymatic, physiological, and pathological processes across different organs and systems in the body [23].

Vitamin D deficiency is widely recognized as a common metabolic or endocrine irregularity [21]. A deficiency of vitamin D in children can lead to rickets, whereas in adults, it can cause osteomalacia. Additionally, a lack of vitamin D can result in muscle weakness and pain, with patients often reporting widespread discomfort in both bones and muscles. This deficiency is linked to rising obesity rates, reduced milk intake, and the widespread use of sun protection measures [17, 25, 26]. Severe rickets can induce developmental delays, hypocalcemic seizures, tetanic spasms, cardiomyopathy, dental deformities, irritability, and tiredness in children [18, 26]. A deficiency in vitamin D is associated with various health conditions such as osteoporosis, rheumatoid arthritis, diabetes, asthma, dizziness, epilepsy, depression, and a compromised immune system [13].

Vitamin D Antioxidant Potential

Research indicates that vitamin D suppresses the generation of reactive oxygen species through Nicotinamide Adenine Dinucleotide Phosphate (NADPH) oxidase and boosts antioxidant capacity by increasing the activity of antioxidative enzymes like superoxide dismutase [27]. Moreover, a research investigation revealed that the treatment with vitamin D resulted in a noteworthy increase in general antioxidant capability and heightened glutathione activity, among other metabolic enzymes. Additionally, the administration of vitamin D has demonstrated its ability to safeguard individuals with diabetes from vascular issues associated with oxidative stress [13].

Vitamin D Supplementation

Vitamin D2 and D3 are available in dietary supplements. Vitamin D2 is created by exposing ergosterol in yeast to UV radiation, whereas vitamin D3 is typically produced by irradiating 7-dehydrocholesterol, which is derived from lanolin found in sheep wool. Vitamin D3 sourced from lichen is also available in an animal-free form. Both vitamin D2 and D3 are effective at raising serum 25(OH)D levels and appear to be equally effective in treating rickets [18].

VITAMIN E

Vitamin E functions as a fat-soluble antioxidant, and it comprises eight isomers within its family. These include four tocotrienols (α-, β-, γ-, and δ-tocotrienol) and four tocopherols (α-, β-, γ-, and δ-tocopherol) [28]. Alpha-tocopherol, a major form of vitamin E, is commonly found in vegetable oils, green leafy vegetables, seeds, and nuts. It is also present in significant amounts in fortified cereals [29, 30]. Vegetable oils are the primary sources of these forms of vitamin E, particularly palm oil and rice bran oil, which contain higher concentrations of tocotrienols. Tocotrienols are also found in grapefruit seed oil, sunflower oil, olive oil, flaxseed oil, poppyseed oil, oats, maize, hazelnuts, buckthorn berry, and rye [31]. The common food oils like palm, corn, rice bran, olive, and peanut oils are the best sources of vitamin E. Conversely, less conventional oils extracted from fruit seeds, tree nuts, and by-products provide creative avenues for acquiring this crucial micronutrient [32].

Vitamin E exerts diverse biological effects that vary with the isoform. Both tocotrienol (Fig. **3A**) and tocopherol (Fig. **3B**) congeners are recognized as powerful scavengers of free radicals. However, chemically, tocopherols possess phytyl sidechains, while tocotrienols feature three carbon-carbon double bonds. The different forms of vitamin E play a crucial role in safeguarding cell membranes abundant in highly unsaturated fatty acids from oxidative damage. *In vivo* investigations have shown that α-tocopherol has higher antioxidant activity than other tocopherol congeners.

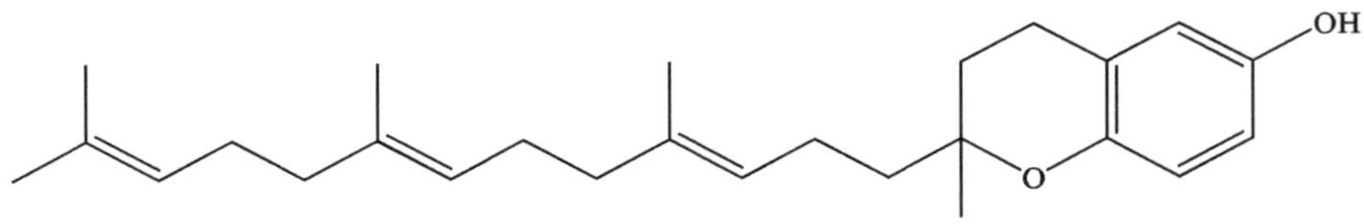

(A)

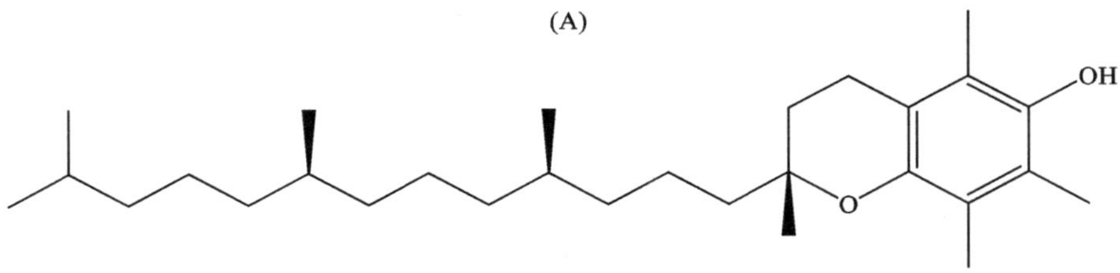

(B)

Fig. (3). Chemical structure of tocotrienol (**A**) and tocopherol (**B**).

Tocotrienols could exhibit stronger antioxidant properties compared to tocopherols, attributed to their shorter side chains that facilitate easier incorporation into cell membranes and the presence of an unsaturated side chain. Nevertheless, it has been suggested that α-tocopherol holds a superior *in vivo* role in neuroprotection due to its significantly higher bioavailability and preferential retention in tissues. Importantly, vitamin E's antioxidant characteristics are not limited to its antioxidant properties; it also has neuroprotective, anti-inflammatory, and cholesterol-lowering properties, as well as the ability to influence gene expression and potentially prevent Alzheimer's disease pathology [33]. Vitamin E's antioxidative qualities have also been discovered to be important in the fight against diseases like cancer, cataracts, asthma, allergies, and diabetes [34]. Vitamin E has been recently discovered to have anti-atherogenic, anti-allergic, anti-cardiovascular, anti-cancer, anti-diabetic, anti-inflammatory, anti-hypertensive, anti-lipidemic, neuroprotective, anti-obesity, and telomerase activity-modulating effects, among other possible health benefits [28]. Placental failure, neuromuscular deficits, hemolytic anaemia, retinopathy, impaired immunity, and increased inflammation are all indications of vitamin E insufficiency [30]. Furthermore, individuals suffering from disorders related to the malabsorption of fat can face an increased risk of developing deficiencies. Symptoms associated with these deficiencies encompass ataxia, skeletal myopathy, retinopathy, peripheral neuropathy, and compromised immune response. Another rare genetic disorder is Ataxia with Vitamin E Deficiency (AVED), characterized by a defect or absence of the alpha-tocopherol transport protein in the liver. People with AVED experience a severe deficiency in vitamin E, leading to nerve damage and a loss of mobility unless they receive substantial doses of additional vitamin E [29].

Vitamin E Antioxidant Potential

The most extensively used and studied dietary antioxidants are vitamin C and vitamin E [35]. Vitamin E's antioxidant activity is derived from the hydroxyl group situated on the aromatic ring of tocopherols, which effectively neutralizes free radicals by donating hydrogen atoms [33, 36]. Furthermore, vitamin E functions as an antioxidant by inhibiting the formation of peroxyl radicals, which are formed when a lipid radical combines with oxygen. Vitamin E interacts with the peroxyl radical, preventing it from attacking polyunsaturated fatty acids during lipid peroxidation. However, this interaction results in the formation of a tocopheroxyl radical, which necessitates reduction by additional antioxidants such as ascorbic acid [30]. Owing to its high levels within the lipid-soluble vitamin category, vitamin E is recognized for regulating the body's redox equilibrium. It is distributed extensively throughout the body, encompassing cell membranes and lipoproteins [28].

Vitamin E Supplementation

Vitamin E supplementation is not indicated for non-deficient children or adults on a regular basis. If a deficiency is discovered or if a person has a disease that causes low or missing vitamin E levels, oral supplementation is available over the counter [36]. While there are "mixed" formulations incorporating various tocopherols and even tocotrienols, the majority of vitamin E supplements primarily consist of alpha-tocopherol. To extend the shelf life of alpha-tocopherol in dietary supplements and fortified foods while maintaining its antioxidant effectiveness, it is commonly esterified. Esters like alpha-tocopheryl acetate and succinate are hydrolyzed and absorbed in a way similar to alpha-tocopherol [29].

VITAMIN K

Vitamin K is a type of fat-soluble vitamin present in certain foods and can also be obtained through dietary supplements. It is the general name for a series of substances having the chemical formula 2-methyl-1,4-naphthoquinone [37]. The name "vitamin K" comes from the German word "koagulation," which means "blood clotting," and it is also known as a blood-clotting factor. Vitamin K comes in three forms: K1, K2, and K3, also known as phylloquinone (Fig. **4A**), menaquinone (Fig. **4B**), and menadione (Fig. **4C**), respectively. K1, the most common form, plays a vital role in photosynthesis in plants. K2 is derived from K1, and K3 is produced by bacteria and other microorganisms. In the human body, K1 and K3 are converted to K2. While K2 is not found naturally in plants, it is synthesized by bacteria through the conversion of K1 to K2 [13].

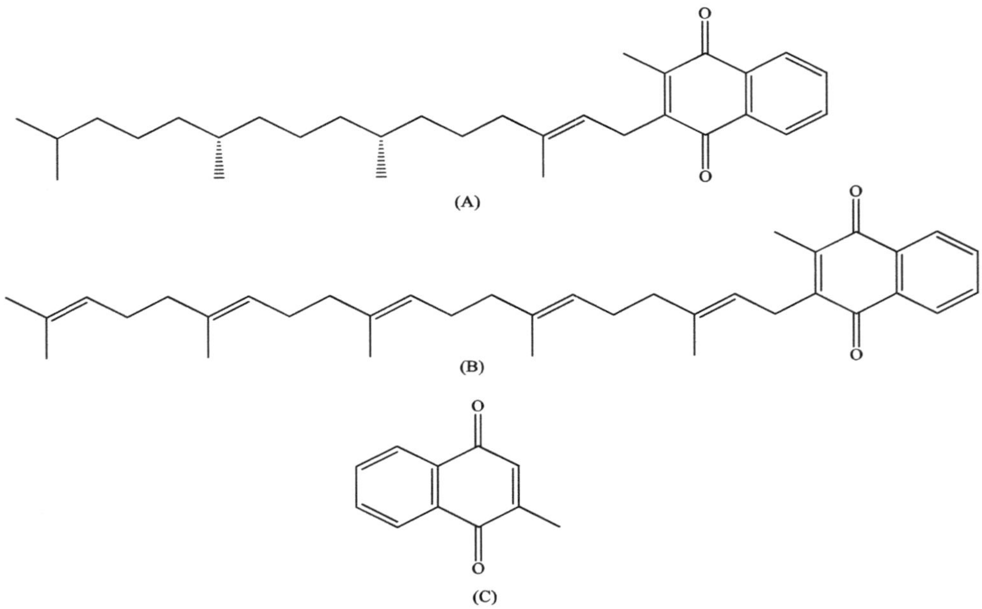

Fig. (4). Chemical structure of phylloquinone (**A**), menaquinone (**B**), and menadione (**C**).

Phylloquinone can be obtained from vegetables, especially green leafy ones, vegetable oils, and certain fruits. Phylloquinone levels are low in meat, dairy products, and eggs, while menaquinones are present in small concentrations. Vitamin K2 is present in meat, eggs, dairy products, fish, as well as fermented plant and animal foods. In contrast, vitamin K3 is not naturally occurring in foods [13, 37].

Vitamin K is a fat-soluble vitamin that influences the body's coagulation pathways. Vitamin K is a nutrient that can be found in foods or taken as a supplement. Vitamin K is required for the production of coagulation factors. It is a cofactor for vitamin K-dependent carboxylation, which is carried out by a number of enzymes. Vitamin K carboxylation causes coagulation factors to bind calcium ions, making the cascade pathways much easier to follow. Vitamin K shortage affects the coagulation process, causing bleeding problems. Vitamin K insufficiency has been related to osteoporosis and cystic fibrosis in recent research [37, 38].

Vitamin K insufficiency is considered clinically significant only when there is a substantial increase in prothrombin time due to a reduction in blood prothrombin activity. As a result, bleeding and haemorrhage are the most common symptoms of vitamin K insufficiency; however, these symptoms only occur in severe cases. A lack of vitamin K might hinder the mineralization of bones and potentially contribute to osteoporosis since vitamin K is essential for the carboxylation of osteocalcin within the bone [37]. Vitamin K deficiency in newborns can occur due to a combination of inherited issues with vitamin K-dependent clotting factors, inadequate dietary absorption, chronic health conditions, or it can be caused by medicine [39].

Vitamin K Antioxidant Potential

Vitamin K has been found to prevent the activation of 12-lipoxygenase during oxidative damage to developing oligodendrocytes caused by arachidonic acid. This is important because the activation of 12-lipoxygenase, an enzyme involved in arachidonic acid metabolism, plays a critical role in producing reactive oxygen species in the body [40]. Phylloquinone (vitamin K1) and menaquinone 4 (MK4), a type of vitamin K, protect developing oligodendrocytes and immature neurons by mitigating oxidative damage and reducing the production of reactive oxygen species that result from glutathione depletion [13]. The preventative and potent effectiveness of this naturally occurring vitamin, with no documented clinical adverse effects, presents a potential therapeutic use in addressing perinatal hypoxic/ischemic brain injury. This application aims to prevent oxidative damage to undifferentiated oligodendrocytes [41].

Vitamin K Supplementation

Most multivitamin/multimineral supplements include vitamin K. Vitamin K is also available in standalone dietary supplements, which may contain only vitamin K or be combined with other nutrients like calcium, magnesium, and/or vitamin D. Vitamin K1 can be found as either phylloquinone or phytonadione (a synthetic form of vitamin K1), whereas vitamin K2 is offered in supplements as MK-4 or MK-7 [37].

SUMMARY

Fat-soluble vitamins are important nutrients that play a crucial role in maintaining various physiological functions such as vision, bone health, immune response, blood clotting, and antioxidant defense. Fat-soluble vitamins are stored in the body, allowing the body to maintain reserves that can be drawn upon when dietary intake is inadequate. The antioxidant properties of certain fat-soluble vitamins, particularly Vitamin E, help protect cells from oxidative stress, which is linked to various chronic diseases. Sufficient intake of fat-soluble vitamins is essential for overall health, and deficiencies can lead to severe health issues, including night blindness, rickets, weakened immunity, and bleeding disorders. Individuals with specific health conditions, such as fat malabsorption disorders, may be at a higher risk for both deficiencies and the effects of toxicity. To ensure sufficient intake, a balanced diet rich in diverse food sources obtained from plants and animals, such as green leafy vegetables, dairy, fish, and fortified foods, is recommended. Continuing research on these vitamins helps to understand their therapeutic potential and broader health benefits, highlighting their importance in nutraceuticals.

CASE STUDIES AND PRACTICE QUESTIONS

Case 1: *A 4-year-old boy is brought to the clinic by his mother, who reports that he has difficulty seeing in low light and has dry, scaly skin. Dietary history reveals that he primarily eats rice and consumes very little fruit or vegetables.*

Discussion Questions

a. What is the medical condition the boy is suffering from?
b. Which vitamin deficiency is most likely responsible for this condition?
c. List dietary sources of this vitamin that can help manage or prevent the condition.
d. Explain the antioxidant role of the vitamin that is deficient in this child.

Case 2: *A 40-year-old male presents with complaints of back pain, loss of height, and postural changes, including a stooped or hunched appearance. He reports avoiding sunlight and regularly using heavy sunscreen due to sensitive skin.*

Discussion Questions

a. What is the medical condition the patient is suffering from?
b. Which vitamin synthesis is affected due to the reduced sunlight exposure?
c. List dietary sources of the vitamin that is deficient in this patient.
d. Explain the antioxidant role of a vitamin that is deficient in this patient.

Case 3: *A 50-year-old male smoker presents with complaints of fatigue and muscle cramps. Laboratory results reveal elevated markers of oxidative stress. His diet lacks nuts, seeds, and vegetable oils.*

Discussion Questions

a. Which vitamin is likely insufficient in this case?
b. Describe the antioxidant role of the vitamin that is deficient in this case.
c. List dietary sources of the deficient vitamin that can help manage or prevent this patient's condition.

Case 4: *A 65-year-old man comes to the clinic with frequent nosebleeds and easy bruising. He also complains of fatigue and has noticed more skin spots and delayed healing after small cuts. He has been on long-term antibiotic treatment for a recent infection and reports a poor diet consisting mainly of toast and tea. He is a long-time smoker. Blood tests show prolonged clotting time with a normal platelet count and elevated markers of oxidative stress.*

Discussion Questions

a. What is the most likely vitamin deficiency in this patient?
b. How might long-term antibiotic use contribute to this patient's condition?
c. What is the connection between smoking and elevated oxidative stress in this patient?
d. Suggest dietary and lifestyle changes to help manage this patient's condition.

REFERENCES

[1] Stevens SL. Fat-soluble vitamins. Nurs Clin North Am 2021; 56(1): 33-45. [http://dx.doi.org/10.1016/j.cnur.2020.10.003] [PMID: 33549284]

[2] Borel P. CHAPTER 3 - Nutrigenetic effect on intestinal absorption of fat-soluble microconstituents (vitamins a, e, d and k, carotenoids and phytosterols). In: Barbosa-Cánovas G, Mortimer A, Lineback D, Spiess W, Buckle K, Colonna P, Eds. Global Issues in Food Science and Technology. San Diego: Academic Press 2009; pp. 31-42. https://www.sciencedirect.com/science/article/pii/B978012374124000003X [http://dx.doi.org/10.1016/B978-0-12-374124-0.00003-X]

[3] Reddy P, Jialal I. Biochemistry, fat soluble vitamins. StatPearls. Treasure Island, FL: StatPearls Publishing 2022. Internet http://www.ncbi.nlm.nih.gov/books/NBK534869/

[4] Engelking LR. Vitamin A. In: Engelking LR, Ed. Textbook of Veterinary Physiological Chemistry. 3rd ed. Boston: Academic Press 2015; pp. 282-7. https://www.sciencedirect.com/science/article/pii/B978012391909050044X [http://dx.doi.org/10.1016/B978-0-12-391909-0.50044-X]

[5] Albahrani AA, Greaves RF. Fat-soluble vitamins: clinical indications and current challenges for chromatographic measurement. Clin Biochem Rev 2016; 37(1): 27-47. [PMID: 27057076]

[6] Office of Dietary Supplements - Vitamin A [Internet]. [cited 2022 Mar 20]. Available from: https://ods.od.nih.gov/factsheets/VitaminA-HealthProfessional/

[7] Soares MM, Silva MA, Garcia PPC, *et al.* Efect of vitamin A suplementation: a systematic review 2019. [http://dx.doi.org/10.1590/1413-81232018243.07112017]

[8] Chea EP, Lopez MJ, Milstein H, Vitamin A. StatPearls. Treasure Island, FL: StatPearls Publishing 2022. Internet http://www.ncbi.nlm.nih.gov/books/NBK482362/

[9] Hombali AS, Solon JA, Venkatesh BT, Nair NS, Peña-Rosas JP. Fortification of staple foods with vitamin A for vitamin A deficiency. Cochrane Libr 2019; 2019(5): CD010068. [http://dx.doi.org/10.1002/14651858.CD010068.pub2] [PMID: 31074495]

[10] Olson JM, Ameer MA, Goyal A. Vitamin A toxicity. StatPearls. Treasure Island, FL: StatPearls Publishing 2022. Internet http://www.ncbi.nlm.nih.gov/books/NBK532916/

[11] Hodge C, Taylor C. Vitamin A deficiency. StatPearls. Treasure Island, FL: StatPearls Publishing 2022. Internet http://www.ncbi.nlm.nih.gov/books/NBK567744/

[12] Olson JALLEN. Vitamin A and carotenoids as antioxidants in a physiological context. J Nutr Sci Vitaminol (Tokyo) 1993; 39 (Suppl.): S57-65. [http://dx.doi.org/10.3177/jnsv.39.Supplement_S57] [PMID: 8164068]

[13] Sinbad OO, Folorunsho AA, Olabisi OL, Ayoola OA, Temitope EJ. Vitamins as Antioxidants. Journal of Food Science and Nutrition Research 2019; 2(3): 214-35.

[14] Dawson M. The importance of vitamin A in nutrition. Curr Pharm Des 2000; 6(3): 311-25. [http://dx.doi.org/10.2174/1381612003401190] [PMID: 10637381]

[15] Palace VP, Khaper N, Qin Q, Singal PK. Antioxidant potentials of vitamin A and carotenoids and their relevance to heart disease. Free Radic Biol Med 1999; 26(5-6): 746-61. [http://dx.doi.org/10.1016/S0891-5849(98)00266-4] [PMID: 10218665]

[16] Office of Dietary Supplements - Vitamin A and Carotenoids [Internet]. [cited 2022 Apr 23]. Available from: https://ods.od.nih.gov/factsheets/VitaminA-HealthProfessional/

[17] Chauhan K, Shahrokhi M, Huecker MR, Vitamin D. StatPearls. Treasure Island, FL: StatPearls Publishing 2022. Internet http://www.ncbi.nlm.nih.gov/books/NBK441912/

[18] Office of Dietary Supplements - Vitamin D [Internet]. [cited 2022 Mar 20]. Available from: https://ods.od.nih.gov/factsheets/VitaminD-HealthProfessional/

[19] Wilson LR, Tripkovic L, Hart KH, Lanham-New SA. Vitamin D deficiency as a public health issue: using vitamin D_2 or vitamin D_3 in future fortification strategies. Proc Nutr Soc 2017; 76(3): 392-9. [http://dx.doi.org/10.1017/S0029665117000349] [PMID: 28347378]

[20] Aguilar Shea AL, Muñoz Moreno-Arrones O, Palacios Martínez D, Vaño-Galván S. Vitamina D para la práctica diaria. Semergen 2020; 46(6): 406-10. [http://dx.doi.org/10.1016/j.semerg.2020.02.008] [PMID: 32234285]

[21] Pfotenhauer KM, Shubrook JH, Vitamin D. Vitamin D deficiency, its role in health and disease, and current supplementation recommendations. Journal of Osteopathic Medicine 2017; 117(5): 301-5. [http://dx.doi.org/10.7556/jaoa.2017.055] [PMID: 28459478]

[22] Benedik E. Sources of vitamin D for humans. Int J Vitam Nutr Res 2021. [PMID: 34658250]

[23] Dominguez LJ, Farruggia M, Veronese N, Barbagallo M, Vitamin D. Vitamin D sources, metabolism, and deficiency: available compounds and guidelines for its treatment. Metabolites 2021; 11(4): 255. [http://dx.doi.org/10.3390/metabo11040255] [PMID: 33924215]

[24] Kühn J, Schröter A, Hartmann BM, Stangl GI. Cocoa and chocolate are sources of vitamin D_2. Food Chem 2018; 269: 318-20. [http://dx.doi.org/10.1016/j.foodchem.2018.06.098] [PMID: 30100440]

[25] Amrein K, Scherkl M, Hoffmann M, *et al.* Vitamin D deficiency 2.0: an update on the current status worldwide. Eur J Clin Nutr 2020; 74(11): 1498-513. [http://dx.doi.org/10.1038/s41430-020-0558-y] [PMID: 31959942]

[26] Sizar O, Khare S, Goyal A, Givler A. Vitamin D deficiency. StatPearls. Treasure Island, FL: StatPearls Publishing 2022. Internet http://www.ncbi.nlm.nih.gov/books/NBK532266/

[27] Kim DH, Meza CA, Clarke H, Kim JS, Hickner RC. Vitamin D and endothelial function. Nutrients 2020; 12(2): 575. [http://dx.doi.org/10.3390/nu12020575] [PMID: 32098418]

[28] Miyazawa T, Burdeos GC, Itaya M, Nakagawa K, Miyazawa T, Vitamin E. Vitamin E: regulatory redox interactions. IUBMB Life 2019; 71(4): 430-41. [http://dx.doi.org/10.1002/iub.2008] [PMID: 30681767]

[29] Office of Dietary Supplements - Vitamin E [Internet]. [cited 2022 Mar 21]. Available from: https://ods.od.nih.gov/factsheets/VitaminE-HealthProfessional/

[30] Traber MG, Vitamin E. Vitamin E. Adv Nutr 2021; 12(3): 1047-8. [http://dx.doi.org/10.1093/advances/nmab019] [PMID: 33684201]

[31] Ahsan H, Ahad A, Siddiqui WA. A review of characterization of tocotrienols from plant oils and foods. J Chem Biol 2015; 8(2): 45-59. [http://dx.doi.org/10.1007/s12154-014-0127-8] [PMID: 25870713]

[32] Shahidi F, Pinaffi-Langley ACC, Fuentes J, Speisky H, de Camargo AC. Vitamin E as an essential micronutrient for human health: Common, novel, and unexplored dietary sources. Free Radic Biol Med 2021; 176: 312-21. [http://dx.doi.org/10.1016/j.freeradbiomed.2021.09.025] [PMID: 34610363]

[33] Browne D, McGuinness B, Woodside JV, McKay GJ. Vitamin E and alzheimer's disease: what do we know so far? Clin Interv Aging 2019; 14: 1303-17. [http://dx.doi.org/10.2147/CIA.S186760] [PMID: 31409980]

[34] Rizvi S, Raza ST, Ahmed F, Ahmad A, Abbas S, Mahdi F. The role of vitamin e in human health and some diseases. Sultan Qaboos Univ Med J 2014; 14(2): 157-65. [http://dx.doi.org/10.18295/2075-0528.1566] [PMID: 24790736]

[35] Forman HJ, Zhang H. Targeting oxidative stress in disease: promise and limitations of antioxidant therapy. Nat Rev Drug Discov 2021; 20(9): 689-709. [http://dx.doi.org/10.1038/s41573-021-00233-1] [PMID: 34194012]

[36] Medina J, Gupta V, Vitamin E. StatPearls. Treasure Island, FL: StatPearls Publishing 2022. Internet http://www.ncbi.nlm.nih.gov/books/NBK557737/

[37] Office of Dietary Supplements - Vitamin K [Internet]. [cited 2022 Mar 21]. Available from: https://ods.od.nih.gov/factsheets/VitaminK-HealthProfessional/

[38] Imbrescia K, Moszczynski Z, Vitamin K. StatPearls. Treasure Island, FL: StatPearls Publishing 2022. Internet http://www.ncbi.nlm.nih.gov/books/NBK551578/

[39] Eden RE, Coviello JM. Vitamin K deficiency. StatPearls. Treasure Island, FL: StatPearls Publishing 2022. Internet http://www.ncbi.nlm.nih.gov/books/NBK536983/

[40] Li J, Wang H, Rosenberg PA. Vitamin K prevents oxidative cell death by inhibiting activation of 12-lipoxygenase in developing oligodendrocytes. J Neurosci Res 2009; 87(9): 1997-2005. [http://dx.doi.org/10.1002/jnr.22029] [PMID: 19235890]

[41] Li J, Lin JC, Wang H, *et al.* Novel role of vitamin k in preventing oxidative injury to developing oligodendrocytes and neurons. J Neurosci 2003; 23(13): 5816-26. [http://dx.doi.org/10.1523/JNEUROSCI.23-13-05816.2003] [PMID: 12843286]

CHAPTER 4

Therapeutic Uses of Macronutrients in the Healthcare System

Arunachalam Muthuraman[1,*], **Yuvaraj Sivamani**[2] and **Sumitha Elayaperumal**[3]

[1] *Pharmacology, Toxicology, and Basic Health Sciences Unit, Faculty of Pharmacy, AIMST University, Jalan Bedong-Semeling, Bedong 08100, Kedah, Malaysia*

[2] *Department of Pharmaceutical Chemistry, Crescent School of Pharmacy, B.S. Abdur Rahman Crescent Institute of Science and Technology, Vandalur – 600048, Chennai, Tamil Nadu, India*

[3] *Department of Biotechnology and Bioinformatics, JSS Academy of Higher Education and Research, Mysore, Karnataka, India*

Abstract: The macronutrients, such as carbohydrates, proteins, fats, and lipids, act as nutritive components of food, and they supply the energy for the body's demands. Macronutrients help in maintaining the body's structure and functions of various systems. Large amounts of macronutrients are required for day-to-day life functions. Furthermore, it is an essential nutrient for a healthy lifestyle and body homeostasis functions. Besides, it plays a vital role in various body functions with multiple biological and pharmacological actions. The outcomes of macronutrients vary with age, sex, fitness goals, pre-existing health conditions, and the daily intake amount of macronutrients. The role of these essential macronutrients in the Healthcare system for various ailments needs to be addressed to achieve better outcomes. However, the clear correlation of macronutrients in the clinical Healthcare system remains to be explored. Hence, this book chapter discusses the functional actions, mechanisms, and beneficial effects of macronutrients.

Keywords: Aerobic metabolism, Body-building elements, Macronutrient deficiency, Mediterranean diet, Tissue repair.

INTRODUCTION

Macronutrients are the types of nutrients that are used in the largest amounts, like carbohydrates, protein, and fats [1]. The nutritive components of food in macronutrients are essential for the body's energy demand and maintenance of

* **Corresponding author Arunachalam Muthuraman:** Pharmacology, Toxicology, and Basic Health Sciences Unit, Faculty of Pharmacy, AIMST University, Jalan Bedong-Semeling, Bedong 08100, Kedah, Malaysia; E-mail: muthuraman.a@aimst.edu.my

Mukesh Singh Sikarwar, Arunachalam Muthuraman & Sohrab A. Shaikh (Eds.)

body structure and system functions [2]. They are also involved in body growth, metabolism, and other body functions [3, 4]. The metabolism process is a major part of energy production, and it processes the body's building blocks (nutrients) that are required for day-to-day life. [5]. Macronutrients support the abundant calories, whereas they vary depending on the source of food and the person's condition. One gram of carbohydrates or proteins is supposed to make four calories; moreover, one gram of fat provides nine calories of energy [6, 7]. The details of macronutrients about carbohydrates, protein, and fats are described in the following sections.

CARBOHYDRATES AS MACRONUTRIENTS

Carbohydrates are the primary source of body energy. It is utilized by muscles and provides abundant energy to muscles and the central nervous system with the influence of movement and exercise [8, 9]. The energy production from carbohydrates is 45-65% of calories per day. Moreover, the amount depends upon the individual's health status and conditions [9]. The carbohydrate-based energy is produced in the form of glucose and enters all tissues and cells. Further, it undergoes multiple steps in the metabolism process, leading to the production of energy in the form of Adenosine Triphosphate (ATP). This metabolism process undergoes the aerobic and anaerobic processes [8, 10]. In metabolic pathways, it is entered into the glycolysis, the Krebs cycle, and the electron transport chain pathways [11, 12]. However, the production of energy is also raised with hexose monophosphate (HMP) shunt pathways. The HMP shunt is also referred to as the pentose phosphate pathway. It is a unique pathway involved in the production of essential energy-producing bio-compounds, *i.e.*, Ribose-5-phosphate (R5P) and Nicotinamide Adenine Dinucleotide Phosphate (NADPH) [13, 14]. In addition, these glucose metabolic products are shunted off the process and can support the production of energy compounds (glucose) from amino acids (protein) and fats (gluconeogenesis pathway). These gluconeogenesis and HMP pathways are also known as anabolic pathways [15]. Carbohydrate-derived energy mainly occurs in high-energy-utilizing tissues like the brain, kidneys, central nervous system, and muscles [16, 17]. Furthermore, the excess carbohydrates are stored in the muscles and liver in the form of glycogen [18, 19]. The primary sources of carbohydrates (macronutrients) are wheat, bread, maize, rice, potatoes, sugar cane, banana, honey, beans, nuts, and seeds [20].

Furthermore, carbohydrates are classified into three major categories based on their sugar group arrangements: monosaccharides, disaccharides, and polysaccharides [21]. Both mono- and disaccharides are known as simple sugars and are easily utilized by the body tissue, which elevates the blood sugar level rapidly [13]. Hence, diabetic patients are recommended to avoid this kind of carbohydrate. Examples include sugar, honey, sweet fruits, and sugar cane [22]. However, polysaccharides are a complex form of carbohydrates. It is broken down into simple sugar forms in the body. Examples are starch and cellulose [21]. It is commonly consumed by diabetic patients without dietary restrictions [23]. Thus, appropriate intake of carbohydrate macronutrients contributes to a healthy body condition, aids in the regulation of blood glucose content in individuals with diabetes, and supports overall metabolic health [24, 25].

Carbohydrate abnormalities also affect the Healthcare system, like lactose intolerance, sucrase deficiency, fructose malabsorption, and congenital carbohydrate intolerances [26, 27]. Lactose intolerance is a kind of carbohydrate macronutrient deficiency disorder. Lactase enzymes are present in the jejunum and cleave the milk sugar, *i.e.*, lactose. Sometimes it disappears in the weaning age [28]. The disappearance effects occur gradually, whereas the process is faster in age-onset conditions. Rarely do these enzymes disappear in early childhood and late adulthood. The absence of lactase leads to abnormal conditions in the body, and it is referred to as lactose intolerance [29]. These changes are mostly identified in white people due to biological abnormalities. Furthermore, this lactase intolerance effect persists throughout life, and it is also known as lactase persistence. In this case, the consumption of milk and lactose-containing products causes diarrhea, cramping, bloating, and flatulence-like gastrointestinal disorders [30]. Moreover, these problems are overcome with the consumption of small amounts of lactose-containing products in a day, plant-based non-dairy beverages, and lactase-treated dairy products [31, 32]. Similarly, sucrase deficiency is a carbohydrate macronutrient-related problem [33]. It is rare in the Healthcare system, and it is documented in adult patients with renal calculi [34, 35].

Further, these sucrase deficiency conditions are common in Human Immunodeficiency Virus (HIV) affected patients, *i.e.*, 31% of the HIV-infected population has a sucrase deficiency problem [36]. Fructose malabsorption also causes gastrointestinal problems like cramps, bloating, and osmotic diarrhea [27]. Further, they are not responding to medications and surgical interventions [37, 38]. The malabsorption of fructose-like problems is similar to the problem of consuming concentrated amounts of sugar, *i.e.*, beverages with high-fructose corn syrup, whereas these problematic effects do not occur when eating sufficient quantities of fruits [39]. Fructose malabsorption appears with fructose intake exceeding 25 grams per meal. These levels were reduced to around 15 grams in those who already have functional bowel disease [40]. Congenital carbohydrate intolerances are also rare, but they can cause life-threatening effects. In this case, all kinds of malnutrition problems, like alactasia (total absence of lactase), glucose-galactose malabsorption, and sucrase-maltase deficiency [41].

PROTEINS AS MACRONUTRIENTS

Proteins are involved in the various processes of body growth and functions. Further, it supports the structural building of the tissue, including blood plasma, cell membranes, muscle, hair, skin, nails, bones, ligaments, and tendons [42]. Further, it is also employed in the hormonal, enzymatic, and metabolic parts of the functions and supports the maintenance of acid-base balance [43]. The daily dietary allowance of protein is 0.8 grams of protein per kilogram of body weight. If a person weighs 150 pounds, then 54 grams of protein per day is recommended [44]. Similar to carbohydrates, the daily requirements of proteins vary depending on the daily activity level, age, medical conditions, and expected healthcare goals [45]. Protein is widely distributed in the body. It supports the body's growth, building, and repair of damaged tissues, and protects muscle mass, especially in a person with lean body mass [46]. Proteins are composed of a group of amino acids, and these amino acids act as building blocks of protein with peptide bonds [47]. Amino acids are classified into two types, *i.e.*, non-essential amino acids and essential amino acids [48]. The non-essential amino acids can be synthesized within the body. It means not required in the daily dietary intake, whereas the essential amino acids are needed *via* dietary products [49, 50]. Further, essential amino acids can be used by the body tissue directly or can be transformed into the non-essential form of amino acid. The protein-rich dietary sources are poultry, meat, fish, cheese, egg, and milk, including by-products of animal-based foods [51, 52]. It has an enriched form of essential amino acids. Even plant proteins also have all the required essential amino acids, like soy, nuts, beans, seeds, lentils, grains, vegetables, and fruits [52, 53]. Proteins play a good role in maintaining the body and also support maintaining good health from disease [54]. The protein package makes a greater difference in our health. The intake of healthy proteins like nuts, beans, fish, and poultry reduces the risk of multiple diseases and premature death, with heart disease, diabetes, cancer, bone health, and obesity [48, 55 - 57].

The regular consumption of small amounts of red meat (1.5 ounces of processed red meat) increases the (20%) risk of heart disease and stroke more than other diseases [58], whereas healthy proteins, *i.e.*, soy foods, beans, nuts, fish, and poultry, reduce these cardiovascular risks [59, 60]. Furthermore, plant sources of protein strongly decrease the risk of cardiovascular disorders. The primary reasons for plant-based healthy proteins are that they are more unsaturated [60, 61]. It reduces the Low-Density Lipoprotein (LDL) and does not contain additional cholesterol [61]. Moreover, the source of proteins is also contributing to further complications with diabetes risk factors like glucose and Advanced Glycation End products (AGE) [62]. Experimentally, red meat proteins cause a higher risk of type-2 diabetes (12%), whereas the consumption of legumes, nuts, and poultry reduces the risk (16% to 35%) in diabetic patients [63 - 65]. Furthermore, the risk is increased by around 32% with the consumption of processed red meat proteins. The primary reason for processed red meat-associated risk is due to the adaptation of the frequent and high-temperature methods of the cooking process [66]. In juvenile or insulin-dependent diabetes, type-1 diabetes is observed in cow's milk proteins and enhances the development of diabetes in babies (predisposition to diabetes) [67, 68]. However, the research reports remain inconclusive.

Cancer disease conditions, the source of proteins, and their quantity are responsible for the complication [69]. About 10% and 16% of cancer death risks are due to red meat or processed red meat, respectively [70]. According to a World Health Organization (WHO) report, the consumption of processed red meat can be a carcinogen to human beings. Furthermore, the consumption of processed meat is also responsible for the progression of colorectal cancer, stomach cancer, pancreatic cancer, and prostate cancer [71]. Moreover, the high consumption of red meat in the adolescent stage causes 22% of premenopausal breast cancer (1.5 servings of red meat per day) [72]. However, this risk was lower with the consumption of nuts, legumes, and poultry [73]. The reason for this risk is again due to the high-temperature application of red meat for grilling, which potentially causes cancer, and it is similar to polycyclic aromatic hydrocarbons and heterocyclic amines associated with cancer progression [74]. Additionally, the researchers also revealed that a protein diet like sausage, bacon, and salami, including red meat, is known to cause a higher risk of premature death, and it is reduced with plant foods based on higher protein intake, with a reduction of the risk factor of premature death [75, 76].

Bone is one of the calcium-containing tissues. Protein digestion enhances the release of acids and enters the bloodstream. This blood acidity is normally neutralized by the calcium ions as a buffering action [77]. The abundant consumption of proteins elevates the levels of blood acidity and requires lots of calcium for neutralizing this elevated acidity. The additional calcium ions are pulled from the bones and affect bone health [78]. Weight control is another problem with protein macronutrients [79]. Normally, healthy dietary protein is good for health, disease prevention, and weight control [80]. However, unhealthy proteins accumulate with changes in diet and lifestyle and subsequently raise body weight, leading to obesity [81]. The consumption of red and processed meat is contributing an extra one pound every four years. However, the intake of more nuts and plant-based proteins reduces the risk of gaining a pound every four years [82]. Further, the chicken with skin and regular cheese also enhances a greater level of weight gain [83]. The dietary sources of yogurt, walnuts, peanut butter, chicken without skin, and seafood are reducing the weight gain process [84, 85].

FATS AS MACRONUTRIENTS

Fats are one more macronutrient that acts as an energy reserve source; insulates and protects all vital organs; and also absorbs and transports fat-soluble vitamins from a dietary source [86]. 20-35% of the daily production of calories is from fat, and less than 10% of daily calories are from saturated fat. Vitally, dietary fats are very important for maintaining the health and proper function of various parts of the body [87]. Dietary fat, as a macronutrient, comes from various forms in the diet. Nowadays, dietary fats are low-carbohydrate and high-fat diets like the keto diet [88]. Dietary fats are in saturated and/or unsaturated form, and they provide nine calories per gram of fat [89]. However, the quality, health benefits, and risks of dietary fats vary in different types of dietary fats like trans fats, triglycerides, and mono- and polyunsaturated fats [88].

Saturated fats are obtained from animal sources like meat and dairy products; some of the fats are from plant sources like coconut oil. The chemistry of saturated fat consists of carbon chains with the bonding of hydrogen [87]. The properties of saturated fats, such as lard, include being solid at room temperature. However, sometimes saturated fats are also available in other forms like coconut oil, butter, ghee, cheese, cured sausages, and bacon [90]. The excess consumption of saturated fats is known to cause obesity in adults [91]. However, a low saturated fat diet like the Mediterranean diet is known to promote good health [92]. Trans fats are also known as trans fatty acids. It is formed when liquid vegetable oils are heated. In this case, extra hydrogen atoms are bound to the empty spaces of carbon atom chains in vegetable oil. This process is also known as hydrogenation [93]. The spaces of carbon chains are present in unsaturated fats, whereas saturated oils are full of hydrogen atoms. This saturation of hydrogen atoms makes the stable solid form of fats. The higher temperature application of vegetable oil in fast food restaurants has been changed to partially hydrogenated oil if not changed frequently, as regular oil [94]. Furthermore, these trans fats are also present in margarine and olive oil. The purpose of the hydrogenation of vegetable oil is to make it more stable and have less chance of going rancid [95]. However, trans fats are bad for health, and they cause the risk of various cardiovascular diseases due to the elevation of 'bad' cholesterol (LDL) and reduction of the 'good' cholesterol (HDL: high-density lipoprotein) [94]. These trans fats increase the risk of cardiac disease and cerebrovascular disorders like stroke [94]. Even the unprocessed form of trans fats, like olive oil, is also known to prevent the inflammation associated with cancer and chronic diseases [96, 97].

Triglycerides are other forms of fat macronutrients, and they are found in the blood. Blood triglycerides are one of the energy sources of the body [98]. Normally, calories are used due to the needs of our day-to-day life. The excess calories are converted and stored in the form of blood triglycerides, followed by storage in fat cells. Poor diet and inactivity have a great impact on blood triglyceride levels. The higher levels of blood triglyceride are one of the major biomarkers in the progression of cardiovascular disease [99]. The lower levels of blood triglyceride with daily 30 minutes of cardiovascular exercise and a balanced diet support the good health of the cardiovascular system. The normal triglyceride level is > 150 milligrams per deciliter (mg/dL). If it is increased, the triglyceride levels >150 to 199 mg/dL need more attention to improve the health status. Even an emergency condition occurs when the triglyceride level rises above 200 mg/dL [100]. Monounsaturated fats are liquid fats, and they have unsaturated double-bonded carbon atom chains. It promotes 'good' cholesterol production and reduces the levels of 'bad' cholesterol. The primary role of monounsaturated fats is to regulate the balance of HDL and LDL cholesterol [101]. The major monounsaturated fats are olive oil, peanut oil, canola oil, avocados, pecan nuts, and pumpkin seeds. Besides, the consumption of monounsaturated fatty acids is supported to maintain positive cardiometabolic actions *via* the promotion of HDL cholesterol and reduction of inflammation [102]. Polyunsaturated fats contain a large number of double bonds in the carbon chain with empty spaces for hydrogen. Polyunsaturated fats like omega-3 and omega-6 fatty acids are found in numerous sources of animal and plant-based products. The sources of polyunsaturated fats are walnuts, soybeans, sunflower oil, flaxseeds, salmon, herring, tuna, trout, and mackerel [103]. The omega-3 and omega-6 forms of polyunsaturated fats are reported to produce good health, whereas higher content of these fats is contributing to the progression of cardiovascular diseases, cancer, and inflammatory diseases [104, 105]. Most of the results documented that polyunsaturated fats like omega-3 and omega-6 improve cardiovascular and neurovascular functions, including cognitive functions [106]. Omega-3 supplementation is also recommended for those who do not eat oily fish once or twice a week. Further, the intake of oily fish improves 40% of cognitive function *via* activation of brain cells [107]. Moreover, these polyunsaturated fats can't be made by our system. Hence, the daily intake of omega-3 and omega-6 is essential for maintaining healthy body conditions. The summary of triangle links of macronutrients is illustrated in Fig. (**1**), and the details of functional benefits, mechanisms, and net effects of macronutrients are tabulated in Table **1**.

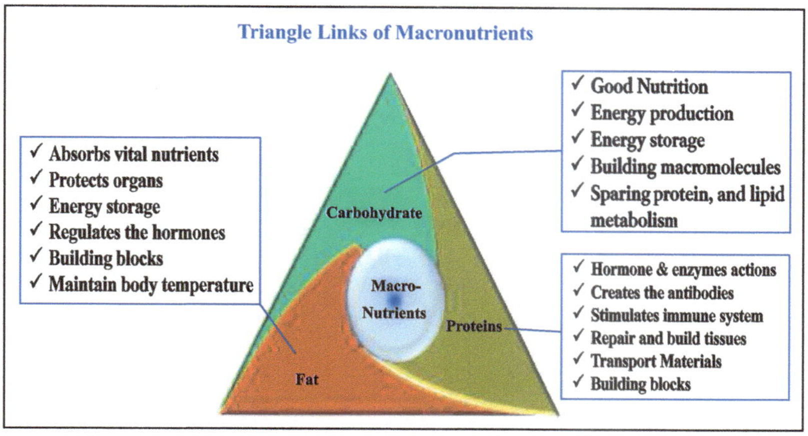

Fig. (1). The summary of the triangle links of macronutrients.

Table 1. The details of functional benefits, mechanisms, and net effects of macronutrients.

Macronutrients	Functional Benefits	Mechanisms	Net Effects
Carbohydrate (Raise the glucose, lactose, sucrose, and ribose concentration)	Supports high energy production and tissue functions.	• Enhance aerobic metabolism. • Activate the respiratory chain (Electron Transport Chain) function for energy production. • Raise the proliferation of fibroblasts and reduce the differentiation of keratinocytes.	• Cell energy and functional regulation. • Tissue repair. • Wound healing. • Diabetes mellitus [8, 10 - 12, 37, 38].
Proteins (Produced by amino acids and peptide bond linkage)	Makes body-building elements. Produce the functional elements of cell proliferation.	• Raise collagen synthesis. • Increase nitric oxide production. • Regulation of the cell signaling process *via* gene expression.	• Enhance the cell and body growth. • Prevents aging. • Wound healing. • Prevents protein deficiency. • Improves neuro-immune functions [43, 50, 80, 108].
Fats and Lipids (Cholesterol, fatty acids, sphingosine-1-phosphate, Ceramide-1-phosphate)	Acts as a body-building component. Supports immune functions. Act for vitamin storage. Regulates the temperature of the body.	• Occupy the cell membrane components. • Interfere with the cellular signaling process. • Enhance the neuronal lipid carrier functions.	• Maintain the cell permeability barrier functions. • Either raise or decrease the apoptosis process. • Regulates the risk of obesity. • Enhance the cell immunity functions [89, 91, 99, 101].

SUMMARY

Macronutrients are considered essential nutrients for a healthy lifestyle and body functions. Even, it is regularly needed and required in large amounts for day-to-day life functions. All three types of macronutrients (carbohydrates, proteins, and fats) play vital roles in our body functions with different biological actions. The better outcome of macronutrients varies based on age, sex, fitness goals, and pre-existing health conditions. These factors influence the daily intake amount of macronutrients. Of course, the additional nutrients are also essential for the Healthcare system, such as micronutrients and essential fatty acids. The detailed description of additional nutrients is provided in the following chapters.

CASE STUDIES AND PRACTICE QUESTIONS

Case 1: *A 38-year-old woman has a body fat content of about 52.2% and a BMI of 48.2 kg/m2, and was seeking medical treatment for obesity. She also suffered from a severe abdominal hernia and was not qualified for bariatric surgery for this condition. After examination, a decision was made to begin with a multi-pronged treatment using a natural dietary supplement. After 23 months of treatment, she had lost 38 kg of body weight and normalized fat percentage.*

Discussion Questions

a. What are the roles of the dietary fibre functions?
b. How does LDL cholesterol increase the risk of CHD?
c. Why is HDL known as good cholesterol?
d. What is the importance of body mass index (BMI) measurement in obesity?
e. Which one of the natural dietary supplements is useful for this obese patient?

Case 2: *A 25-year-old female suffers from autoimmune disease and Coeliac disease. Her current dietary plan is causing macronutrient deficiency-associated symptoms like bouts of diarrhea, constipation, bloating, and pain. Additionally, according to the Muslim faith, she is unable to consume pork products. This is hypothesized due to her symptoms, low fibre diet, and associated coeliac disease, whereby she avoids carbohydrate foods which supply fibre because many of these also contain gluten (e.g.,* wheat, rye, barley).

Discussion Questions

a. List the dietary fiber-containing carbohydrate.
b. Write the role of natural sources of lipids in preventing Diverticular disease?

c. How to regulate the positive energy balance for this patient?
d. Which one of the natural dietary supplements is useful for autoimmune disease and coeliac disease?

Case 3: *A 72-year-old female uses black tea and white toast for breakfast, canned fruit and a small muffin for lunch, and frozen potpie for dinner. She had trouble chewing and a poor appetite for the past few years. She doesn't drink milk due to too phlegmy and complains of 'no thirst for water'. She is also trying to treat her constipation with Metamucil, and she also has a gas problem.*

Discussion Questions

a. List macronutrient inadequate problems and specify a food supplement for this patient.
b. List the reasons for her present meal pattern and include the suggestion to improve her hydration status and alleviate constipation.
c. Recommend the TWO additional macronutrient suggestions for this patient.
d. How to improve the dehydration of this patient with macronutrient selections.

MCQs Questions

1. Which one of the following metabolites is the biologically active form of vitamin E?
   A. RRR-γ-tocopherol
   B. RRR-α-tocopherol
   C. All-rac α-tocopherol
   D. All-rac α-tocotrienol

2. Which one of the following functions is produced by body proteins?
   A. Insulate the body.
   B. Prevent constipation.
   C. Provide heat and energy.
   D. Growth and repair of body cells.

3. Which one of the following types of fats is found in foods that come from animals?
   A. Trans fat
   B. Saturated fat
   C. Unsaturated fat
   D. Monounsaturated fat

4. Which one of the following quantities is the recommended daily intake of fat for adults?
   A. Not more than 20 grams
   B. Not more than 50 grams
   C. Not more than 70 grams
   D. Not more than 100 grams

5. Which one of the following functions is produced by body fats?
   A. Aid in digestion.
   B. Insulate the body.
   C. Prevent constipation.
   D. Prevent the waste removal.

Answers: 1) A; 2) D; 3) B; 4) C; 5) B

REFERENCES

[1] Pahwa H, Sharan K. Food and nutrition as modifiers of the immune system: A mechanistic overview. Trends Food Sci Technol 2022; 123: 393-403. [http://dx.doi.org/10.1016/j.tifs.2022.03.017]

[2] Venn BJ. Macronutrients and human health for the 21st century. Vol. 12. Nutrients 2020; 12(8): 2363. [http://dx.doi.org/10.3390/nu12082363] [PMID: 32784664]

[3] Gerrits WJJ. Symposium review: Macronutrient metabolism in the growing calf. J Dairy Sci 2019; 102(4): 3684-91. [http://dx.doi.org/10.3168/jds.2018-15261] [PMID: 30415852]

[4] Savarino G, Corsello A, Corsello G. Macronutrient balance and micronutrient amounts through growth and development. Ital J Pediatr 2021; 47(1): 109. [http://dx.doi.org/10.1186/s13052-021-01061-0] [PMID: 33964956]

[5] Wali JA, Solon-Biet SM, Freire T, Brandon AE. Macronutrient determinants of obesity, insulin resistance and metabolic health. Biology (Basel) 2021; 10(4): 336. [http://dx.doi.org/10.3390/biology10040336] [PMID: 33923531]

[6] Srimiati M, Agestika L. The substitution of fresh Moringa leaves and Moringa leaves powder on organoleptic and proximate characteristics of pudding. Amerta Nutrition 2022; 6(2): 164-72. [http://dx.doi.org/10.20473/amnt.v6i2.2022.164-172]

[7] Sizer F, Whitney E. Nutrition: Concepts and controversies. Cengage Learning 2022.

[8] Hargreaves M, Spriet LL. Skeletal muscle energy metabolism during exercise. Nat Metab 2020; 2(9): 817-28. [http://dx.doi.org/10.1038/s42255-020-0251-4] [PMID: 32747792]

[9] Alghannam AF, Ghaith MM, Alhussain MH. Regulation of energy substrate metabolism in endurance exercise. Vol. 18. Int J Environ Res Public Health 2021; 18(9): 4963. [http://dx.doi.org/10.3390/ijerph18094963] [PMID: 34066984]

[10] Henselmans M, Bjørnsen T, Hedderman R, Vårvik FT. The effect of carbohydrate intake on strength and resistance training performance: A systematic review. Nutrients 2022; 14(4): 856. [http://dx.doi.org/10.3390/nu14040856] [PMID: 35215506]

[11] Stojkovski K. What is the difference between aerobic metabolism *vs* anaerobic metabolism? 2022.

[12] Hussain Y. Effects of phytonutrients in various metabolic pathways. The Role of Phytonutrients in

Metabolic Disorders. Elsevier 2022; pp. 35-66.
[http://dx.doi.org/10.1016/B978-0-12-824356-5.00009-6]

[13] Salih KJ, Sabir DK, Abdoul HJ. Glycolysis regulation to maintain blood glucose homeostasis. Kurdistan Journal of Applied Research 2022; pp. 114-24.

[14] Wamelink M, Williams M. Disorders of the pentose phosphate pathway and polyol metabolism. Physician's Guide to the Diagnosis, Treatment, and Follow-Up of Inherited Metabolic Diseases. Springer 2022; pp. 701-12.
[http://dx.doi.org/10.1007/978-3-030-67727-5_40]

[15] Evans RD, Heather LC. Human metabolism: Pathways and clinical aspects. Surgery (Oxford). 2022.

[16] Choi JH, Kim MS. Homeostatic regulation of glucose metabolism by the central nervous system. Endocrinol Metab (Seoul) 2022; 37(1): 9-25.
[http://dx.doi.org/10.3803/EnM.2021.1364] [PMID: 35255598]

[17] Penticoff HB, Fortin JS. Toxic/metabolic diseases of the nervous system. Neurobiology of Brain Disorders. Elsevier 2023; pp. 379-401.
[http://dx.doi.org/10.1016/B978-0-323-85654-6.00040-X]

[18] Scanes CG. Carbohydrate metabolism. Sturkie's avian physiology. Elsevier 2022; pp. 593-625.
[http://dx.doi.org/10.1016/B978-0-12-819770-7.00005-0]

[19] Korlimarla A, Gibson R, Kishnani PS. Glycogen storage diseases. Nutrition Management of Inherited Metabolic Diseases. Springer 2022; pp. 349-62.
[http://dx.doi.org/10.1007/978-3-030-94510-7_25]

[20] Palma-Morales M, Mateos A, Rodríguez J, Casuso RA, Huertas JR. Food made us human: Recent genetic variability and its relevance to the current distribution of macronutrients. Nutrition 2022; 101: 111702.
[http://dx.doi.org/10.1016/j.nut.2022.111702] [PMID: 35700591]

[21] Chaudhary S, Jain VP, Jaiswar G. The composition of polysaccharides: monosaccharides and binding, group decorating, polysaccharides chains. Innovation in Nano-Polysaccharides for Eco-sustainability. Elsevier 2022; pp. 83-118.
[http://dx.doi.org/10.1016/B978-0-12-823439-6.00005-2]

[22] Zidan D, Azlan A. Non-Centrifugal sugar (NCS) and health: A review on functional components and health benefits. Appl Sci (Basel) 2022; 12(1): 460.
[http://dx.doi.org/10.3390/app12010460]

[23] Liu H, Wang S, Yang L, Song H, Zhou D. Polysaccharides from soybean hulls and their functional activities. Phytochemicals in Soybeans. CRC Press 2022; pp. 285-300.
[http://dx.doi.org/10.1201/9781003030294-12]

[24] Isa ZM, Ismail NH, Tamil AM, *et al.* Pattern of macronutrients intake among type-2 diabetes mellitus (T2DM) patients in Malaysia. 2022.

[25] Korkut S, Köse Çetinkaya A, Işık Ş, *et al.* Macronutrient composition of colostrum in mothers with gestational diabetes mellitus. Breastfeed Med 2022; 17(4): 322-5.
[http://dx.doi.org/10.1089/bfm.2021.0209] [PMID: 35143337]

[26] Hasan Al-bayati DAA, MJ AL-Khateeb DS. The effects of thyroid hormones and their abnormalities on intestinal and hepatic glucose metabolism. Scholars International Journal of Biochemistry 2021; 4(3): 26-36.
[http://dx.doi.org/10.36348/sijb.2021.v04i03.002]

[27] Benardout M, Le Gresley A, ElShaer A, Wren SP. Fructose malabsorption: causes, diagnosis and treatment. Br J Nutr 2022; 127(4): 481-9.
[http://dx.doi.org/10.1017/S0007114521001215] [PMID: 33818329]

[28] Catanzaro R, Sciuto M, Marotta F. Lactose intolerance: An update on its pathogenesis, diagnosis, and

treatment. Nutr Res 2021; 89: 23-34.
[http://dx.doi.org/10.1016/j.nutres.2021.02.003] [PMID: 33887513]

[29] Katoch GK, Nain N, Kaur S, Rasane P. Lactose intolerance and its dietary management: An update. Journal of the American Nutrition Association 2022; 41(4): 424-34.
[http://dx.doi.org/10.1080/07315724.2021.1891587] [PMID: 33831336]

[30] Mullen A. Crisis and chronic selection of lactase persistence. Nat Food 2022; 3(8): 564.
[http://dx.doi.org/10.1038/s43016-022-00583-y]

[31] Nowak JK, Dybska E, Dworacka M, *et al.* Ileal lactase expression associates with lactase persistence genotypes. Nutrients 2021; 13(4): 1340.
[http://dx.doi.org/10.3390/nu13041340] [PMID: 33920682]

[32] Toca MDC, Fernández A, Orsi M, Tabacco O, Vinderola G. Lactose intolerance: myths and facts. An update. Arch Argent Pediatr 2022; 120(1): 59-66.
[PMID: 35068123]

[33] Lenhart A, Chey WD, Eswaran S. Sucrase-isomaltase deficiency: hiding in plain sight? Curr Treat Options Gastroenterol 2021; 19(3): 500-8.
[http://dx.doi.org/10.1007/s11938-021-00357-8]

[34] Andersen MK, Skotte L, Jørsboe E, *et al.* Loss of sucrase-isomaltase function increases acetate levels and improves metabolic health in greenlandic cohorts. Gastroenterology 2022; 162(4): 1171-1182.e3.
[http://dx.doi.org/10.1053/j.gastro.2021.12.236] [PMID: 34914943]

[35] Dahl NK, Goldfarb DS. Nutritional prevention and treatment of urinary tract stones. Nutritional Management of Renal Disease. Elsevier 2022; pp. 685-97.
[http://dx.doi.org/10.1016/B978-0-12-818540-7.00046-X]

[36] Gericke B, Amiri M, Naim HY. The multiple roles of sucrase-isomaltase in the intestinal physiology. Mol Cell Pediatr 2016; 3(1): 2.
[http://dx.doi.org/10.1186/s40348-016-0033-y] [PMID: 26812950]

[37] Budd AN, Wood B, Zheng W, Rong LQ. Perioperative management of direct oral anticoagulants in cardiac surgery: Practice recommendations based on current evidence. J Cardiothorac Vasc Anesth 2022; 36(11): 4141-9.
[http://dx.doi.org/10.1053/j.jvca.2022.07.016] [PMID: 35965231]

[38] Sirrs S, Fabbro E, Sechi A, Group SAMMTCW. Training competencies in adult metabolic medicine: A survey of working adult metabolic medicine physicians. JIMD Rep 2022; 63(5): 468-74.
[http://dx.doi.org/10.1002/jmd2.12312] [PMID: 36101815]

[39] Cano A, Alcalde C, Belanger-Quintana A, *et al.* Vitamin C and folate status in hereditary fructose intolerance. Eur J Clin Nutr 2022; 76(12): 1733-9.
[http://dx.doi.org/10.1038/s41430-022-01178-3] [PMID: 35854131]

[40] Jung S, Bae H, Song WS, Jang C. Dietary fructose and fructose-induced pathologies. Annu Rev Nutr 2022; 42(1): 45-66.
[http://dx.doi.org/10.1146/annurev-nutr-062220-025831] [PMID: 35995049]

[41] Boyer SW, Johnsen C, Morava E. Nutrition interventions in congenital disorders of glycosylation. Trends Mol Med 2022; 28(6): 463-81.
[http://dx.doi.org/10.1016/j.molmed.2022.04.003] [PMID: 35562242]

[42] Goldsmith JA, Holman ME, Puri P, Khalil RE, Ennasr AN, Gorgey AS. The interaction of macronutrients and body composition among individuals with chronic spinal cord injury. Br J Nutr 2022; (Jun): 1-12.
[PMID: 35738897]

[43] Holovakha VI, Mostovyi EV, Sliusarenko AO, Piddubnyak OV, Suslova NI, Matsinovich MS. Macronutrient status and indicators of acid-alkaline blood balance in cats with chronic renal failure. Regul Mech Biosyst 2020; 11(2): 266-71.

[http://dx.doi.org/10.15421/022039]

[44] Wu G. Dietary protein intake and human health. Food Funct 2016; 7(3): 1251-65.
[http://dx.doi.org/10.1039/C5FO01530H] [PMID: 26797090]

[45] Lourida I, Boer JMA, Teh R, *et al.* Association of daily physical activity and sedentary behaviour with protein intake patterns in older adults: A multi-study analysis across five countries. Nutrients 2021; 13(8): 2574.
[http://dx.doi.org/10.3390/nu13082574] [PMID: 34444732]

[46] Carbone JW, Pasiakos SM. Dietary protein and muscle mass: translating science to application and health benefit. Nutrients 2019; 11(5): 1136.
[http://dx.doi.org/10.3390/nu11051136] [PMID: 31121843]

[47] Tan Y, Wu H, Wei T, Li X. Chemical protein synthesis: advances, challenges, and outlooks. J Am Chem Soc 2020; 142(48): 20288-98.
[http://dx.doi.org/10.1021/jacs.0c09664] [PMID: 33211477]

[48] Lippi I, Perondi F, Pierini A, *et al.* Essential and non-essential amino acids in dogs at different stages of chronic kidney disease. Vet Sci 2022; 9(7): 331.
[http://dx.doi.org/10.3390/vetsci9070331] [PMID: 35878348]

[49] Lopez MJ, Mohiuddin SS. Biochemistry, essential amino acids 2020.

[50] Azhar G, Wei JY, Schutzler SE, *et al.* Daily consumption of a specially formulated essential amino acid-based dietary supplement improves physical performance in older adults with low physical functioning. J Gerontol A Biol Sci Med Sci 2021; 76(7): 1184-91.
[http://dx.doi.org/10.1093/gerona/glab019] [PMID: 33475727]

[51] Cartoni Mancinelli A, Mattioli S, Twining C, *et al.* Poultry meat and eggs as an alternative source of n-3 long-chain polyunsaturated fatty acids for human nutrition. Nutrients 2022; 14(9): 1969.
[http://dx.doi.org/10.3390/nu14091969] [PMID: 35565936]

[52] Yano H, Fu W. Effective use of plant proteins for the development of "New" foods 2022.
[http://dx.doi.org/10.3390/foods11091185]

[53] Kumar M, Tomar M, Punia S, *et al.* Plant-based proteins and their multifaceted industrial applications. Lebensm Wiss Technol 2022; 154: 112620.
[http://dx.doi.org/10.1016/j.lwt.2021.112620]

[54] Zhang C, Guan X, Yu S, Zhou J, Chen J. Production of meat alternatives using live cells, cultures and plant proteins. Curr Opin Food Sci 2022; 43: 43-52.
[http://dx.doi.org/10.1016/j.cofs.2021.11.002]

[55] Post A, Kremer D, Groothof D, *et al.* Amino acid homeostasis and fatigue in chronic hemodialysis patients. Nutrients 2022; 14(14): 2810.
[http://dx.doi.org/10.3390/nu14142810] [PMID: 35889768]

[56] Aggarwal R, Bains K. Protein, lysine and vitamin D: critical role in muscle and bone health. Crit Rev Food Sci Nutr 2022; 62(9): 2548-59.
[http://dx.doi.org/10.1080/10408398.2020.1855101] [PMID: 33290094]

[57] Wang D, Ye J, Shi R, *et al.* Dietary protein and amino acid restriction: Roles in metabolic health and aging-related diseases. Free Radic Biol Med 2022; 178: 226-42.
[http://dx.doi.org/10.1016/j.freeradbiomed.2021.12.009] [PMID: 34890767]

[58] Kim MN, Lo CH, Corey KE, *et al.* Red meat consumption, obesity, and the risk of nonalcoholic fatty liver disease among women: Evidence from mediation analysis. Clin Nutr 2022; 41(2): 356-64.
[http://dx.doi.org/10.1016/j.clnu.2021.12.014] [PMID: 34999330]

[59] Lin SP, Chen CM, Wang KL, Wu KL, Li SC. Association of dietary fish and n-3 unsaturated fatty acid consumption with diabetic nephropathy from a district hospital in Northern Taiwan. Nutrients 2022; 14(10): 2148.

[http://dx.doi.org/10.3390/nu14102148] [PMID: 35631289]

[60] Feingold KR. The effect of diet on cardiovascular disease and lipid and lipoprotein levels. Endotext 2021. [Internet]

[61] Sekhar S, Makaram Ravinarayan S, Kashmer D Yu A, *et al.* Are we nuts over coconuts? Studying the effects of coconut oil on low-density lipoprotein and cardiovascular diseases: A systematic review. Cureus 2022; 14(4): e24212.
[http://dx.doi.org/10.7759/cureus.24212] [PMID: 35637823]

[62] Steenbeke M, De Decker I, Marchand S, *et al.* Dietary advanced glycation end products in an elderly population with diabetic nephropathy: An exploratory investigation. Nutrients 2022; 14(9): 1818.
[http://dx.doi.org/10.3390/nu14091818] [PMID: 35565786]

[63] Zhao Z, Deng X, Jia J, *et al.* Angiopoietin-like protein 8 (betatrophin) inhibits hepatic gluconeogenesis through PI3K/Akt signaling pathway in diabetic mice. Metabolism 2022; 126: 154921.
[http://dx.doi.org/10.1016/j.metabol.2021.154921] [PMID: 34715116]

[64] Sanders LM, Wilcox ML, Maki KC. Red meat consumption and risk factors for type 2 diabetes: a systematic review and meta-analysis of randomized controlled trials. Eur J Clin Nutr 2022; 1-10.
[PMID: 35513448]

[65] Hosseinpour-Niazi S, Hadaegh F, Mirmiran P, Daneshpour MS, Mahdavi M, Azizi F. Effect of legumes in energy reduced dietary approaches to stop hypertension (DASH) diet on blood pressure among overweight and obese type 2 diabetic patients: a randomized controlled trial. Diabetol Metab Syndr 2022; 14(1): 72.
[http://dx.doi.org/10.1186/s13098-022-00841-w] [PMID: 35562742]

[66] Omofuma OO, Steck SE, Olshan AF, Troester MA. The association between meat and fish intake by preparation methods and breast cancer in the Carolina Breast Cancer Study (CBCS). Breast Cancer Res Treat 2022; 193(1): 187-201.
[http://dx.doi.org/10.1007/s10549-022-06555-x] [PMID: 35275284]

[67] Girdhar K, Huang Q, Chow IT, *et al.* A gut microbial peptide and molecular mimicry in the pathogenesis of type 1 diabetes. Proc Natl Acad Sci USA 2022; 119(31): e2120028119.
[http://dx.doi.org/10.1073/pnas.2120028119] [PMID: 35878027]

[68] Singh NK. Dry heated Cow's Milk protein and it's immunogenicity. Int J Innov Res Sci Eng Technol 2021; 7(12): 25-33.

[69] Ford KL, Arends J, Atherton PJ, *et al.* The importance of protein sources to support muscle anabolism in cancer: An expert group opinion. Clinical nutrition (Edinburgh, Scotland) 2022; 41(1): 192-201.

[70] Fuhrman J. The hidden dangers of fast and processed food. Am J Lifestyle Med 2018; 12(5): 375-81.
[http://dx.doi.org/10.1177/1559827618766483] [PMID: 30283262]

[71] Doe JE, Boobis AR, Cohen SM, *et al.* A new approach to the classification of carcinogenicity. Arch Toxicol 2022; 96(9): 2419-28.
[http://dx.doi.org/10.1007/s00204-022-03324-z] [PMID: 35701604]

[72] Farvid MS, Stern MC, Norat T, *et al.* Consumption of red and processed meat and breast cancer incidence: A systematic review and meta-analysis of prospective studies. Int J Cancer 2018; 143(11): 2787-99.
[http://dx.doi.org/10.1002/ijc.31848] [PMID: 30183083]

[73] Jin S, Je Y. Nuts and legumes consumption and risk of colorectal cancer: a systematic review and meta-analysis. Eur J Epidemiol 2022; 37(6): 569-85.
[http://dx.doi.org/10.1007/s10654-022-00881-6] [PMID: 35622305]

[74] Bulanda S, Janoszka B. Consumption of thermally processed meat containing carcinogenic compounds (Polycyclic aromatic hydrocarbons and heterocyclic aromatic amines) *versus* a risk of some cancers in humans and the possibility of reducing their formation by natural food additive. Int J Environ Res Public Health 2022; 19(8): 4781.

[http://dx.doi.org/10.3390/ijerph19084781] [PMID: 35457645]

[75] Milešević J, Vranić D, Gurinović M, *et al.* The intake of phosphorus and nitrites through meat products: A health risk assessment of children aged 1 to 9 years old in serbia. Nutrients 2022; 14(2): 242.
[http://dx.doi.org/10.3390/nu14020242] [PMID: 35057423]

[76] Kamal N, Ilowefah MA, Hilles AR, *et al.* Genesis and mechanism of some cancer types and an overview on the role of diet and nutrition in cancer prevention. Molecules 2022; 27(6): 1794.
[http://dx.doi.org/10.3390/molecules27061794] [PMID: 35335158]

[77] Jaziri AA, Shapawi R, Mohd Mokhtar RA, Md Noordin WN, Huda N. Biochemical analysis of collagens from the bone of lizardfish (*Saurida tumbil* Bloch, 1795) extracted with different acids. PeerJ 2022; 10: e13103.
[http://dx.doi.org/10.7717/peerj.13103] [PMID: 35310170]

[78] Gholami F, Naghshi S, Samadi M, Rasaei N, Mirzaei K. Dietary acid load and bone health: A systematic review and meta-analysis of observational studies. Vol. 9. Front Nutr 2022; 9: 869132.
[http://dx.doi.org/10.3389/fnut.2022.869132] [PMID: 35600825]

[79] Lim JJ, Liu Y, Lu LW, Barnett D, Sequeira IR, Poppitt SD. Does a higher protein diet promote satiety and weight Loss independent of carbohydrate content? An 8-week low-energy diet (LED) intervention. Nutrients 2022; 14(3): 538.
[http://dx.doi.org/10.3390/nu14030538] [PMID: 35276894]

[80] Ogilvie AR, Schlussel Y, Sukumar D, Meng L, Shapses SA. Higher protein intake during caloric restriction improves diet quality and attenuates loss of lean body mass. Obesity (Silver Spring) 2022; 30(7): 1411-9.
[http://dx.doi.org/10.1002/oby.23428] [PMID: 35538903]

[81] Marcelin G, Clément K. The multifaceted progenitor fates in healthy or unhealthy adipose tissue during obesity. Rev Endocr Metab Disord 2021; 22(4): 1111-9.
[http://dx.doi.org/10.1007/s11154-021-09662-0] [PMID: 34105090]

[82] Langyan S, Yadava P, Khan FN, Dar ZA, Singh R, Kumar A. Sustaining protein nutrition through plant-based foods. Front Nutr 2022; 8: 772573.
[http://dx.doi.org/10.3389/fnut.2021.772573] [PMID: 35118103]

[83] Betancourt-Núñez A, Torres-Castillo N, Martínez-López E, *et al.* Emotional eating and dietary patterns: Reflecting food choices in people with and without abdominal obesity. Nutrients 2022; 14(7): 1371.
[http://dx.doi.org/10.3390/nu14071371] [PMID: 35405983]

[84] Liaset B, Øyen J, Jacques H, Kristiansen K, Madsen L. Seafood intake and the development of obesity, insulin resistance and type 2 diabetes 2019.https://www.cambridge.org/core/article/seafood-intake-and-the-development-of-obesity-insulin-resistance-and-type-2-diabetes/9E470BE8B7957D9281A6E9BB79AA072D
[http://dx.doi.org/10.1017/S0954422418000240]

[85] Liu X, Li Y, Guasch-Ferré M, *et al.* Changes in nut consumption influence long-term weight change in US men and women 2019.
[http://dx.doi.org/10.1136/bmjnph-2019-000034]

[86] Agah S, Aminianfar A, Hassanzadeh Keshteli A, *et al.* Association between dietary macronutrient intake and symptoms in uninvestigated dyspepsia: Evidence from a population-based, cross-sectional study. Nutrients 2022; 14(13): 2577.
[http://dx.doi.org/10.3390/nu14132577] [PMID: 35807757]

[87] Meijaard E, Abrams JF, Slavin JL, Sheil D. Dietary fats, human nutrition and the environment: Balance and sustainability. Front Nutr 2022; 9: 878644.
[http://dx.doi.org/10.3389/fnut.2022.878644] [PMID: 35548568]

[88] Naude CE, Brand A, Schoonees A, Nguyen KA, Chaplin M, Volmink J. Low-carbohydrate *versus* balanced-carbohydrate diets for reducing weight and cardiovascular risk. Cochrane Database Syst Rev 2022; 1(1): CD013334.
[PMID: 35088407]

[89] Bhandari P, Sapra A. Low fat diet 2020.

[90] Hewlings S. Coconuts and health: Different chain lengths of saturated fats require ifferent consideration. J Cardiovasc Dev Dis 2020; 7(4): 59.
[http://dx.doi.org/10.3390/jcdd7040059] [PMID: 33348586]

[91] Wuni R, Adela Nathania E, Ayyappa AK, *et al.* Impact of lipid genetic risk score and saturated fatty acid intake on central obesity in an Asian Indian population. Nutrients 2022; 14(13): 2713.
[http://dx.doi.org/10.3390/nu14132713] [PMID: 35807893]

[92] Castaldi S, Dembska K, Antonelli M, Petersson T, Piccolo MG, Valentini R. The positive climate impact of the Mediterranean diet and current divergence of Mediterranean countries towards less climate sustainable food consumption patterns. Sci Rep 2022; 12(1): 8847.
[http://dx.doi.org/10.1038/s41598-022-12916-9] [PMID: 35614126]

[93] Bhat S, Maganja D, Huang L, Wu JHY, Marklund M. Influence of heating during cooking on *Trans* fatty acid content of edible oils: a systematic review and meta-analysis. Nutrients 2022; 14(7): 1489.
[http://dx.doi.org/10.3390/nu14071489] [PMID: 35406103]

[94] Pipoyan D, Stepanyan S, Stepanyan S, *et al.* The effect of trans fatty acids on human health: Regulation and consumption patterns. Foods (Basel, Switzerland) 2021; 10.

[95] Tatematsu K, Miyazawa D, Saito Y, Okuyama H, Ohara N. Fully hydrogenated canola oil extends lifespan in stroke-prone spontaneously hypertensive rats. Lipids Health Dis 2021; 20(1): 102.
[http://dx.doi.org/10.1186/s12944-021-01540-7] [PMID: 34511125]

[96] Majumder D, Debnath M, Sharma KN, *et al.* Olive oil consumption can prevent non-communicable diseases and COVID-19: A review. Curr Pharm Biotechnol 2022; 23(2): 261-75.
[http://dx.doi.org/10.2174/1389201022666210412143553] [PMID: 33845735]

[97] Silveira EA, Rosa LPS, de Resende DP, *et al.* Positive effects of extra-virgin olive oil supplementation and DietBra on inflammation and glycemic profiles in adults with type 2 diabetes and class II/III obesity: A randomized clinical trial. Front Endocrinol (Lausanne) 2022; 13: 841971.
[http://dx.doi.org/10.3389/fendo.2022.841971] [PMID: 35586621]

[98] Yeh JH, Tung YT, Yeh YS, Chien YW. Effects of dietary fatty acid composition on lipid metabolism and body fat accumulation in ovariectomized rats. Nutrients 2021; 13(6): 2022.
[http://dx.doi.org/10.3390/nu13062022] [PMID: 34208400]

[99] Song Y, Jensen MD. Red blood cell triglycerides—a unique pool that incorporates plasma-free fatty acids and relates to metabolic health. J Lipid Res 2021; 62: 100131.
[http://dx.doi.org/10.1016/j.jlr.2021.100131] [PMID: 34619142]

[100] Jung MH, Yi SW, An SJ, *et al.* Associations between the triglyceride-glucose index and cardiovascular disease in over 150,000 cancer survivors: a population-based cohort study. Cardiovasc Diabetol 2022; 21(1): 52.
[http://dx.doi.org/10.1186/s12933-022-01490-z] [PMID: 35429972]

[101] Hendriksen RB, van der Gaag EJ. Effect of a dietary intervention including minimal and unprocessed foods, high in natural saturated fats, on the lipid profile of children, pooled evidence from randomized controlled trials and a cohort study. PLoS One 2022; 17(1): e0261446.
[http://dx.doi.org/10.1371/journal.pone.0261446] [PMID: 34986194]

[102] Haldar S, Ponnalagu S, Osman F, *et al.* Increased consumption of unsaturated fatty acids improves body composition in a hypercholesterolemic chinese population. Front Nutr 2022; 9: 869351.
[http://dx.doi.org/10.3389/fnut.2022.869351] [PMID: 35548564]

[103] Mariamenatu AH, Abdu EM. Overconsumption of omega-6 polyunsaturated fatty acids (PUFAs) *versus* deficiency of omega-3 PUFAs in modern-day diets: The disturbing factor for their "Balanced antagonistic metabolic functions" in the human body. J Lipids 2021; 2021: 1-15. [http://dx.doi.org/10.1155/2021/8848161] [PMID: 33815845]

[104] Saini RK, Keum YS. Omega-3 and omega-6 polyunsaturated fatty acids: Dietary sources, metabolism, and significance — A review. Life Sci 2018; 203: 255-67. [http://dx.doi.org/10.1016/j.lfs.2018.04.049] [PMID: 29715470]

[105] Visioli F, Agostoni C. Omega 3 fatty acids and health: The little we Know after all these years. Vol. 14. Nutrients 2022; 14(2): 239. [http://dx.doi.org/10.3390/nu14020239]

[106] Mora I, Arola L, Caimari A, Escoté X, Puiggròs F. Structured long-chain omega-3 fatty acids for improvement of cognitive function during aging. Int J Mol Sci 2022; 23(7): 3472. [http://dx.doi.org/10.3390/ijms23073472] [PMID: 35408832]

[107] Teisen MN, Vuholm S, Niclasen J, *et al.* Effects of oily fish intake on cognitive and socioemotional function in healthy 8–9-year-old children: the FiSK Junior randomized trial. Am J Clin Nutr 2020; 112(1): 74-83. [http://dx.doi.org/10.1093/ajcn/nqaa050] [PMID: 32529206]

[108] Ruiz A, Quintela-López T, Sánchez-Gómez MV, Gaminde-Blasco A, Alberdi E, Matute C. Mitochondrial division inhibitor 1 disrupts oligodendrocyte Ca^{2+} homeostasis and mitochondrial function. Glia 2020; 68(9): 1743-56. [http://dx.doi.org/10.1002/glia.23802] [PMID: 32060978]

CHAPTER 5

Therapeutic Uses of Micronutrients in the Healthcare System

Khian Giap Lim[1], **Venkata Rathina Kumar Thigarajan**[2] and **Arunachalam Muthuraman**[3,*]

[1] *Clinical Pharmacy and Pharmacy Practice Unit, Faculty of Pharmacy, AIMST University, Jalan Bedong-Semeling, Bedong, 08100, Kedah, Malaysia*

[2] *Department of Pharmacognosy, College of Pharmacy, Madurai Medical College, Madurai - 625020, India*

[3] *Pharmacology, Toxicology, and Basic Health Sciences Unit, Faculty of Pharmacy, AIMST University, Jalan Bedong-Semeling, Bedong 08100, Kedah, Malaysia*

Abstract: Micronutrients are considered vitamins and minerals that are needed for the body to function in smaller amounts. The impact of micronutrients on the body's health and homeostasis is very critical. The deficiencies of micronutrients readily cause severe health impairments and even cause life-threatening conditions. The requirement for micronutrients depends upon the various influencing factors, such as absorption and excretion of nutrients. Micronutrient deficiency is associated with various disorders, and the requirements of micronutrients are variable based on the person's disease conditions and health status. Furthermore, pre-existing health conditions like sex, age, and fitness are also major factors in micronutrient requirements for essential body functions. The common principles of micronutrient actions are free radical scavenging and regulation of natural killer cells to prevent various disease progressions like cancer, Alzheimer's, and heart disease. However, the strong relationship between micronutrients and their uses in clinical conditions needs to be explored. Hence, this book chapter is focused on discussing the beneficial effects of micronutrients in the management of various ailments in patients.

Keywords: Amino acids, Free radical scavenger, Neurodegenerative disorders, Non-enzymatic antioxidants, Oil supplements.

INTRODUCTION

Micronutrients are an essential part of a healthy life after the use of macronutrients. Micronutrients are needed in very small quantities daily in our

* **Corresponding author Arunachalam Muthuraman:** Pharmacology, Toxicology, and Basic Health Sciences Unit, Faculty of Pharmacy, AIMST University, Bedong 08100, Kedah, Malaysia.; E-mail: muthuraman.a@aimst.edu.my

diet. It covers vitamins and minerals [1]. The major vitamins and their functions in the Healthcare process are described in chapters 2 and 3. This chapter is focused on essential minerals as micronutrients for a better Healthcare process. Micronutrients play a role in healthy body development, the prevention of disease, and maintaining well-being [2]. Moreover, these micronutrients are not produced in the body except for vitamin D. Hence, the supplements of micronutrients are essential in the diet. Worldwide, half of the younger children (< 5 years of age) are suffering from vitamin and mineral deficiencies [3]. The deficiencies of micronutrients are playing a role in devastating consequences. The details of various micronutrients like calcium, potassium, sodium, iron, zinc, magnesium, cobalt, chromium, coenzyme Q10 (CoQ10), iodine, and selenium are discussed in the following sections [4].

CALCIUM IN THE HEALTHCARE SYSTEM

Calcium is one of the essential micronutrients. In a cellular system, it acts as a secondary messenger for the cell signaling process. The abundant quantity is present in bones and teeth [5]. Furthermore, it also enhances the functions of the nervous system, cardiovascular system, and other organ functions. The recommended calcium levels for adults are 1,000 milligrams per day, and post-menopausal women need 1,200 mg per day [6]. Good sources of calcium are dairy products, legumes, and green and leafy vegetables. Moreover, calcium is important for maintaining the structure of bones and teeth. It also supports making normal body movements with tissue that is strong, rigid, and flexible [7]. Calcium nutrients are available in different forms, as free ions and bound forms. The free ion forms of calcium are present in the extracellular fluid, cell cytosol, and circulatory system [8]. Besides, it helps to make the constriction and dilation of blood vessels, muscular functions, blood clotting, neuronal impulse transmission, and hormone secretion [9, 10]. The transport of calcium ions occurs with active transport and passive diffusion in the intestinal mucosa [11]. In lower concentrations of calcium, it undergoes active transport, whereas passive diffusion occurs when the calcium ion concentration is raised [12]. In addition, the calcium reservoir, *i.e.*, bone, releases the calcium to maintain the cellular and circulatory calcium homeostasis process [13]. Calcium in bone and teeth is stored in the form of calcium hydroxyapatite and calcium phosphate [14]. It also helps to cure the bone *via* bone remodeling with bone growth, and repair [15].

The lower amount of calcium causes the weakening of bones and teeth. The deficiency of calcium leads to tingling and abnormal cardiac rhythm, and sometimes causes life-threatening conditions, whereas a large quantity of calcium leads to kidney stones, reduced absorption of other minerals, and constipation [16, 17]. The altered levels of calcium affect the various levels of the health system.

Calcium deficiency can raise bone weakness, the fragility of bones, and osteoporosis [18]. In addition to that, calcium deficiency is also responsible for rickets in children and multiple bone disorders in adults. In rickets conditions, the growth of cartilage bones is not mineralized and leads to the irreversible modification of the skeletal structure [19]. Chronic calcium deficiency leads to osteomalacia with defects of bone mineralization [4]. Normally, the symptoms of hypocalcemia are rising neuromuscular irritability, perioral numbness, tingling of hands and feet, and muscle spasms [20]. In severe conditions, calcium deficiency shows renal calcification, tissue injury, brain calcification, cataracts, congestive heart failure, paresthesia, seizures, coma, and neurological behavioural abnormalities like depression and bipolar disorders [2]. Hence, the balanced micronutrient calcium is needed from an individual's birth to the end of their life.

POTASSIUM IN THE HEALTHCARE SYSTEM

Potassium ions are essential for a variety of body functions. It is mainly involved in the healthy functions of the kidneys, heart, muscles, and nervous system [21]. It is also involved in the cellular membrane potential and structural regulatory functions. The recommended dose of potassium for adults is 4,700 milligrams per day [22]. The sources of potassium are bananas, coconut water, dried fruit, avocados, beans, and lentils [23]. The lower amount of potassium causes high blood pressure, stroke, and kidney stones, whereas a large amount of potassium produces harmful effects in patients with kidney disease [21]. The altered levels of these micronutrients, *i.e.*, potassium, affect the body's health. Besides, potassium helps to regulate body fluid, impulse transmission, and muscular contractions [24]. In a healthy body, about 98% of potassium is present in cells. Further, 80% is present in muscular cells, and 20% is present in bones, liver, and red blood cells [25]. Normally, potassium is present in the body in the form of electrolytes (positive charge) [26]. Furthermore, the lower and/or higher levels of potassium electrolytes affect many crucial functions [27].

Potassium deficiency causes hypertension, risk of kidney stones, altered bone turnover, excretion of urinary calcium ions, and changes in salt sensitivity. In severe conditions, potassium deficiency causes hypokalemia with the use of diuretics and other medications [28]. The symptoms of mild hypokalemia are constipation, muscle weakness, fatigue, and malaise, whereas moderate to severe hypokalemia conditions are shown as polyuria, encephalopathy with renal disease, glucose intolerance, paralysis of muscular tissue, respiratory dysfunction, and cardiac arrhythmias [29 - 31]. Moreover, chronic high hypokalemia can cause life-threatening problems like muscular contractions and cardiac dysfunctions. In addition, hypokalemia also contributes to magnesium depletion, which leads to the risk of cardiac arrhythmias *via* reduction of intracellular potassium ion concentrations in cardiomyocytes [32]. Potassium inadequacy also affects inflammatory bowel diseases (Crohn's disease and ulcerative colitis) [29]. The major fact is that potassium is secreted within the colon and facilitates the balanced absorption of potassium. However, potassium secretion increases in inflammatory bowel diseases and also enhances the excretion of potassium due to chronic diarrhea conditions [4].

Moreover, certain diuretics like thiazide diuretics are used for the treatment of hypertension and raise the urinary excretion of potassium, which leads to hypokalemia. Paradoxically, potassium-sparing diuretics do not cause potassium excretion, whereas they raise the levels of potassium, leading to hyperkalemia [21]. Further, heavy doses of laxatives and multiple doses of enemas also produce hypokalemia by raising the potassium excretion in stool [33]. Besides, the changes in potassium levels are also involved in the pathogenesis of hypertension, stroke, kidney stones, bone health, and type-2 diabetes [34]. The intake of potassium levels supports the reduction of blood pressure *via* dilation of blood vessels, urinary excretion of sodium, and reduction of plasma volume [35]. Further, it also enhances the absorption of other nutrients like magnesium and calcium, which reduces blood pressure. Low potassium intakes cause impairment of calcium reabsorption in the kidney and raise the urinary calcium, leading to hypercalciuria and kidney stones [36]. Besides, the excess consumption of potassium contained in fruits and vegetables raises bone mineral density and improves bone health [37, 38].

The lower intakes of potassium and lower concentration of serum and/or urinary potassium levels raise the risk of insulin resistance, fasting glucose, and type-2 diabetes [30]. The impairment of urinary excretion of potassium occurs due to chronic kidney disease, usage of angiotensin-converting enzyme inhibitors, and potassium-sparing diuretics, leading to hyperkalemia [39, 40]. This hyperkalemia condition may be asymptomatic, whereas the severe condition shows heart palpitations, paralysis, muscle weakness, paresthesias, and cardiac arrhythmias [41, 42]. Hence, the balanced micronutrient potassium is needed for better health and an extended lifestyle care system.

SODIUM IN THE HEALTHCARE SYSTEM

Sodium is another electrolyte, and it is an essential micronutrient for nerve and muscle functions. Further, it regulates the body's fluid levels. The recommended intake level of sodium for an adult is 2,300 mg per day [43]. This quantity is around one teaspoon of table salt. Table salt is made up of sodium and chloride ions, and it is obtained from seawater. Sometimes, the intake of one teaspoon of table salt raises the sodium level in the body due to the presence of sodium in other foods like salted meat and fish [44]. The intake of low levels of sodium leads to hyponatremia, which indicates fatigue, lethargy, and confusion [45]. However, the intake of high levels of sodium causes hypertension and raises the risk of cardiovascular disease and stroke [46]. Normally, hypertensive and kidney disease patients are advised to take less sodium salt and salted foods [47]. Furthermore, it is involved in the regulation of cellular ion balance of other micronutrients like calcium and potassium [48].

Sodium ions are essential for fluid balance and maintaining cellular homeostasis. Sodium is referred to as the "fluid matrix" of the body. For several decades, the amount of dietary sodium has contributed to maintaining homeostasis [49]. The intake of high dietary sodium or a decline in sodium causes salt-sensitive blood pressure. Further, no alteration of blood pressure when sodium restriction is made, and it is considered salt-resistant blood pressure [50]. In addition, the overloading of sodium raises the extracellular volume and causes hypertension with renal dysfunction and chronic kidney disease [51]. The impairment of hormonal systems like the renin-angiotensin-aldosterone system is also sensitized with sodium manipulation *via* activation of angiotensin II type-1 receptors in renal and non-renal vascular tissue, and the central nervous system [52, 53]. In peripheral vascular smooth muscle tissue, resistance is also involved in the blood pressure response with an elevation of expanded dietary sodium intake [54]. The high dietary sodium also enhances the central sympathetic outflow, leading to an elevation in blood pressure *via* modest elevations of plasma sodium ions [55]. Hence, the balanced administration of sodium micronutrients is needed for a better healthcare system.

IRON IN THE HEALTHCARE SYSTEM

Iron is a primary micronutrient, and it is involved in many body functions like growth, metabolism, and immunity. It is also a major component of hemoglobin and myoglobin. It is responsible for transporting oxygen throughout the body tissues [56]. The deficiency of iron is commonly known as anemia. Sometimes iron deficiency-associated anemia is lethal. According to the WHO, iron-deficiency anemia is the most common nutritional deficiency worldwide [57]. It mainly affects aged school children and pregnant women. Even though it has risen by 30 to 40 percent in industrialized countries [58]. The major sources of iron are heme from meat, minerals from plants, and iron-fortified foods [56]. Moreover, the iron from heme is not affected by other dietary products to raise the bioavailability of iron in the blood. However, the non-heme types of iron show less bioavailability and are also affected by other foods [59]. Normally, vegetarians readily absorb 14 to 18% of the iron in their diets, whereas non-vegetarians absorb 5 to 12% of the iron in their diets [60]. Besides, vitamin C, poultry, and fish with non-heme iron foods enhance the bioavailability of iron. Further, some foods and beverages, like soy and tea, also affect iron absorption [59]. The daily intake of iron is 18 milligrams for age 4 children and older people [61].

Iron deficiencies are common in infants, young children, teenage girls, and pregnant women, including premenopausal women [62]. Furthermore, iron supplements are reducing the absorption levels of certain medications like levodopa and levothyroxine [63, 64]. Similarly, certain drugs also reduce iron absorption, like proton pump inhibitors [65]. Hence, the discussion of iron supplementation and other foods and medication recommendations needs to be considered by healthcare professionals. Furthermore, the long-lasting detrimental effects of iron are also shown in the dysfunction of cognitive ability and neuronal development [66]. Further, it is a severe risk in people with cancer, chronic blood loss, chronic disease, chronic infections, autoimmune disease, frequent blood donors, heart failure, and gastrointestinal disorders [67, 68]. The common symptoms of iron deficiency are dizziness, weakness, fatigue, headache, swollen tongue, pale skin, and fingernails [69]. However, the toxic levels of iron (60 milligrams of iron per kilogram of body weight) are causing abdominal cramps, nausea, vomiting, constipation, organ failure, and probably death [70]. Sometimes patients with hemochromatosis (a genetic disorder) have a higher risk of iron toxicity with iron overload [71]. Hence, iron requirements vary from person to person. Therefore, the exact recommendation of iron supplements needs to be considered carefully by healthcare providers. Currently, iron-fortified wheat flour is made mandatory in 83 countries to raise the iron intake for a healthy life. Hence, a balanced iron supplement is essential for a better healthcare system.

ZINC IN THE HEALTHCARE SYSTEM

Zinc is one of the essential trace elements in micronutrients. It is needed to maintain the Healthcare system. Zinc is present in all types of cells throughout the body. The primary function of zinc is to be the body's defensive system [72]. It also plays a key role in cell divisions, cell growth, wound healing, and the breakdown of carbohydrates [73]. Moreover, zinc is also needed for the functions of smell and taste [74]. Besides, during pregnancy and infancy, zinc is an essential component for the growth and development of the child [75]. Zinc also supports enhancing insulin actions [76]. Zinc also reduces the risk of the common cold *via* the promotion of the immune system. It is also involved in the prevention of infectious diseases like malaria, diarrhea, and pneumonia [77].

The animal sources of zinc are beef, lamb, pork, and fish (low levels). Even the dark meat of a chicken has a large amount of zinc [78]. Plant sources like legumes, nuts, whole grains, and yeast also possess zinc [79]. Zinc is used in various multivitamin and mineral supplement preparations in the form of zinc gluconate, zinc sulfate, and zinc acetate [80]. Further, zinc is an over-the-counter medicine like cold lozenges, nasal sprays, and gels [81]. Zinc deficiency affects about 17.3% of the population globally. Moreover, the supplements of zinc prevent childhood diarrhea, premature birth, and the reduction of respiratory infections [77, 82]. It even supports the growth and weight gain of infants and young children. Physiologically, it also supports healthy immune cell function, body cell growth, wound repair, and the expression of healthy proteins [83, 84]. When low levels of zinc lead to skin soreness, loss of hair, diarrhea, and changes in taste and smell. Further, excess zinc can cause diarrhea, abdominal cramps, vomiting, and headaches [85, 86]. Even excessive intakes of zinc also cause copper and/or iron deficiency [87]. Hence, the balanced zinc supplement is essential for a better healthcare system.

MAGNESIUM IN THE HEALTHCARE SYSTEM

Magnesium is also considered a micronutrient component. It has a big role in the maintenance of overall Healthcare. It helps to prevent and mitigate chronic disorders. In addition, it makes the bones very strong and reduces the complication of neurovascular unit dysfunctions associated with symptoms like migraine, headache, and fatigue [88, 89]. Magnesium is important for the human body's function. The low level of magnesium produces nausea, tiredness, weakness, restless legs, and sleep disturbance. Further, the large amount of magnesium causes digestive and heart problems [90]. The major sources of magnesium are spinach, eggs, beans, peanuts, pumpkin seeds, apples, and brown rice [91, 92]. The recommended dose of magnesium for adult females is 320 mg per day, and adult males need 420 mg of magnesium per day [93].

Magnesium is also essential for multiple metabolic pathways like blood sugar control, blood pressure control, energy production, protein synthesis, muscle contraction, and nerve functions. In the nervous system, magnesium prevents neuronal excitability [94, 95]. Excitation of neuron cells is responsible for multiple neurological disorders like epilepsy, neuropathic pain, drug addiction, anxiety, depression, Parkinson's disease, and Alzheimer's disease [96]. The intake of magnesium is known to reduce severe pain sensation, depression, anxiety, migraine, and cognitive disorders [97]. Further, it involves a variety of enzymatic reactions. It also helps in the production of energy [98]. It even reduces the risk of heart disease with the action of calcium and vitamin D. The deficiency of magnesium is known to raise cardiovascular disease by supplementation of calcium and vitamin D, whereas the administration of calcium and vitamin D enhances the magnesium-associated cardioprotective actions [99]. Hence, a balanced magnesium supplement is essential for a better Healthcare system.

COBALT IN THE HEALTHCARE SYSTEM

Cobalt micronutrient is a part of vitamin B-12. It is present in red blood cells and supports the process of erythropoiesis. Further, it is also involved in the healthy maintenance of the nervous system [100]. The actions of cobalt are similar to those of manganese and zinc micronutrients. In addition, cobalt can replace the manganese action for activation of a variety of enzymes and also replace some of the zinc-dependent biochemical reactions [101]. Hence, they are called activators of biochemical reactions. It is also involved in part of the metabolic pathways, *i.e.*, the biotin-dependent Krebs cycle [102, 103]. The recommended dose of cobalt for an adult is 5 to 8 micrograms per day. Trace amounts of cobalt are present in most foods in the form of vitamin B-12 [104]. Thus, vitamin B-12 is the only source of cobalt micronutrients.

The deficiency of cobalt is also indicated as vitamin B-12 deficiency. The common symptoms of cobalt deficiency are anemia, especially pernicious anemia. In addition, cobalt deficiency also showed severe tiredness, numbness, and tingling of hands and feet [105]. The latter lower level of cobalt causes nerve dysfunction [104]. It is exposed in humans in multiple ways, such as drinking water, breathing air, and eating food. Even though it is also contacted and exposed to the skin to cause dermatitis and hypersensitive reactions [106]. The higher concentrations of cobalt are causing organ damage [107]. Inhalation of cobalt smoke and particles affects the lungs, leading to asthma, pneumonia, and heart disease. Further, it causes vomiting, nausea, vision problems, and thyroid dysfunction [108, 109]. Besides, the radioactive cobalt isotopes are causing diarrhea, hair loss, bleeding, sterility, coma, and death [110]. Hence, a safer and more balanced dose of cobalt intake is recommended daily for a better healthcare system.

CHROMIUM IN THE HEALTHCARE SYSTEM

Chromium is also an essential micronutrient, and it is present in various foods. Two main forms of chromium exist, *i.e.*, trivalent chromium and hexavalent chromium. A trivalent form of chromium is present in food and supplements, and it does not produce any toxic effects [111]. However, the hexavalent form of chromium is present in industrial pollution, and it is known to produce organ toxicity. The inhalation form of chromium hexavalent causes carcinogenic actions [112, 113]. Chromium physiologically enhances insulin actions [114]. Further, it supports the absorption and metabolism of carbohydrates, proteins, and fats [115]. However, the absorption of chromium is supported by vitamin B3, *i.e.*, niacin, and vitamin C. Chromium is present in a wide range of foods like bran cereals, whole grains, broccoli, green beans, potatoes, apples, bananas, beef, poultry, egg yolks, fish, coffee, brewer's yeast, and red wine [116]. Chromium deficiency is rarely caused by a reduction of gut absorption and is excreted *via* urine with the influence of a diet containing highly refined sugar. The excess loss of chromium content can cause abnormalities in strenuous exercise, pregnancy, and lactating women, and infections and trauma associated with physical stress [117]. Chronic chromium deficiency causes malnutrition [118]. Further, a higher intake of chromium also causes adverse effects and renal and hepatic toxicity [119].

Chromium regulates blood glucose levels by enhancing the action of the insulin hormone in type 2 diabetes mellitus patients. The intake of chromium also corrects glucose intolerance in animals and humans [120, 121]. Further, diabetic patients show the lowest level of blood chromium content. Clinically, chromium supplementation improves insulin sensitivity and glucose metabolism in diabetes patients [122]. Chromium supplement also suppresses the appetite, breaks down fat, stimulates heat production, and slightly increases calorie usage [123, 124]. Furthermore, the supplement of chromium interferes with various medications like insulin, proton pump inhibitors, corticosteroids, beta-blockers, and nonsteroidal anti-inflammatory drugs [125, 126]. Hence, a safer and balanced dose of chromium is recommended for better improvement of the health system.

COQ10 IN THE HEALTHCARE SYSTEM

CoQ10 is also known as ubiquinone and ubiquinol. It is a fat-soluble quinone molecule and structurally similar to the vitamin K molecule. It possesses an effective antioxidant role readily fused with vitamin E and produces the potential free radical scavenging actions [127]. It is essential for energy (ATP, adenosine-triphosphate) production *via* the mitochondrial electron transport chain reaction (respiratory chain) [128]. Our body readily synthesizes CoQ10 from the tyrosine amino acid. CoQ10 exists in two forms, *i.e.*, ubiquinone and ubiquinol [129]. Ubiquinone is an oxidized form with 864 molecular weight, whereas ubiquinol is a reduced form with 866 molecular weight [130]. Further, the ubiquinol structure has two more hydrogen molecules. Ubiquinone and ubiquinol are involved in the oxidation-reduction reaction and rapidly interchange their forms in cells, lymph, and the blood depending on the needs of cellular functions [131]. The primary dietary sources of CoQ10 are oily fish like salmon and tuna fish; organ meats like liver; and whole grains [132]. The recommended intake of CoQ10 micronutrients is 90–200 mg per day. In some conditions, it is recommended at higher dosages of 300–600 mg [131]. Further, it is well-tolerated and safer for use by a variety of people. The ideal dose of CoQ10 for adults is 100-200 mg per day [133].

It also prevents lipid peroxidation and oxygen radicals associated with damage to deoxyribonucleic acids (DNA) [128]. CoQ10 also neutralizes heavy metals, improves energy synthesis and the development of healthy immune functions, and prevents mitochondrial disorders, radiation injury, hypertension, cancer, obesity, diabetes, Parkinson's disease, gastric ulcers, migraine, kidney failure, and muscular dystrophy, including aging [132, 134, 135]. The common risk of CoQ10 is rare and mild nausea, diarrhea, and heartburn. Sometimes it causes the risk of heart failure, liver problems, diabetes, low blood sugar, and hypotension [136]. The CoQ10 interacts with blood thinners and thyroid medications [137, 138]. Further, CoQ10 supplements are advised for children and pregnant and breastfeeding women [139, 140]. Hence, the balanced CoQ10 micronutrient is essential for a better Healthcare system.

IODINE IN THE HEALTHCARE SYSTEM

Iodine is also an important micronutrient for the Healthcare system. Iodine is essential for the synthesis of thyroid hormones like thyroxine (T4) and triiodothyronine (T3). Iodine is required for pregnancy health and infant growth and development [141]. Further, it also supports neuronal growth and cognitive performance [142]. About 75% of total body iodine is stored in the thyroid gland, and it helps in the synthesis of thyroid hormones, which are essential for physiological processes like body growth, metabolism, reproductive function, bone formation, neural development, and tissue repair functions [143, 144]. The source of iodine is mainly seawater salt, iodine-rich foods like baked cod, low-fat yogurt, fat milk, white bread, shrimp, macaroni, and tuna [145, 146]. The recommended dose for children from 0-6 months is 110 mcg per day; for children from 7-12 months is 130 mcg per day; for children aged 1-8 is 90 mcg per day; for ages 9-13 is 120 mcg per day, and for ages>14 is 150 mcg per day [147]. Moreover, pregnant and lactating women require 220 mcg and 290 mcg, respectively [148].

The deficiency of iodine develops due to inadequate iodine intake and excess urinary iodine excretion. The loss of iodine causes cretinism with severe mental and physical retardations [149]. Further, it also raises the risk of thyroid cancer (goiter) and rarely causes breast, prostate, endometrial, and ovarian cancers. Moreover, the imbalance of iodine and thyroid hormone causes infertility in women and autoimmune disease [146, 150]. The most serious side effects of iodine deficiency cause fetal damage, low birth weight, and decreased child survival, including the negative performance of cognitive function, impaired speech, and reading ability [149]. Iodine intake prevents the development of thyroid disorders, neuronal impairments, fibrocystic breast disease, and skin inflammations [151]. However, the chronic and excessive intake of iodine and iodine-rich foods is known to cause nausea, diarrhea, a runny nose, headache, and a metallic taste [152]. Hence, the balanced iodine supplement is essential for a better healthcare system.

SELENIUM IN THE HEALTHCARE SYSTEM

Selenium is a trace mineral and acts as a micronutrient. It needs only a small amount for body functions. It helps the various enzymes and proteins function. The selenium-based proteins, *i.e.*, selenoproteins, help to prevent DNA damage and infections [153]. It is also employed in the reproduction process and metabolism of thyroid hormones. Further, it is stored in muscular tissue and thyroid glands [154]. Selenium-associated selenoproteins have an antioxidant role in the prevention of cell damage [155]. The major sources of selenium are Brazil nuts, spinach, oats, baked beans, Tuna, ham, and macaroni [156]. The recommended daily intake of selenium for adult men and women is 55 mcg of selenium; pregnant and lactating women need 60 and 70 mcg of selenium per day, respectively [157]. The maximum tolerable dose of selenium for adults, pregnant, and lactating women is 400 mcg per day, whereas this amount is exceeded and can cause harmful effects [157, 158]. The lower level of selenium produces cardiac disease, infertility in men, and arthritis [153].

The deficiency of selenium causes the Keshan disease and Kashin-Beck disease. Keshan disease is a type of cardiomyopathy. Kashin-Beck disease is a form of osteoarthritic disorder. The common symptoms of selenium deficiency are nausea, vomiting, headaches, altered mental state, confusion, lethargy, seizures, and coma [159]. In contrast, a large amount of selenium causes brittle hair and nails, hair loss, skin rashes, muscular tremors, stomach upset, garlic breath, respiratory distress, heart attack, and kidney failure [157, 158]. The antioxidant actions of selenium-associated proteins help prevent oxidative stress in various chronic disorders *via* the breakdown of peroxides and inflammatory proteins [160]. These antioxidant and anti-inflammatory proteins protect the cell membranes and keep the non-sticky conditions of blood platelets [161]. However, clinical trials revealed mixed results regarding cardiovascular disease [162]. Moreover, the role of selenium increases the immune functions and fights against infectious diseases like HIV, influenza, and hepatitis C infections, whereas the effects on auto-immune thyroid diseases are not clear [163 - 165]. Further, selenium prevents the loss of muscle mass and muscle dysfunctions associated with aging [166]. Hence, the balanced selenium supplement is essential for a better healthcare system. The summary of micronutrients is illustrated in Fig. (**1**), and the details of functional benefits and deficiency effects of micronutrients are tabulated in Table **1**.

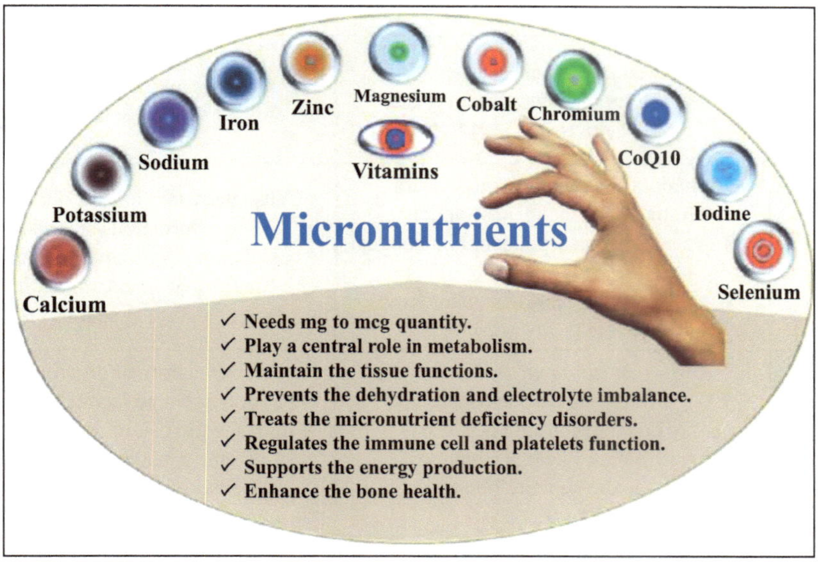

Fig. (1). The summary of micronutrients.

Table 1. The details of the functional benefits and deficiency effects of micronutrients.

Micronutrients	Functional Benefits	Deficiency
Calcium	√ Dilates the blood vessels. √ Supports blood clotting. √ Transmit the cell and neuronal impulse. √ Supports the secretion of hormones.	√ Weakening the bones and teeth. √ The fragility of bones and osteoporosis. √ Rickets in children [9, 10, 18, 19].
Potassium	√ Cellular membrane potential and structural regulatory functions. √ Regulates the body fluid, impulse transmission, and muscular contractions.	√ Altered bone turnover. Hypertension and stroke. √ Polyuria, encephalopathy, glucose intolerance, and paralysis [22, 29 - 31].
Sodium	√ Enhance nerve and muscle functions. √ Regulates the body's fluid levels. √ Acid is the "fluid matrix" of the body.	√ Hyponatremia causes fatigue, lethargy, and confusion [43, 45, 49].
Iron	√ Regulates the oxygen-carrying capacity of heme. √ Supports the control of respiration. √ Improves cognitive ability *via* neuronal development [62, 167].	√ Cause the anemic syndrome. √ Raise the risk of cancers and infections. √ Cause weakness, fatigue, swollen tongue, pale skin, and fingernails [56, 62, 66, 69].
Zinc	√ Protects from infections and phototoxicity. √ Enhance the body's defensive action. √ Supports the functions of smell and taste [72, 74, 77].	√ Cause atopic dermatitis, skin soreness, loss of hair, diarrhea, and changes in taste and smell. √ Develops childhood diarrhea, premature birth, and respiratory infections [77, 82].

(Table 1) cont.....

Micronutrients	Functional Benefits	Deficiency
Magnesium	√ Makes the bones strong. √ Regulates the neurovascular unit functions [88, 89].	√ Cause the neuronal excitability. √ Develops migraine, headache, fatigue, severe pain, and cognitive dysfunction [94, 95, 168].
Cobalt	√ Maintaining the nervous system. √ Replace the manganese actions. √ Replace the zinc-dependent biochemical reactions. √ Involves the biotin-dependent Krebs cycle [100 - 103].	√ Cause the vitamin B-12 deficiency causes pernicious anemia. √ Develop severe tiredness, numbness, tingling of limbs, dermatitis, and hypersensitive reactions [105, 106].
Chromium	√ Break down the fat. √ Raise the calorie usage. √ Enhances insulin actions. √ Stimulates heat production. √ Suppresses the appetite sensation [114, 115, 124].	√ Cause abnormal organ functions in pregnant and lactating women. √ Enhance the risk of infections, traumatic injury, and physical stress. √ Causes malnutrition and glucose intolerance [117, 122, 169].
CoenzymeQ10	√ Prevents oxidative stress and improves energy production. √ Involved in oxidation-reduction reactions. √ Essential for pregnant and breastfeeding women [127, 128, 140].	√ It causes mild nausea, diarrhea, and heartburn. √ Alters the heart and liver functions. √ Accelerate the progression of diabetes [136].
Iodine	√ Essential for the synthesis of thyroid hormones. √ Supports pregnancy health, infant growth and development, and cognitive performance. √ Improves the metabolism, reproductive function, bone formation, and tissue repair functions [141 - 143, 170].	√ Causes cretinism. √ Raises the risk of thyroid, breast, prostate, endometrial, and ovarian cancers. √ Imbalance the fertility and immune functions, and cause damage to the fetus, leading to low birth weight. √ Impairs cognitive function, speech, and reading ability [146, 149, 150].
Selenium	√ Useful for the prevention and treatment of psoriasis and UV irradiation-induced tissue damage. √ Improve the reproductive health and metabolic function of thyroid hormones. √ Stored in the muscular tissue and the thyroid gland. √ Prevents DNA damage and infections [153, 155, 171].	√ Causes the Keshan disease and Kashin-Beck disease. √ Forms osteoarthritic disorders. √ Induces headaches, mental confusion, lethargy, seizures, and coma. √ Causes blood disorders like blood coagulation and cardiovascular disease [157, 159, 162].

SUMMARY

Micronutrients are essential nutrients, such as macronutrients, for better health and body functions. Macronutrients cover carbohydrates, proteins, and fats, whereas micronutrients cover the essential vitamins and minerals. The body needs both types of nutrients to maintain healthy functions. Normally, macronutrients are needed more than micronutrients. The measurable quantity of macronutrients is the grams (g) range, and micronutrients are needed in the range of mg to mcg. The requirement of both macronutrients and micronutrients depends on the number of influencing factors involved in the absorption and excretion of nutrients. Normally, micronutrients are regularly needed in the smallest amounts to maintain a better health system. However, the recommendation of micronutrients is variable based on the person's disease conditions and health status. It varies based on pre-existing health conditions, sex, age, and fitness. All micronutrients are essential for the proper management of body functions. The common action of micronutrients is antioxidants, which prevent various diseases like cancer, Alzheimer's, and heart disease.

CASE STUDIES AND PRACTICE QUESTIONS

Case 1: *A 29-year-old professional woman has a family history of osteoporosis. She has 62 Kg and is 168 cm tall. She eats a varied diet that has meat, fish, and poultry. She also consumes 2 cups of low-fat milk for most of the days. She drinks a small glass of orange juice every morning and typically eats 2 cups of vegetables daily. Further, she also takes a daily multi-vitamin that contains 10,000 IU of vitamin A.*

Discussion Questions

a. How much vitamin A does this patient need each day?
b. What is the formula involved in the conversion of vitamin A for her supplement into Retinol Activity Equivalents (RAE) units?
c. Calculate the milligrams of vitamin A to find the required RAE units?
d. Based on her history, what are the reasons involved in avoiding excessive intakes of vitamin A as a dietary supplement?

Case 2: *A 25-year-old adult woman has the following lunch meal plans, and discuss the following questions based on these meal plans.*

Lunch #1	*Lunch #2*	*Lunch #3*
Beef and bean burrito (1) *Mexican white rice (1 cup)* *Bottled water (350 mL)*	*Hamburger – plan –small (1)* *French fries – Medium (1)* *Diet cola (350 mL)*	*Wheat bread slices (2)* *Peanut butter – chunky (1 tsp)* *Jam (1 tsp)* *Low-fat yogurt (1 cup)* *Grapes (1 cup)* *Raw broccoli (1 cup)*

Discussion Questions

a. What are the Dietary Reference Intakes (DRIs) of riboflavin, folate, vitamin B_{12}, and vitamin C for a non-pregnant woman?
b. Which meal plan is most useful for the achievement of DRIs of riboflavin, folate, vitamin B_{12}, and vitamin C?
c. Which one of the above lunch meal plans has the highest to meet the DRIs?
d. What changes can be made to these meal plans to improve the DRIs nutrient plans?

Case 3: *A 28-year-old pregnant woman in the second trimester of pregnancy. She reached out to the physician and complained of fatigue, dizziness, and pale skin. The physician suggests making the lab test, and the test results revealed that low levels of hemoglobin indicate iron-deficiency anemia. She also expressed occasional leg cramps and symptoms of lactose intolerance.*

Discussion Questions

a. Which vitamins and minerals are important for this pregnant woman?
b. What is the balanced meal (carbohydrate, protein, and fats) recommended for the pregnant woman?
c. Identify the key micronutrients required for the pregnant woman.
d. What is the normal iron requirement for the pregnant woman?
e. What is the iron-folic acid combination suitable for the pregnant woman?

MCQs Questions

1. Which one of the following properties is CORRECT pertaining to vitamin A?
   A. Macro mineral
   B. Trace element
   C. Fat-soluble vitamin
   D. Water-soluble vitamin

2. Which one of the following conditions is CORRECT pertaining to vitamin D?
   A. Scurvy
   B. Osteoporosis
   C. Night Blindness
   D. Haemochromatosis

3. Which one of the following elements acts as an antioxidant and has a synergic effect with vitamin E?
   A. Iron

B. Iodine
C. Copper
D. Selenium

4. Which one of the following diseases is caused by micronutrient malnutrition?
   A. Goiter
   B. Obesity
   C. Diabetes
   D. Protein-energy malnutrition

5. Identify the major sources of vitamins.
   A. Animal fats, industrial sauces, sweets, and precooked food.
   B. Starchy vegetables, cereals, grains, rice, and bread.
   C. Beef, poultry, fish, eggs, dairy products, and beans.
   D. Most of the fruits and vegetables.

Answers: 1) C; 2) B; 3) D; 4) A; 5) D

REFERENCES

[1] Shenkin A. The key role of micronutrients. Clin Nutr 2006; 25(1): 1-13. [http://dx.doi.org/10.1016/j.clnu.2005.11.006] [PMID: 16376462]

[2] Quigg A. Micronutrients. In: Borowitzka MA, Beardall J, Raven JA, editors. The Physiology of microalgae. cham: springer international publishing; 2016. p. 211–31. (Developments in Applied Phycology).

[3] Castela Forte J, Gannamani R, Folkertsma P, Kanthappu S, van Dam S, Wolffenbuttel BHR. A pilot study on the prevalence of micronutrient imbalances in a dutch general population cohort and the effects of a digital lifestyle program. Nutrients 2022; 14(7): 1426. [http://dx.doi.org/10.3390/nu14071426] [PMID: 35406037]

[4] Broadley M, Brown P, Cakmak I, Rengel Z, Zhao F. Function of nutrients: micronutrients. In: Marschner P, Ed. Marschner's Mineral Nutrition of Higher Plants. 3rd ed. San Diego: Academic Press 2012; pp. 191-248. [http://dx.doi.org/10.1016/B978-0-12-384905-2.00007-8]

[5] Narayanam H, Chinni SV, Samuggam S. The Impact of micronutrients-Calcium, Vitamin D, Selenium, Zinc in cardiovascular health: a mini review. Front Physiol 2021; 12: 742425. [http://dx.doi.org/10.3389/fphys.2021.742425] [PMID: 34566703]

[6] How Much Calcium Does an Indian Postmenopausal Woman Need MM. J Midlife Health 2022; 13(1): 9-14. [http://dx.doi.org/10.4103/jmh.jmh_70_22] [PMID: 35707304]

[7] Beal T, Ortenzi F. Priority micronutrient density in foods. Front Nutr 2022; 9: 806566. [http://dx.doi.org/10.3389/fnut.2022.806566] [PMID: 35321287]

[8] Prot-Bertoye C, Lievre L, Houillier P. The importance of kidney calcium handling in the homeostasis of extracellular fluid calcium. Pflugers Arch 2022; 474(8): 885-900. [http://dx.doi.org/10.1007/s00424-022-02725-4] [PMID: 35842482]

[9] Spitzer V, Maggini S. Phytosterols and micronutrients for heart health. Bioactive food as dietary interventions for cardiovascular disease: Bioactive Foods in Chronic Disease States. 2012; 393.

[10] Huskisson E, Maggini S, Ruf M. The influence of micronutrients on cognitive function and performance. J Int Med Res 2007; 35(1): 1-19. [http://dx.doi.org/10.1177/147323000703500101] [PMID: 17408051]

[11] Beto JA. The role of calcium in human aging. Clin Nutr Res 2015; 4(1): 1-8. [http://dx.doi.org/10.7762/cnr.2015.4.1.1] [PMID: 25713787]

[12] Ayu Agbecha . Gastrointestinal and renal regulation of calcium metabolism. International Journal of Frontline Research in Life Science 2022; 1(1): 005-23. [http://dx.doi.org/10.56355/ijfrls.2022.1.1.0003]

[13] Morciano G, Rimessi A, Patergnani S, *et al.* Calcium dysregulation in heart diseases: Targeting calcium channels to achieve a correct calcium homeostasis. Pharmacol Res 2022; 177: 106119. [http://dx.doi.org/10.1016/j.phrs.2022.106119] [PMID: 35131483]

[14] Hernández-Ruiz KL, López-Cervantes J, Sánchez-Machado DI, Martínez-Macias MR, Correa-Murrieta MA, Sanches-Silva A. Hydroxyapatite recovery from fish byproducts for biomedical applications. Sustain Chem Pharm 2022; 28: 100726. [http://dx.doi.org/10.1016/j.scp.2022.100726]

[15] Takeyama H, Maruta M, Sato T, *et al.* Fabrication of bioresorbable hydroxyapatite bone grafts through the setting reaction of calcium phosphate cement. Dent Mater J 2022; 41(6): 882-8. [http://dx.doi.org/10.4012/dmj.2022-045] [PMID: 36002294]

[16] Lloyd T, Andon MB, Rollings N, *et al.* Calcium supplementation and bone mineral density in adolescent girls. JAMA 1993; 270(7): 841-4. [http://dx.doi.org/10.1001/jama.1993.03510070063037] [PMID: 8340983]

[17] Shlisky J, Mandlik R, Askari S, *et al.* Calcium deficiency worldwide: prevalence of inadequate intakes and associated health outcomes. Ann N Y Acad Sci 2022; 1512(1): 10-28. [http://dx.doi.org/10.1111/nyas.14758] [PMID: 35247225]

[18] Wilson-Barnes SL, Lanham-New SA, Lambert H. Modifiable risk factors for bone health & fragility fractures. Best Pract Res Clin Rheumatol 2022; 36(3): 101758. [http://dx.doi.org/10.1016/j.berh.2022.101758] [PMID: 35750569]

[19] Charoenngam N, Ayoub D, Holick MF. Nutritional rickets and vitamin D deficiency: consequences and strategies for treatment and prevention. Expert Rev Endocrinol Metab 2022; 17(4): 351-64. [http://dx.doi.org/10.1080/17446651.2022.2099374] [PMID: 35852141]

[20] Signs V. Muscle spasms in a patient with a history of thyroidectomy. rapid response events in the critically ill-e-book: a case-based approach to inpatient medical emergencies. 2022; 344.

[21] Kim BS, Yi H, Chun J, Cha CJ. Genome sequence of type strain of Staphylococcus aureus subsp. aureus. Gut Pathog 2014; 6(1): 6. [http://dx.doi.org/10.1186/1757-4749-6-6] [PMID: 24628867]

[22] Tang J, Tang O. Introductory chapter: potassium in human health. Potassium in Human Health 2022; p. 3. [http://dx.doi.org/10.5772/intechopen.94820]

[23] Marrero A, Mattei J. Reclaiming traditional, plant-based, climate-resilient food systems in small islands. Lancet Planet Health 2022; 6(2): e171-9. [http://dx.doi.org/10.1016/S2542-5196(21)00322-3] [PMID: 35150626]

[24] Lee J-Y, Shin C, Baik I. Longitudinal associations between micronutrient consumption and leukocyte telomere length 2017. [http://dx.doi.org/10.1111/jhn.12403]

[25] Tchounwou PB, Udensi UK. Potassium homeostasis, oxidative stress, and human disease. Int J Clin Exp Physiol 2017; 4(3): 111-22. [http://dx.doi.org/10.4103/ijcep.ijcep_43_17] [PMID: 29218312]

[26] Plovanich M, Weng QY, Mostaghimi A. Low usefulness of potassium monitoring among healthy young women taking spironolactone for acne. JAMA Dermatol 2015; 151(9): 941-4. [http://dx.doi.org/10.1001/jamadermatol.2015.34] [PMID: 25796182]

[27] McDonough AA, Fenton RA. Potassium homeostasis: sensors, mediators, and targets. Pflugers Arch 2022; 474(8): 853-67. [http://dx.doi.org/10.1007/s00424-022-02718-3] [PMID: 35727363]

[28] Kurtz TW, Pravenec M, DiCarlo SE. Mechanism-based strategies to prevent salt sensitivity and salt-induced hypertension 2022. [http://dx.doi.org/10.1042/CS20210566]

[29] Cheung JY, Bonventre J V, Malis CD, Leaf A. Calcium and Ischemic Injury 2009. [http://dx.doi.org/10.1056/NEJM198606263142604]

[30] Coregliano-Ring L, Goia-Nishide K, Rangel ÉB. Hypokalemia in diabetes mellitus setting. Medicina (Kaunas) 2022; 58(3): 431. [http://dx.doi.org/10.3390/medicina58030431] [PMID: 35334607]

[31] Sardar Z, Waheed KAF, Javed MA, Akhtar F, Bokhari SRA. Clinical and etiological spectrum of hypokalemic periodic paralysis in a tertiary care hospital in pakistan. Cureus 2019; 11(1): e3921. [http://dx.doi.org/10.7759/cureus.3921] [PMID: 30931192]

[32] Makinouchi R, Machida S, Matsui K, Shibagaki Y, Imai N. Severe hypokalemia in the emergency department: A retrospective, single-center study. Health Sci Rep 2022; 5(3): e594. [http://dx.doi.org/10.1002/hsr2.594] [PMID: 35509383]

[33] Diebakate-Scordamaglia L, Voican CS, Perlemuter G. Iatrogenic constipation in gastrointestinal surgery. J Visc Surg 2022; 159(1) (Suppl.): S51-7. Available from: https://www.sciencedirect.com/science/article/ pii/S1878788621002083 [http://dx.doi.org/10.1016/j.jviscsurg.2021.12.003] [PMID: 35172956]

[34] Johnson LS, Mattsson N, Sajadieh A, Wollmer P, Söderholm M. Serum potassium is positively associated with stroke and mortality in the large, population-based malmö preventive project cohort. Stroke 2017; 48(11): 2973-8. [http://dx.doi.org/10.1161/STROKEAHA.117.018148] [PMID: 28974633]

[35] Song DY, Youn J, Kim K, Sung J, Lee JE. Urinary sodium and potassium levels and blood pressure in population with high sodium intake. Nutrients 2020; 12(11): 3442. [http://dx.doi.org/10.3390/nu12113442] [PMID: 33182633]

[36] Hanna RM, Ahdoot RS, Kalantar-Zadeh K, Ghobry L, Kurtz I. Calcium Transport in the Kidney and Disease Processes. Front Endocrinol (Lausanne) 2022; 12: 762130. [http://dx.doi.org/10.3389/fendo.2021.762130] [PMID: 35299844]

[37] New SA. Intake of fruit and vegetables: implications for bone health. Proc Nutr Soc 2003; 62(4): 889-99. [http://dx.doi.org/10.1079/PNS2003310] [PMID: 15018489]

[38] Ha J, Kim SA, Lim K, Shin S. The association of potassium intake with bone mineral density and the prevalence of osteoporosis among older Korean adults. Nutr Res Pract 2020; 14(1): 55-61. [http://dx.doi.org/10.4162/nrp.2020.14.1.55] [PMID: 32042374]

[39] Chang AR, Sang Y, Leddy J, *et al.* Antihypertensive medications and the prevalence of hyperkalemia in a large health system 2016. [http://dx.doi.org/10.1161/HYPERTENSIONAHA.116.07363]

[40] Landolfo M, Di Rosa MV, Gasparotto L, Marchese A, Biolo G. Hyperkalemia: do you forget something? Intern Emerg Med 2022. [http://dx.doi.org/10.1007/s11739-022-03073-y] [PMID: 35969317]

[41] Cohn JN, Kowey PR, Whelton PK, Prisant LM. New guidelines for potassium replacement in clinical

practice: a contemporary review by the National Council on Potassium in Clinical Practice. Arch Intern Med 2000; 160(16): 2429-36.
[http://dx.doi.org/10.1001/archinte.160.16.2429] [PMID: 10979053]

[42] Tavares J, Mosca S, do Sameiro Faria M, Mota C. Hypokalemia and hyperkalemia: Two sides of the same coin. Nascer E Crescer-Birth and Growth Medical Journal 2022; 31(2): 137-47.

[43] Kumar I, Gautam M. Excessive intake of micronutrients in rural population of Uttar Pradesh state. Science Progress and Research 2022; 2(2): 583-7. [SPR].
[http://dx.doi.org/10.52152/spr/2022.174]

[44] Gupta PD, Pushkala K. Two white enemies: Salt and sugar. Journal of Cell and Tissue Research 2022; 22(2): 7203-23.

[45] Mosmiller AC. Water intoxication: Current developments in hyponatremia. 2022.

[46] Messerli FH, O'Donnell M, Mente A, Yusuf S. Settling the controversy of salt substitutes and stroke: sodium reduction or potassium increase? Eur Heart J 2022; 43(35): 3365-7.
[http://dx.doi.org/10.1093/eurheartj/ehac160] [PMID: 35923132]

[47] Burnier M Sr. Nutritional management of sodium, chloride, and water in kidney disease and kidney failure. Nutritional Management of Renal Disease. Elsevier 2022; pp. 313-28.
[http://dx.doi.org/10.1016/B978-0-12-818540-7.00038-0]

[48] Cheteu Wabo TM, Wu X, Sun C, *et al.* Association of dietary calcium, magnesium, sodium, and potassium intake and hypertension: a study on an 8-year dietary intake data from the National Health and Nutrition Examination Survey. Nutr Res Pract 2022; 16(1): 74-93.
[http://dx.doi.org/10.4162/nrp.2022.16.1.74] [PMID: 35116129]

[49] Noda M, Matsuda T. Central regulation of body fluid homeostasis. Proc Jpn Acad, Ser B, Phys Biol Sci 2022; 98(7): 283-324.
[http://dx.doi.org/10.2183/pjab.98.016] [PMID: 35908954]

[50] Felder RA, Gildea JJ, Xu P, *et al.* Inverse salt sensitivity of blood pressure: mechanisms and potential relevance for prevention of cardiovascular disease. Curr Hypertens Rep 2022; 24(9): 361-74.
[http://dx.doi.org/10.1007/s11906-022-01201-9] [PMID: 35708819]

[51] Borrelli S, Provenzano M, Gagliardi I, *et al.* Sodium intake and chronic kidney disease. Int J Mol Sci 2020; 21(13): 4744.
[http://dx.doi.org/10.3390/ijms21134744] [PMID: 32635265]

[52] Perrin EC, South AM. Correlation between kidney sodium and potassium handling and the renin-angiotensin-aldosterone system in children with hypertensive disorders. Pediatr Nephrol 2022; 37(3): 633-41.
[http://dx.doi.org/10.1007/s00467-021-05204-7] [PMID: 34499251]

[53] Ma K, Gao W, Xu H, Liang W, Ma G. Role and mechanism of the renin-angiotensin-aldosterone system in the onset and development of cardiorenal syndrome. J Renin Angiotensin Aldosterone Syst 2022; 2022: 3239057.
[http://dx.doi.org/10.1155/2022/3239057] [PMID: 35111237]

[54] Hill MA, Jaisser F, Sowers JR. Role of the vascular endothelial sodium channel activation in the genesis of pathologically increased cardiovascular stiffness. Cardiovasc Res 2022; 118(1): 130-40.
[http://dx.doi.org/10.1093/cvr/cvaa326] [PMID: 33188592]

[55] Ralph AF, Grenier C, Costello HM, *et al.* Activation of the sympathetic nervous system promotes blood pressure salt-sensitivity in C57BL6/J mice. Hypertension 2021; 77(1): 158-68.
[http://dx.doi.org/10.1161/HYPERTENSIONAHA.120.16186] [PMID: 33190558]

[56] Skolmowska D, Głąbska D, Kołota A, Guzek D. Effectiveness of dietary interventions to treat iron-deficiency anemia in women: a systematic review of randomized controlled trials. Nutrients 2022; 14(13): 2724.
[http://dx.doi.org/10.3390/nu14132724] [PMID: 35807904]

[57] Kumar SB, Arnipalli SR, Mehta P, Carrau S, Ziouzenkova O. Iron deficiency anemia: efficacy and limitations of nutritional and comprehensive mitigation strategies. Nutrients 2022; 14(14): 2976. [http://dx.doi.org/10.3390/nu14142976] [PMID: 35889932]

[58] Mezzano J, Namirembe G, Ausman LM, *et al.* Effects of iron and vitamin a levels on pregnant women and birth outcomes: complex relationships untangled using a birth cohort study in uganda. Matern Child Health J 2022; 26(7): 1516-28. [http://dx.doi.org/10.1007/s10995-022-03387-5] [PMID: 35239084]

[59] Piskin E, Cianciosi D, Gulec S, Tomas M, Capanoglu E. Iron absorption: factors, limitations, and improvement methods. ACS Omega 2022; 7(24): 20441-56. [http://dx.doi.org/10.1021/acsomega.2c01833] [PMID: 35755397]

[60] Singhdeo S, Kaur J, Singh J, Borah A. Survey on dietary habit, consumption of iron rich food and awareness in females. Pharma Innovation Journal 2022; SP-11(6): 944-7.

[61] Puga AM, Samaniego-Vaesken ML, Montero-Bravo A, Ruperto M, Partearroyo T, Varela-Moreiras G. Iron supplementation at the crossroads of nutrition and gut microbiota: the state of the art. Nutrients 2022; 14(9): 1926. [http://dx.doi.org/10.3390/nu14091926] [PMID: 35565894]

[62] Abd Rahman R, Idris IB, Isa ZM, Rahman RA, Mahdy ZA. The prevalence and risk factors of iron deficiency anemia among pregnant women in malaysia: a systematic review. Front Nutr 2022; 9: 847693. [http://dx.doi.org/10.3389/fnut.2022.847693] [PMID: 35495961]

[63] Kron A, Del Giudice ME, Sholzberg M, *et al.* Daily *versus* every other day oral iron supplementation in patients with iron deficiency anemia (DEODO): study protocol for a phase 3 multicentered, pragmatic, open-label, pilot randomized controlled trial. Pilot Feasibility Stud 2022; 8(1): 98. [http://dx.doi.org/10.1186/s40814-022-01042-y] [PMID: 35509085]

[64] D'Alessandro C, Benedetti A, Di Paolo A, Giannese D, Cupisti A. Interactions between food and drugs, and nutritional status in renal patients: a narrative review. Nutrients 2022; 14(1): 212. [http://dx.doi.org/10.3390/nu14010212]

[65] Gifford AH, Sanville JL, Sathe M, Heltshe SL, Goss CH. Use of proton pump inhibitors is associated with lower hemoglobin levels in people with cystic fibrosis. Pediatr Pulmonol 2021; 56(7): 2048-56. [http://dx.doi.org/10.1002/ppul.25431] [PMID: 33860641]

[66] Cecilia A, Patricio P, Donna C, *et al.* Cognitive control inhibition networks in adulthood are impaired by early iron deficiency in infancy. Neuroimage Clin 2022; 35: 103089. [http://dx.doi.org/10.1016/j.nicl.2022.103089] [PMID: 35753235]

[67] Hamodi LE, Naji AS, Ismael SH. Factors associated with anemia in women of reproductive age in iraqi females sample 2022. [http://dx.doi.org/10.36740/WLek202201203]

[68] Manceau H, Ausseil J, Masson D, *et al.* Neglected comorbidity of chronic heart failure: iron deficiency. Nutrients 2022; 14(15): 3214. [http://dx.doi.org/10.3390/nu14153214] [PMID: 35956390]

[69] Paul P, Maiti D, Adhikary T. Iron deficiency anemia-An updated overview. International Journal of Research in Pharmacy and Pharmaceutical Sciences 2021; 6(4): 28-33.

[70] Gowan J, Roller L. Disease state management: Iron deficiency with or without anaemia. AJP. Australas J Pharm 2022; 103(1214): 110-7.

[71] Baschant U, Altamura S, Steele-Perkins P, *et al.* Iron effects *versus* metabolic alterations in hereditary hemochromatosis driven bone loss. Trends Endocrinol Metab 2022; 33(9): 652-63. [http://dx.doi.org/10.1016/j.tem.2022.06.004] [PMID: 35871125]

[72] Ho E, Wong CP, King JC. Impact of zinc on DNA integrity and age-related inflammation. Free Radic

Biol Med 2022; 178: 391-7.
[http://dx.doi.org/10.1016/j.freeradbiomed.2021.12.256] [PMID: 34921929]

[73] Praharaj S, Skalicky M, Maitra S, *et al.* Zinc biofortification in food crops could alleviate the zinc malnutrition in human health. Molecules 2021; 26(12): 3509.
[http://dx.doi.org/10.3390/molecules26123509] [PMID: 34207649]

[74] Wessels I, Rolles B, Slusarenko AJ, Rink L. Zinc deficiency as a possible risk factor for increased susceptibility and severe progression of Corona Virus Disease 19. Br J Nutr 2022; 127(2): 214-32.
[http://dx.doi.org/10.1017/S0007114521000738] [PMID: 33641685]

[75] Agedew E, Tsegaye B, Bante A, *et al.* Zinc deficiency and associated factors among pregnant women's attending antenatal clinics in public health facilities of Konso Zone, Southern Ethiopia. PLoS One 2022; 17(7): e0270971.
[http://dx.doi.org/10.1371/journal.pone.0270971] [PMID: 35797387]

[76] Nazem MR, Asadi M, Adelipour M, Jabbari N, Allameh A. Zinc supplementation ameliorates type 2 diabetes markers through the enhancement of total antioxidant capacity in overweight patients. Postgrad Med J 2022.
[PMID: 37137539]

[77] Batool N, Shaikh S, Chohan MN. Clinical effectiveness of prophylactic zinc on growth, pneumonia and diarrhea in children less than 1 year. JLUMHS 2021; 20(1): 26-30.
[http://dx.doi.org/10.22442/jlumhs.2021.00646]

[78] Forouzesh A, Forouzesh F, Samadi Foroushani S, Forouzesh A. A new method for calculating zinc content and determining appropriate zinc levels in foods. SSRN 4133664.2022;
[http://dx.doi.org/10.2139/ssrn.4133664]

[79] Liao F, Lilay GH, Castro PH, Azevedo H, Assunção AGL. Regulation of the zinc deficiency response in the legume model *Medicago truncatula.* Front Plant Sci 2022; 13: 916168.
[http://dx.doi.org/10.3389/fpls.2022.916168] [PMID: 35845702]

[80] Wai W, Landy K. Does oral zinc supplementation, started at the onset of cold symptoms, decrease symptom duration in adults and children? Evidence-Based Practice 2021; 24(1): 14-5.
[http://dx.doi.org/10.1097/EBP.0000000000000851]

[81] Hemilä H, Fitzgerald JT, Petrus EJ, Prasad A. Zinc acetate lozenges may improve the recovery rate of common cold patients: an individual patient data meta-analysis. Open Forum Infect Dis 2017; 4(2): ofx059.
[http://dx.doi.org/10.1093/ofid/ofx059] [PMID: 28480298]

[82] Durrani AM, Parveen H. Zinc deficiency and its consequences during pregnancy. Microbial Biofertilizers and Micronutrient Availability 2022; pp. 69-82.
[http://dx.doi.org/10.1007/978-3-030-76609-2_3]

[83] Brion LP, Heyne R, Lair CS. Role of zinc in neonatal growth and brain growth: review and scoping review. Pediatr Res 2021; 89(7): 1627-40.
[http://dx.doi.org/10.1038/s41390-020-01181-z] [PMID: 33010794]

[84] Wessels I, Fischer HJ, Rink L. Update on the multi-layered levels of zinc-mediated immune regulation. Seminars in Cell and Developmental Biology. Elsevier 2021; pp. 62-9.
[http://dx.doi.org/10.1016/j.semcdb.2020.11.005]

[85] Tang W, Liu H, Ooi TC, Rajab NF, Cao H, Sharif R. Zinc carnosine: Frontiers advances of supplement for cancer therapy. Biomed Pharmacother 2022; 151: 113157.
[http://dx.doi.org/10.1016/j.biopha.2022.113157] [PMID: 35605299]

[86] Shah ED. Zinc deficiency and intestinal permeability in the context of rational diagnostic and drug development for diarrhea-predominant irritable bowel syndrome digestive diseases and sciences. Springer 2022; pp. 1-2.

[87] Munie S, Pintavorn P. Erythropoietin-resistant anemia secondary to zinc-induced Hypocupremia in a

hemodialysis patient. Case Rep Nephrol Dial 2021; 11(2): 167-75.
[http://dx.doi.org/10.1159/000512612] [PMID: 34327219]

[88] Sreenivasamurthy SA, Akhter FF, Akhter A, Su Y, Zhu D. Cellular mechanisms of biodegradable zinc and magnesium materials on promoting angiogenesis. Biomaterials Advances 2022; 139: 213023.
[http://dx.doi.org/10.1016/j.bioadv.2022.213023] [PMID: 35882117]

[89] Chambers PW. Long Covid, Short Magnesium. OAlib 2022; 9(5): 1-25.
[http://dx.doi.org/10.4236/oalib.1108736]

[90] dos Santos LR, Melo SRS, Severo JS, *et al.* Cardiovascular diseases in obesity: what is the role of magnesium? Biol Trace Elem Res 2021; 199(11): 4020-7.
[http://dx.doi.org/10.1007/s12011-020-02528-7] [PMID: 33389619]

[91] Martiniakova M, Babikova M, Mondockova V, Blahova J, Kovacova V, Omelka R. The role of macronutrients, micronutrients and flavonoid polyphenols in the prevention and treatment of osteoporosis. Nutrients 2022; 14(3): 523.
[http://dx.doi.org/10.3390/nu14030523] [PMID: 35276879]

[92] Abbas A, Rajagopal V, Huang SJ. Magnesium metal matrix composites and their applications. Magnesium Alloys Structure and Properties 2021.

[93] Arias-Fernández L, Struijk EA, Caballero FF, *et al.* Prospective association between dietary magnesium intake and physical performance in older women and men. Eur J Nutr 2022; 61(5): 2365-73.
[http://dx.doi.org/10.1007/s00394-022-02808-z] [PMID: 35122152]

[94] Barbagallo M, Veronese N, Dominguez LJ. Magnesium in aging, health and diseases. Nutrients 2021; 13(2): 463.
[http://dx.doi.org/10.3390/nu13020463] [PMID: 33573164]

[95] Hosseini Dastgerdi A, Ghanbari Rad M, Soltani N. The therapeutic effects of magnesium in insulin secretion and insulin resistance. Adv Biomed Res 2022; 11(1): 54.
[http://dx.doi.org/10.4103/abr.abr_366_21] [PMID: 35982863]

[96] Cantone M, Lanza G, Ranieri F, Opie GM, Terranova C. Non-invasive brain stimulation in the study and modulation of metaplasticity in neurological disorders. Front Neurol 2021; 12: 721906.
[http://dx.doi.org/10.3389/fneur.2021.721906] [PMID: 34276553]

[97] Zhang J, Mai CL, Xiong Y, *et al.* The causal role of magnesium deficiency in the neuroinflammation, pain hypersensitivity and memory/emotional deficits in ovariectomized and aged female mice. J Inflamm Res 2021; 14: 6633-56.
[http://dx.doi.org/10.2147/JIR.S330894] [PMID: 34908863]

[98] Barbagallo M, Veronese N, Dominguez LJ. Magnesium in type 2 diabetes mellitus, obesity, and metabolic syndrome. Nutrients. MDPI 2022; Vol. 14: p. 714.

[99] Patel UH, Jagrit NN, Madole MB, Panchal SS. Correlation of magnesium and calcium in the management of cardiac arrhythmia: Perspectives for better outcome. Adesh University Journal of Medical Sciences & Research 2021; 3(2): 85-90.
[http://dx.doi.org/10.25259/AUJMSR_19_2021]

[100] Maio N, Zhang DL, Ghosh MC, Jain A, SantaMaria AM, Rouault TA. Mechanisms of cellular iron sensing, regulation of erythropoiesis and mitochondrial iron utilization. Seminars in Hematology. Elsevier 2021; pp. 161-74.
[http://dx.doi.org/10.1053/j.seminhematol.2021.06.001]

[101] Nies DH. How is a zinc ion correctly allocated to a zinc-dependent protein? Microbial Metabolism of Metals and Metalloids. Springer 2022; pp. 579-660.
[http://dx.doi.org/10.1007/978-3-030-97185-4_19]

[102] Dasgupta A. Immunoassay design and biotin interference. Adv Clin Chem 2022; 109: 165-83.
[http://dx.doi.org/10.1016/bs.acc.2022.03.005] [PMID: 35953126]

[103] Yoshii K, Hosomi K, Sawane K, Kunisawa J. Metabolism of dietary and microbial vitamin B family in the regulation of host immunity. Front Nutr 2019; 6: 48.
[http://dx.doi.org/10.3389/fnut.2019.00048] [PMID: 31058161]

[104] Gómez-Arnaiz S, Tate RJ, Grant MH. Cobalt neurotoxicity: transcriptional effect of elevated cobalt blood levels in the rodent brain. Toxics 2022; 10(2): 59.
[http://dx.doi.org/10.3390/toxics10020059] [PMID: 35202246]

[105] Wolffenbuttel BHR, Wouters HJCM, Heiner-Fokkema MR, van der Klauw MM. The many faces of cobalamin (vitamin B_{12}) deficiency. Mayo Clin Proc Innov Qual Outcomes 2019; 3(2): 200-14.
[http://dx.doi.org/10.1016/j.mayocpiqo.2019.03.002] [PMID: 31193945]

[106] Bregnbak D, Thyssen JP, Zachariae C, Menné T, Johansen JD. Association between cobalt allergy and dermatitis caused by leather articles – a questionnaire study. Contact Dermat 2015; 72(2): 106-14.
[http://dx.doi.org/10.1111/cod.12319] [PMID: 25407465]

[107] Simonsen LO, Harbak H, Bennekou P. Cobalt metabolism and toxicology—A brief update. Sci Total Environ 2012; 432: 210-5.
[http://dx.doi.org/10.1016/j.scitotenv.2012.06.009] [PMID: 22732165]

[108] Lison D. Cobalt. Handbook on the Toxicology of Metals. Elsevier 2022; pp. 221-42.
[http://dx.doi.org/10.1016/B978-0-12-822946-0.00008-8]

[109] Crutsen JRW, Koper MC, Jelsma J, *et al.* Prosthetic hip-associated cobalt toxicity: a systematic review of case series and case reports. EFORT Open Rev 2022; 7(3): 188-99.
[http://dx.doi.org/10.1530/EOR-21-0098] [PMID: 35298414]

[110] Biswal J, Pant HJ, Sharma VK, Joseph A, Ananthanarayanan A. Preparation and characterization of cobalt-60 glass microspheres for radioactive particle tracking applications 2022.
[http://dx.doi.org/10.1016/j.apradiso.2022.110249]

[111] Alvarez CC, Bravo Gómez ME, Hernández Zavala A. Hexavalent chromium: Regulation and health effects. J Trace Elem Med Biol 2021; 65: 126729.
[http://dx.doi.org/10.1016/j.jtemb.2021.126729] [PMID: 33610058]

[112] Zhao Y, Hao D, Zhang H, Wang J, Liu C. Selenium-enriched yeast relieves hexavalent chromium toxicity by inhibiting nf-κb signaling pathway in broiler spleens. Animals (Basel) 2022; 12(2): 146.
[http://dx.doi.org/10.3390/ani12020146] [PMID: 35049769]

[113] Singh D, Singh CK, Singh D, *et al.* Glycine betaine modulates chromium (VI)-induced morpho-physiological and biochemical responses to mitigate chromium toxicity in chickpea (Cicer arietinum L.) cultivars. Sci Rep 2022; 12(1): 8005.
[http://dx.doi.org/10.1038/s41598-022-11869-3] [PMID: 35568714]

[114] Wolosowicz M, Prokopiuk S, Kaminski TW. Recent advances in the treatment of insulin resistance targeting molecular and metabolic pathways: fighting a losing battle? Medicina (Kaunas) 2022; 58(4): 472.
[http://dx.doi.org/10.3390/medicina58040472] [PMID: 35454311]

[115] Staniek HZ, Król E, Wójciak RW. The interactive effect of high doses of chromium(iii) and different iron(iii) levels on the carbohydrate status, lipid profile, and selected biochemical parameters in female wistar rats. Nutrients 2020; 12(10): 3070.
[http://dx.doi.org/10.3390/nu12103070] [PMID: 33050015]

[116] Rondanelli M, Faliva MA, Barrile GC, *et al.* Nutrition, physical activity, and dietary supplementation to prevent bone mineral density loss: a food pyramid. Nutrients 2021; 14(1): 74.
[http://dx.doi.org/10.3390/nu14010074] [PMID: 35010952]

[117] Marshall NE, Abrams B, Barbour LA, *et al.* The importance of nutrition in pregnancy and lactation: lifelong consequences. Am J Obstet Gynecol 2022; 226(5): 607-32.
[http://dx.doi.org/10.1016/j.ajog.2021.12.035] [PMID: 34968458]

[118] Yao X, Liu R, Li X, *et al.* Zinc, selenium and chromium co-supplementation improves insulin resistance by preventing hepatic endoplasmic reticulum stress in diet-induced gestational diabetes rats. J Nutr Biochem 2021; 96: 108810.
[http://dx.doi.org/10.1016/j.jnutbio.2021.108810] [PMID: 34192590]

[119] Chakraborty R, Renu K, Eladl MA, *et al.* Mechanism of chromium-induced toxicity in lungs, liver, and kidney and their ameliorative agents. Biomed Pharmacother 2022; 151: 113119.
[http://dx.doi.org/10.1016/j.biopha.2022.113119] [PMID: 35613529]

[120] Asbaghi O, Naeini F, Ashtary-Larky D, *et al.* Effects of chromium supplementation on lipid profile in patients with type 2 diabetes: A systematic review and dose-response meta-analysis of randomized controlled trials. J Trace Elem Med Biol 2021; 66: 126741.
[http://dx.doi.org/10.1016/j.jtemb.2021.126741] [PMID: 33813266]

[121] Yao X, Huang S, Li Y, *et al.* Transgenerational effects of zinc, selenium and chromium supplementation on glucose homeostasis in female offspring of gestational diabetes rats. J Nutr Biochem 2022; 110: 109131.
[http://dx.doi.org/10.1016/j.jnutbio.2022.109131] [PMID: 36028097]

[122] Asbaghi O, Naeini F, Ashtary-Larky D, *et al.* Effects of chromium supplementation on blood pressure, body mass index, liver function enzymes and malondialdehyde in patients with type 2 diabetes: A systematic review and dose-response meta-analysis of randomized controlled trials. Complement Ther Med 2021; 60: 102755.
[http://dx.doi.org/10.1016/j.ctim.2021.102755] [PMID: 34237387]

[123] Tsang C, Taghizadeh M, Aghabagheri E, Asemi Z, Jafarnejad S. A meta-analysis of the effect of chromium supplementation on anthropometric indices of subjects with overweight or obesity. Clin Obes 2019; 9(4): e12313.
[http://dx.doi.org/10.1111/cob.12313] [PMID: 31115179]

[124] Anton SD, Morrison CD, Cefalu WT, *et al.* Effects of chromium picolinate on food intake and satiety. Diabetes Technol Ther 2008; 10(5): 405-12.
[http://dx.doi.org/10.1089/dia.2007.0292] [PMID: 18715218]

[125] Ramamoorthy S, Cidlowski JA. Corticosteroids. Rheum Dis Clin North Am 2016; 42(1): 15-31, vii.
[http://dx.doi.org/10.1016/j.rdc.2015.08.002] [PMID: 26611548]

[126] Suliburska J, Krejpcio Z, Staniek H, *et al.* The effects of antihypertensive drugs on chromium status, glucose metabolism, and antioxidant and inflammatory indices in spontaneously hypertensive rats. Biol Trace Elem Res 2014; 157(1): 60-6.
[http://dx.doi.org/10.1007/s12011-013-9864-8] [PMID: 24249586]

[127] Sharma A, Fonarow GC, Butler J, Ezekowitz JA, Felker GM. Coenzyme Q10 and heart failure: a state-of-the-art review. Circ Heart Fail 2016; 9(4): e002639.
[http://dx.doi.org/10.1161/CIRCHEARTFAILURE.115.002639] [PMID: 27012265]

[128] Wardhani LFK, Dewi IP, Putra KNS, Andrianto A, Soemantri D. The physiological insight of Coenzyme-Q10 administration in preventing the incidence of reperfusion arrhythmia among patients undergoing coronary artery bypass grafting surgery. J Basic Clin Physiol Pharmacol 2022; 33(6): 695-701.
[http://dx.doi.org/10.1515/jbcpp-2021-0329] [PMID: 35858280]

[129] Sue-Ling CB, Abel WM, Sue-Ling K. Coenzyme Q10 as adjunctive therapy for cardiovascular disease and hypertension: a systematic review. J Nutr 2022; 152(7): 1666-74.
[http://dx.doi.org/10.1093/jn/nxac079] [PMID: 35348726]

[130] Temova Rakuša Ž, Kristl A, Roškar R. Stability of reduced and oxidized coenzyme Q10 in finished products 2021.
[http://dx.doi.org/10.3390/antiox10030360]

[131] Drobnic F, Lizarraga MA, Caballero-García A, Cordova A. Coenzyme Q_{10} supplementation and its

impact on exercise and sport performance in humans: a recovery or a performance-enhancing molecule? Nutrients 2022; 14(9): 1811.
[http://dx.doi.org/10.3390/nu14091811] [PMID: 35565783]

[132] Ayunin Q, Miatmoko A, Soeratri W, Erawati T, Susanto J, Legowo D. Improving the anti-ageing activity of coenzyme Q10 through protransfersome-loaded emulgel. Sci Rep 2022; 12(1): 906.
[http://dx.doi.org/10.1038/s41598-021-04708-4] [PMID: 35042910]

[133] Liang Y, Zhao D, Ji Q, *et al.* Effects of coenzyme Q10 supplementation on glycemic control: A GRADE-assessed systematic review and dose-response meta-analysis of randomized controlled trials. EClinicalMedicine 2022; 52: 101602. Available from: https://www.sciencedirect.com/science/article/pii/ S2589537022003327
[http://dx.doi.org/10.1016/j.eclinm.2022.101602] [PMID: 35958521]

[134] Leurcharusmee P, Sawaddiruk P, Punjasawadwong Y, *et al.* CoenzymeQ10 and ischemic preconditioning potentially prevent tourniquet-induced ischemia/reperfusion in knee arthroplasty, but combined pretreatment possibly neutralizes their beneficial effects. Antioxidants (Basel, Switzerland) 2022; 11(2).

[135] Testai L, Martelli A, Flori L, *et al.* Coenzyme Q_{10}: clinical applications beyond cardiovascular diseases. Nutrients 2021; 13(5): 1697.
[http://dx.doi.org/10.3390/nu13051697] [PMID: 34067632]

[136] Renke G, Pereira MB, Renke A. Coenzyme Q10 for diabetes and cardiovascular disease: useful or useless? Curr Diabetes Rev 2022.
[PMID: 35507785]

[137] Mancini A, Corbo GM, Gaballo A, *et al.* Relationships between plasma CoQ10 levels and thyroid hormones in chronic obstructive pulmonary disease. Biofactors 2005; 25(1-4): 201-4.
[http://dx.doi.org/10.1002/biof.5520250124] [PMID: 16873947]

[138] Landbo C, Almdal TP. [Interaction between warfarin and coenzyme Q10]. Ugeskr Laeger 1998; 160(22): 3226-7.
[PMID: 9621803]

[139] Saini R. Coenzyme Q10: The essential nutrient. J Pharm Bioallied Sci 2011; 3(3): 466-7. Available from: http://www.jpbsonline.org/text.asp?2011/3/3/466/84471
[http://dx.doi.org/10.4103/0975-7406.84471] [PMID: 21966175]

[140] Teran E, Hernandez I, Nieto B, Tavara R, Ocampo JE, Calle A. Coenzyme Q10 supplementation during pregnancy reduces the risk of pre-eclampsia. Int J Gynaecol Obstet 2009; 105(1): 43-5.
[http://dx.doi.org/10.1016/j.ijgo.2008.11.033] [PMID: 19154996]

[141] Chen X, Wu C, Wang Z, *et al.* Iodine nutrition status and thyroid autoimmunity during pregnancy: a cross-sectional study of 4635 pregnant women. Nutr J 2022; 21(1): 7.
[http://dx.doi.org/10.1186/s12937-022-00760-6] [PMID: 35093086]

[142] Choudhry H, Nasrullah M. Iodine consumption and cognitive performance: Confirmation of adequate consumption. Food Sci Nutr 2018; 6(6): 1341-51.
[http://dx.doi.org/10.1002/fsn3.694] [PMID: 30258574]

[143] Ahad F, Ganie SA. Iodine, Iodine metabolism and Iodine deficiency disorders revisited. Indian J Endocrinol Metab 2010; 14(1): 13-7.
[PMID: 21448409]

[144] Gupta S, Shinde RK, Shinde S. Comparison of the outcomes of cadexomer iodine and povidone-iodine ointments in wound management. Cureus 2022; 14(5): e24667.
[http://dx.doi.org/10.7759/cureus.24667] [PMID: 35663699]

[145] Gunnarsdottir I, Dahl L. Iodine intake in human nutrition: a systematic literature review. Food Nutr Res 2012; 56(1): 19731.
[http://dx.doi.org/10.3402/fnr.v56i0.19731] [PMID: 23060737]

[146] Winder M, Kosztyła Z, Boral A, Kocełak P, Chudek J. The impact of iodine concentration disorders on health and cancer. Nutrients 2022; 14(11): 2209.
[http://dx.doi.org/10.3390/nu14112209] [PMID: 35684009]

[147] Vasiljev V, Subotić A, Marinović Glavić M, *et al.* Overview of iodine intake. Southeastern European medical journal 2022; 6(1): 12-20.
[http://dx.doi.org/10.26332/seemedj.v6i1.241]

[148] Plotkin JB, Leung AM. Iodine requirements in pregnancy. Thyroid Diseases in Pregnancy. Springer 2022; pp. 31-43.
[http://dx.doi.org/10.1007/978-3-030-98777-0_3]

[149] Nazeri P, Delshad H. Iodine deficiency/excess and pregnancy outcomes. Thyroid Diseases in Pregnancy. Springer 2022; pp. 17-30.
[http://dx.doi.org/10.1007/978-3-030-98777-0_2]

[150] Brough L. Improving iodine status in lactating women: what works? Curr Nutr Rep 2022; 11(4): 592-9.
[http://dx.doi.org/10.1007/s13668-022-00427-y] [PMID: 35867268]

[151] Aceves C, Mendieta I, Anguiano B, Delgado-González E. Molecular iodine has extrathyroidal effects as an antioxidant, differentiator, and immunomodulator. Int J Mol Sci 2021; 22(3): 1228.
[http://dx.doi.org/10.3390/ijms22031228] [PMID: 33513754]

[152] Southern AP, Jwayyed S. In Treasure Island, FL: Iodine Toxicity 2022.

[153] Barchielli G, Capperucci A, Tanini D. The role of selenium in pathologies: an updated review. Antioxidants 2022; 11(2): 251.
[http://dx.doi.org/10.3390/antiox11020251] [PMID: 35204134]

[154] Kieliszek M, Bano I. Selenium as an important factor in various disease states - a review. EXCLI J 2022; 21: 948-66.
[PMID: 36172072]

[155] Staneviciene I, Sulinskiene J, Sadauskiene I, *et al.* Effect of selenium on the iron homeostasis and oxidative damage in brain and liver of mice. Antioxidants 2022; 11(7): 1216.
[http://dx.doi.org/10.3390/antiox11071216] [PMID: 35883707]

[156] Cardoso BR, Duarte GBS, Reis BZ, Cozzolino SMF. 2017.

[157] Adewale GG, Olajide PA, Omowumi OS, Okunlola DD, Taiwo AM, Adetuyi BO. Toxicological Significance of the Occurrence of Selenium in Foods. World News of Natural Sciences 2022; 44: 63-88.

[158] Karaağaç RM, Pınarlı Ç, Tarlak F. Effects of Selenium Mineral on Health 2022.

[159] Wang H, Li Z, Liu Y, *et al.* Effects of selenoprotein s knockdown on endoplasmic reticulum stress in atdc5 cells and gene expression profiles in hypertrophic chondrocytes. Biol Trace Elem Res 2022; 1-12.
[PMID: 35725994]

[160] Weaver K, Skouta R. The selenoprotein glutathione peroxidase 4: from molecular mechanisms to novel therapeutic opportunities. Biomedicines 2022; 10(4): 891.
[http://dx.doi.org/10.3390/biomedicines10040891] [PMID: 35453641]

[161] Zhang B, Qin Y, Yang L, *et al.* An organic selenium and VEGF-conjugated bioinspired coating promotes vascular healing. Biomaterials 2022; 287: 121654.
[http://dx.doi.org/10.1016/j.biomaterials.2022.121654] [PMID: 35842980]

[162] Zhao D, Domingo-Relloso A, Tellez-Plaza M, *et al.* High level of selenium exposure in the strong heart study: a cause for incident cardiovascular disease? 2022.
[http://dx.doi.org/10.1089/ars.2022.0029]

[163] Rashidi S, Fernández-Rubio C, Mansouri R, *et al.* Selenium and protozoan parasitic infections: selenocompounds and selenoproteins potential. Parasitol Res 2022; 121(1): 49-62. [http://dx.doi.org/10.1007/s00436-021-07400-8] [PMID: 34993638]

[164] Saito Y. Essential trace element selenium and redox regulation-its metabolism, physiological function, and related diseases 2022. [http://dx.doi.org/10.1530/REM-22-0010]

[165] Davcheva DM, Kirova GK, Miteva MZ, *et al.* Serum selenium concentration in patients with autoimmune thyroid disease. Folia Med (Plovdiv) 2022; 64(3): 443-9. [http://dx.doi.org/10.3897/folmed.64.e64997] [PMID: 35856106]

[166] Bao B, Kang Z, Zhang Y, Li K, Xu R, Guo M. Selenium deficiency leads to reduced skeletal muscle cell differentiation by oxidative stress in mice. Biol Trace Elem Res 2022; 1-10. [PMID: 35576098]

[167] Castro-López C, Romero-Luna HE, García HS, Vallejo-Cordoba B, González-Córdova AF, Hernández-Mendoza A. Key stress response mechanisms of probiotics during their journey through the digestive system: a review. Probiotics Antimicrob Proteins 2022; 1-21. [PMID: 36001271]

[168] Zhang W, Liu CY, Ji LN, Wang JG, Investigators A. Age-stratified association of blood pressure with albuminuria and left ventricular hypertrophy in patients with hypertension and diabetes mellitus. Blood Press 2021; 30(3): 180-7. [http://dx.doi.org/10.1080/08037051.2021.1889967] [PMID: 33622108]

[169] Yao YF, Wang ZJ, Jiang RD, *et al.* Protective efficacy of inactivated vaccine against sars-cov-2 infection in mice and non-human primates. Virol Sin 2021; 36(5): 879-89. Available from: https://link.springer.com/10.1007/s12250-021-00376-w [http://dx.doi.org/10.1007/s12250-021-00376-w] [PMID: 33835391]

[170] Sharma M, Gupta PK, Gupta P, Garabadu D. Antinociceptive activity of standardized extract of bacopa monnieri in different pain models of zebrafish. J Ethnopharmacol 2022; 282: 114546. [http://dx.doi.org/10.1016/j.jep.2021.114546] [PMID: 34418512]

[171] Kieliszek M, Bano I, Zare H. A comprehensive review on selenium and its effects on human health and distribution in middle eastern countries. Biol Trace Elem Res 2022; 200(3): 971-87. [http://dx.doi.org/10.1007/s12011-021-02716-z] [PMID: 33884538]

CHAPTER 6

Essential Fatty Acids Benefits in the Healthcare System

Nallupillai Paramakrishnan[1], **Yuvaraj Sivamani**[2], **Sumitha Elayaperumal**[3] and **Arunachalam Muthuraman**[4,*]

[1] *Department of Pharmacognosy, JSS College of Pharmacy, JSS Academy of Higher Education and Research, Mysuru - 570015, Karnataka, India*

[2] *Department of Pharmaceutical Chemistry, Crescent School of Pharmacy, B.S. Abdur Rahman Crescent Institute of Science and Technology, Vandalur – 600048, Chennai, Tamil Nadu, India*

[3] *Department of Biotechnology and Bioinformatics, JSS Academy of Higher Education and Research, Mysore, Karnataka, India*

[4] *Pharmacology, Toxicology, and Basic Health Sciences Unit, Faculty of Pharmacy, AIMST University, Jalan Bedong-Semeling, Bedong 08100, Kedah, Malaysia*

Abstract: The dietary Essential Fatty Acids (EFA), also referred to as Polyunsaturated Fatty Acids (PUFA), include alpha-linolenic acid, Docosahexaenoic Acid (DHA), Eicosapentaenoic Acid (EPA), and linoleic acid. It regulates the immune and central nervous system functions, and also produces various hormones. It is also correlated positively to infant development; reduction of cardiovascular morbidity and mortality; prevention of cancer progression; optimal functioning of the brain and eyes; arthritis; hypertension; and diabetes mellitus. It shows the multiple pharmacological actions *via* β-oxidation for the production of cellular energy currency, *i.e.*, Adenosine Triphosphate (ATP); esterification of cellular lipids into phospholipids, triglycerides, and cholesterol esters; and conversion of the longer chain fatty acids to unsaturated fatty acid products. The clear correlation of dietary EFA for the management of various ailments in multiple clinical conditions remains to be explored. Hence, this book chapter reveals the beneficial effects of dietary EFA in the management of various metabolic and inflammatory disorders, along with the correlation of their mechanism of action.

Keywords: Cytokines, Eicosanoids, Nuclear factor kappa-activated B cells, Peroxisome proliferator-activated receptors, Retinal degeneration, Visual pigments.

* **Corresponding author Arunachalam Muthuraman:** Pharmacology, Toxicology, and Basic Health Sciences Unit, Faculty of Pharmacy, AIMST University, Bedong 08100, Kedah, Malaysia; E-mail: muthuraman.a@aimst.edu.my

Mukesh Singh Sikarwar, Arunachalam Muthuraman & Sohrab A. Shaikh (Eds.)

INTRODUCTION

Essential Fatty Acids (EFAs) are essential for healthy body functions. It is synthesized in the body. EFAs are alpha-linolenic acid, Docosahexaenoic Acid (DHA), Eicosapentaenoic Acid (EPA), and linoleic acid [1]. Generally, EFA is also referred to as Polyunsaturated Fatty Acids (PUFA). EFA is also categorized as two families of omega-3 (ω-3) and omega-6 (ω-6) fatty acids [2]. Omega-3 fatty acids, *i.e.*, alpha-linolenic acid, DHA, and EPA, are composed of a final carbon-carbon double bond in the ω-3 position, whereas ω-6 fatty acids, *i.e.*, linoleic acid, have a carbon-carbon double bond in the ω-6 position [3]. Both ω-3 and ω-6 fatty acids possess physiological transformation in the human body and produce stable energy [1, 4]. The EFA is called a functional food, as it plays a significant role in the improvement of healthy physiological functions. The EFA is important for maintaining the membrane structure and functions. Membranes are mainly incorporated with phospholipids associated with EFA [5, 6]. It is also involved in the regulation of membrane flexibility, fluidity, and permeability with active membrane-bound enzymes and cell-signaling actions [7]. Furthermore, it also regulates the endogenous metabolism and composition of cellular membranes. Thus, increasing ω-3 fatty acids raises the ω-3 fatty acids content in the red blood cells, immune cells, atherosclerotic plaques, and cardiac myocytes [8]. The details of alpha-linolenic acid, DHA, EPA, and linoleic acid have been described in the following sections [9].

PHYSIOLOGICAL FUNCTIONS OF EFA

EFA has pleiotropic actions on cellular functions. Further, it regulates gene expression *via* interactions of transcriptional factors and influences membrane lipid compositions [10]. In addition, both ω-3 and ω-6 fatty acids modulate the expression of fatty acid metabolic and inflammatory proteins *via* interactions of specific transcription factors like Peroxisome Proliferator-activated Receptors (PPARs) and poly(ADP-ribose) glycohydrolase (PARG) actions [11]. It also acts as a hydrophobic hormone-like steroid hormone, and it controls the gene expression and binds directly to PPARs, leading to activation of the transcription factors, *i.e.*, nuclear factor kappa-light-chain-enhancer of activated B cells (NFκB) and sterol regulatory element-binding transcription factor 1 (SREBP-1) [12, 13]. Both are responsible for the transcription of inflammatory proteins. Besides, ω-3 fatty acids suppress the NFκB nuclear content and inhibit the production of eicosanoids and cytokines [14]. It also alters the conservation and recycling of DHA and regulates the retinal degeneration and impairment of visual pigment [15]. In the nervous system, brain phospholipids alter the glucose uptake process *via* cortical astrocytes and enhance synaptic plasticity and memory functions [16].

The details of ω-3 essential fatty acids (alpha-linolenic acid, DHA, and EPA) have been described in the following sections.

ALPHA-LINOLENIC ACID IN THE HEALTHCARE SYSTEM

Alpha-linolenic acid is a type of omega-3 fatty acid, and it is present in various plants like chia seeds, flaxseeds, flaxseed oil, canola oil, mustard oil, tofu, perilla, soy, soybean oil, walnuts, and walnut oils [17]. It is similar to omega-3 fatty acids like DHA and EPA. The recommended intake of alpha-linolenic acid for men is 1.8 to 2.0 g per day and for women 1.4 to 1.5 g per day [18]. It is necessary for growth and development. The intake of alpha-linolenic acid reduces the risk of cardiac disease *via* the reduction of various risk factors like antiplatelet and anti-thrombotic actions [19]. Dietary omega-3 fatty acids like alpha-linolenic acid also prevent the risk of type-2 diabetes mellitus, atherosclerotic events, stroke, and peripheral vascular disease [20 - 22]. Besides, alpha-linolenic acid reduces blood pressure, asthma, and dry eye *via* reduction of inflammation and improves physiological functions [23 - 25]. The benefits of alpha-linolenic acid are improved cognitive and brain health, supporting mood balance, and reducing joint inflammation and pain [26]. Furthermore, the deficiency of alpha-linolenic acid causes reduced vision, inability to walk, pain and weakness in the legs, scaliness of the skin, excessive cholesterol, and inflammation [27, 28].

Moreover, alpha-linolenic acid has interaction properties with various medications like blood-thinning medications (warfarin, clopidogrel, and aspirin) and cholesterol-lowering medications (atorvastatin, rosuvastatin, fluvastatin, lovastatin, simvastatin, and pravastatin) [29, 30]. Experimentally, alpha-linolenic acid is used for the treatment of rheumatoid arthritis, pneumonia, multiple sclerosis, systemic lupus erythematosus, diabetes, renal disease, ulcerative colitis, and Crohn's disease [31, 32]. It also treats skin cancer, chronic obstructive pulmonary disease, migraine, depression, psoriasis, and eczema [33, 34]. The oral dosing of alpha-linolenic acid, *i.e.*, 1.2 to 2 grams per day, prevents coronary heart disease-associated chest pain, heart attack, and heart failure [35, 36].

DHA in the Healthcare System

DHA is one of the major ω-3 fatty acids, and it is found with EPA in cold-water fish like tuna and salmon. It is also present in sardines and herring fish; walnuts, flaxseed, flaxseed oil, canola oil, soy beverages, milk, and yogurt [37]. Physiologically, DHA supports the development of eye and neuronal tissues and leads to the prevention of visual disturbance and attention deficit hyperactivity disorders [38, 39]. Further, it reduces the risk of cardiovascular disease *via* reduction of blood thickness, tissue swelling, and lowering triglycerides in blood levels [40, 41]. Moreover, the DHA reduces the cholesterol and fat deposition in the blood vessels, boosting thinking and memory skills, helping infant and child development, and preventing eye disorders [42, 43]. Besides, it also reduces 40% to 64% of the risk of early preterm births [44]. Hence, in pregnant women, it is recommended to avoid DHA deficiency. The recommended intake of DHA is 1 to 4 grams per day [45]. Oral DHA intake is probably effective in higher levels of cholesterol and fats in the blood vessels. Normally, DHA and EPA together are more effective, whereas a lower level of effects is observed without EPA [46].

Experimentally, it is proven that a higher concentration of DHA is present in the retinal cell membranes, and it conserves and recycles the DHA contents under low levels of ω-3 fatty acid conditions [23]. Further, it is essential for the normal growth, development, and function of the retinal tissue *via* regeneration of visual pigment, *i.e.*, rhodopsin, and the visual transduction process with the conversion of light hitting effect in the retina to visual images in the visual cortex of the brain [47 - 49]. The deficiency of DHA causes permanent abnormalities in retinal functions [50]. Further, DHA deficiency also affects learning disabilities, aggressive hostility, poor visual function, and neural development in the child [51]. Moreover, it also affects the prefrontal cortex damage, neuronal shrinkage, and indices of astrocytes and modulates the multiple limbic structures in the DHA-deficient rat brain [52 - 54]. Further, DHA deficiency is also shown as skin irritation, rashes, acne, brittleness and thinning of the hair, joint pain and stiffness, brain fog, loss of cognitive function, depression, dry eyes, and fatigue [55, 56]. The treatment of ω-3 fatty acids helps the above DHA deficiency-associated health problems [57]. However, DHA is known to cause the following side effects: mild stomach and intestinal cramps, and an increased chance of bleeding and blood clotting [58]. In this case, 200-300 mg DHA per day is recommended for the improvement of the health of pregnant and breastfeeding women [59, 60]. Hence, the intake of DHA with recommended doses is essential for the improvement of the Healthcare system.

EPA in the Healthcare System

EPA is also one of the ω-3 fatty acids, and it is found in cold-water fish like salmon. The major sources of EPA are herring, sardines, tuna, Atlantic salmon, sockeye salmon, trout, rainbow trout, Pacific oysters, and crab [61, 62]. Normally, EPA helps to prevent the risk of cardiac diseases like coronary heart disease, atherosclerosis, and hypertension [63, 64]. The oral intake of EPA also relieves clogged coronary arteries, prevents heart attacks, and reduces blood triglyceride levels [65]. It reduces the risk of neurological disorders like schizophrenia, Alzheimer's disease, and depression; vision impairments like age-related macular degeneration [66]; psoriasis, asthma, cystic fibrosis, diabetes, lung cancer, and prostate cancer [67, 68]. The recommended intake of EPA is 0.03 to 0.06 g per day for the infant. The required intake of EPA is 220 mg per day or 1,250 mg of EPA per week for an adult [69, 70].

EPA is commonly used for attention-deficit hyperactivity disorder for children, depression, cardiac disease, rheumatoid arthritis, menopause, menstrual pain, Raynaud syndrome, Lupus syndrome, type-2 diabetes, obesity, ulcerative colitis, Crohn's disease, osteoarthritis, and osteoporosis *via* reduction of inflammatory protein expression and immune reactions [71, 72]. Further, EPA interacts with blood-thinning medications like warfarin, clopidogrel, and aspirin [73, 74]. Moreover, EPA is also reducing the side effects of cyclosporine [75]. EPA is normally safe, whereas the excess amount of EPA (3 grams per day) intake produces various side effects like nausea, diarrhea, and belching [76]. In severe conditions, a higher dose of EPA slows down the blood clotting process and enhances the chance of bleeding [77]. Hence, the EPA intake is limited to not more than 2 grams per day [78]. Further, EPA needs to take precautions due to its potential for irregular heartbeat, *i.e.*, arrhythmia, in pregnant and breastfeeding women [79]. Further, it also interacts with anti-hypertensive drugs, anticoagulants, and antiplatelet drugs [80]. The deficiencies of EPA-associated symptoms are similar to those of other ω-3 fatty acids (DHA), *i.e.*, heart problems, poor circulation, poor memory, fatigue, dry skin, mood swings, and depression [81, 82]. However, the proper ratio of DHA and EPA intake is essential for maintaining the Healthcare system.

LINOLEIC ACID IN THE HEALTHCARE SYSTEM

Linoleic acid is a ω-6 essential fatty acid, and it is necessary for human health. Moreover, linoleic acid cannot be made by our body system and needs to be obtained through food. Both ω-3 and ω-6 fatty acids contribute to healthy brain function and normal growth and development [83]. Linoleic acid is present in various dietary sources (90%) in the form of ω-6 PUFA [84]. The sources of linoleic acid are safflower, safflower oil, sunflower seeds, sunflower oil, soybean, soybean oil, corn oil, sesame oil, pine nuts, Brazil nuts, pecans, and vegetables [85, 86]. The recommended dose of linoleic acid for adult men is 17 to 20 g per day and for women is 12 to 13 g per day [87]. Linoleic acid has cholesterol-lowering effects and improvement of insulin sensitivity and vascular functions *via* the replacement of saturated fat and reduction of total and Low-Density Lipoprotein (LDL) cholesterol levels [40, 88]. Besides, linoleic acid also helps to improve skin, heart, brain, bone, and reproductive health *via* regulation of blood lipid levels, immune functions, blood clotting, and inflammation [89]. Linoleic acid also acts as a substrate for the synthesis of prostaglandins [90].

Physiologically, it helps to reduce the risk of cardiovascular disease, and brain dysfunction supports skin and hair growth, improves reproductive health, boosts immune functions, and protects bone mineral density [85, 91, 92]. The recommended intake of linoleic acid for an adult is 17 grams per day; for adult women, 12 grams per day, for children, 7 grams per day; and for infants, 4.4 to 4.6 grams per day [93, 94]. The major risk of linoleic acid enhances the arachidonic metabolism associated with prostaglandin and leukotriene molecules, which leads to severe inflammation and serious health complications [95]. It also causes weight gain-associated problems [96]. However, higher linoleic acid-containing foods and supplements are needed to avoid pregnancy and breastfeeding women [97]. The consumption of large amounts of alpha-linolenic acid can raise the risk of kidney disease after post-transplantation and the progression of prostate cancer [98, 99].

It is commonly used for the management of cardiovascular diseases due to the prevention of arrhythmias, decreasing the risk of thrombosis, reducing serum triglyceride levels, slowing atherosclerotic plaque formation, improving endothelial function, and reducing inflammation [17, 85]. The deficiency of linoleic acid leads to visual disturbance, sensory neuropathy, skin hemorrhagic complications, and scalp inflammations [100 - 102]. Hence, the proper usage of linoleic acid is needed for the maintenance of good health conditions in the cardiovascular and neurological systems. The summary of essential fatty acid metabolism pathways and their actions is illustrated in Fig. (**1**).

SUMMARY

The dietary essential fatty acids readily lower the total blood cholesterol and LDL. The experimental evidence supports the use of essential fatty acids, *i.e.*, ω-3 and ω-6, for the amelioration of cardiac and vascular health, including neurological systems. It also reduces the risk of cardio-metabolism with type-2 diabetes mellitus *via* reduction of hypertriglyceridemia and circulatory pro-inflammatory cytokines like tumor necrosis factor-α and Interleukin 6. Lifestyle modifications with dietary essential fatty acids are needed for the improvement of body health from diseases like type-2 diabetes mellitus and cardiovascular problems, and maintaining a healthy lifestyle.

CASE STUDIES AND PRACTICE QUESTIONS

Case 1: *A 30-year-old pregnant woman has a strong sugar craving and consumes a hot fudge sundae. She has a high level of serum glucose content and releases insulin.*

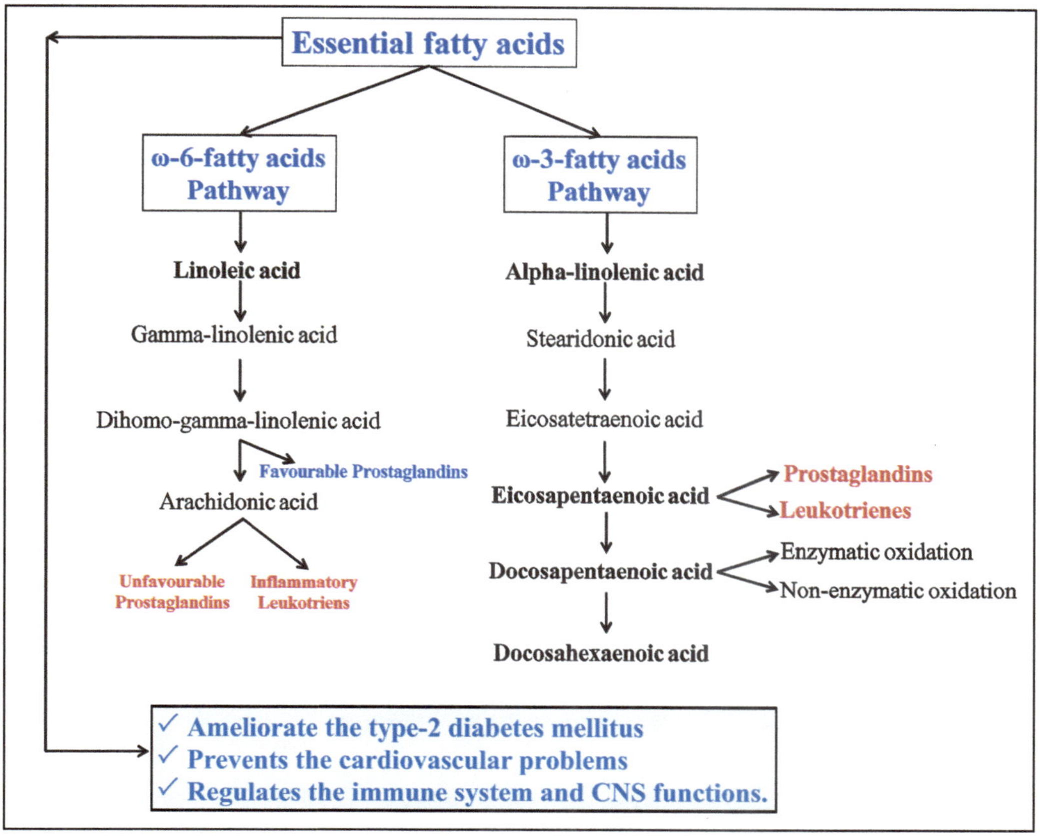

Fig. (1). The summary of essential fatty acids metabolism pathways and their actions.

Discussion Questions

a. What is the role of acetyl-CoA carboxylase in fatty acid biosynthesis?
b. Which mechanism regulates fatty acid biosynthesis?
c. What are the major health benefits of essential fatty acids?
d. Do essential fatty acids reduce inflammation?
e. How much of the EPA affects the inflammatory process?
f. What is the role of a hot fudge sundae in the improvement of insulin sensitivity and reduction of blood sugar levels?

Case 2: *A 24-year-old male patient showed fatigue and weight loss. A laboratory result indicates the elevated levels of FFAs in the blood.*

Discussion Questions

a. Which one of the enzyme deficiencies impairs the triglyceride synthesis?
b. What are the complications caused by elevated levels of blood FFAs?
c. Discuss the connection between the elevated FFAs in the blood and fatigue and weight loss.
d. Do fatty acids help you lose weight?
e. What is the FFA link between obesity and insulin resistance?

Case 3: *A 28-year-old women take the high-carbohydrate diet. A food contains high amounts of added sugars, especially fructose. A laboratory result indicates the rise of triglyceride levels and increases the risk markers of cardiovascular disease.*

Discussion Questions

a. What are the benefits of a high-carbohydrate diet?
b. Which molecule activates the acetyl-CoA carboxylase, leading to the stimulation of the FFAs?
c. Which one of the sources provides a high-calorie diet?
d. What happens when you eat a high-carbohydrate meal?
e. What are the symptoms of high carbohydrates?

MCQs Questions

1. Which one of the following metabolic conversions provides reducing power for fatty acid synthesis (FAS)?
   A. Pyruvate → Acetyl-CoA
   B. Acetyl-CoA → Malonyl-CoA
   C. Glucose-6-Phosphate → 6-Phosphogluconate
   D. Glyceraldehyde-3-Phosphate → 1,3-Bisphosphoglycerate

2. Which one of the following mechanisms is involved in regulating FAS when a person consumes a low-carbohydrate diet?
   A. Repression
   B. Feedback inhibition
   C. Allosteric modification
   D. Covalent modification

3. Which one of the following biochemicals is mostly accumulated in the cytoplasm due to decreased FAS activity?
   A. Acetyl-CoA

B. Citrate-CoA
C. Malonyl-CoA
D. Pyruvate-CoA

4. Which one of the following molecules is essential in the triglyceride synthesis for fatty acid attachment?
A. Fructose-6-Phosphate
B. Glucose-6-Phosphate
C. Glycerol-3-Phosphate
D. Glyceraldehyde-3-Phosphate

5. Which one of the following is the primary role of NADPH in FAS?
A. Activates the FAS
B. Inhibits the acetyl-CoA carboxylase
C. Provides ATP for the condensation reaction
D. Acts as a reducing agent in the chain elongation process

Answers: 1) C; 2) A; 3) C; 4) C; 5) D

REFERENCES

[1] Sardesai VM. The essential fatty acids. Nutr Clin Pract 1992; 7(4): 179-86. [http://dx.doi.org/10.1177/011542659200700417 9] [PMID: 1294887]

[2] Moore SA, Yoder E, Spector AA. Role of the blood-brain barrier in the formation of long-chain ω-3 and ω-6 fatty acids from essential fatty acid precursors. J Neurochem 1990; 55(2): 391-402. [http://dx.doi.org/10.1111/j.1471-4159.1990.tb04150.x] [PMID: 2115069]

[3] Takashima S, Toyoshi K, Yamamoto T, Shimozawa N. Positional determination of the carbon–carbon double bonds in unsaturated fatty acids mediated by solvent plasmatization using LC–MS. Sci Rep 2020; 10(1): 12988. [http://dx.doi.org/10.1038/s41598-020-69833-y] [PMID: 32737371]

[4] Adarme-Vega TC, Thomas-Hall SR, Schenk PM. Towards sustainable sources for omega-3 fatty acids production. Curr Opin Biotechnol 2014; 26: 14-8. [http://dx.doi.org/10.1016/j.copbio.2013.08.003] [PMID: 24607804]

[5] Dyall SC, Balas L, Bazan NG, *et al.* Polyunsaturated fatty acids and fatty acid-derived lipid mediators: Recent advances in the understanding of their biosynthesis, structures, and functions. Prog Lipid Res 2022; 86: 101165. [http://dx.doi.org/10.1016/j.plipres.2022.101165] [PMID: 35508275]

[6] Goulet O, Lamazière A, Abi Nader E, Talbotec C, Wolf C, Lambe C. Erythrocyte fatty acid membrane composition in children on long-term parenteral nutrition enriched with ω-3 fatty acids. Am J Clin Nutr 2022; 115(2): 422-31. [http://dx.doi.org/10.1093/ajcn/nqab263] [PMID: 34582547]

[7] Patel A, Desai SS, Mane VK, *et al.* Futuristic food fortification with a balanced ratio of dietary ω-3/ω-6 omega fatty acids for the prevention of lifestyle diseases. Trends Food Sci Technol 2022; 120: 140-53. [http://dx.doi.org/10.1016/j.tifs.2022.01.006]

[8] Drenjančević I, Pitha J. Omega-3 polyunsaturated fatty acids—vascular and cardiac effects on the cellular and molecular level (narrative review). Int J Mol Sci 2022; 23(4): 2104.

[http://dx.doi.org/10.3390/ijms23042104] [PMID: 35216214]

[9] Cunnane SC. Problems with essential fatty acids: time for a new paradigm? Prog Lipid Res 2003; 42(6): 544-68.
[http://dx.doi.org/10.1016/S0163-7827(03)00038-9] [PMID: 14559071]

[10] Simopoulos AP. Essential fatty acids in health and chronic disease. Am J Clin Nutr 1999; 70(3) (Suppl.): 560S-9S.
[http://dx.doi.org/10.1093/ajcn/70.3.560s] [PMID: 10479232]

[11] Innis SM. Essential fatty acids in growth and development. Prog Lipid Res 1991; 30(1): 39-103.
[http://dx.doi.org/10.1016/0163-7827(91)90006-Q] [PMID: 1771170]

[12] Heshmati J. Effect of omega-3 fatty acid supplementation on gene expression of inflammation, oxidative stress and cardiometabolic parameters: Systematic review and meta-analysis. J Funct Foods 2021; 85: 104619.
[http://dx.doi.org/10.1016/j.jff.2021.104619]

[13] Pham DV, Tilija Pun N, Park PH. Autophagy activation and SREBP-1 induction contribute to fatty acid metabolic reprogramming by leptin in breast cancer cells. Mol Oncol 2021; 15(2): 657-78.
[http://dx.doi.org/10.1002/1878-0261.12860] [PMID: 33226729]

[14] Jalili M, Hekmatdoost A. Dietary ω-3 fatty acids and their influence on inflammation *via* Toll-like receptor pathways. Nutrition 2021; 85: 111070.
[http://dx.doi.org/10.1016/j.nut.2020.111070] [PMID: 33545546]

[15] Gordon W, Jun B. The onset of retinal degeneration in a mutation of membrane-type frizzled protein or adiponectin receptor 1 engages essential fatty acid impairments

[16] Popov A, Brazhe N, Fedotova A, *et al.* A high-fat diet changes astrocytic metabolism to enhance synaptic plasticity and promote exploratory behavior. bioRxiv 2021.

[17] Yuan Q, Xie F, Huang W, *et al.* The review of alpha-linolenic acid: Sources, metabolism, and pharmacology. Phytother Res 2022; 36(1): 164-88.
[http://dx.doi.org/10.1002/ptr.7295] [PMID: 34553434]

[18] Maarafi Z. Consumption of omega-3 fatty acids in american adults. Pomona: California State Polytechnic University 2022.

[19] Stivala S, Gobbato S, Bonetti N, Camici GG, Lüscher TF, Beer JH. Dietary alpha-linolenic acid reduces platelet activation and collagen-mediated cell adhesion in sickle cell disease mice. J Thromb Haemost 2022; 20(2): 375-86.
[http://dx.doi.org/10.1111/jth.15581] [PMID: 34758193]

[20] Jo SH, Han SH, Kim SH, Eckel RH, Koh KK. Cardiovascular effects of omega-3 fatty acids: Hope or hype? Atherosclerosis 2021; 322: 15-23.
[http://dx.doi.org/10.1016/j.atherosclerosis.2021.02.014] [PMID: 33706079]

[21] A Blindauer C, J Stewart A. Changes in plasma free fatty acids associated with type-2 diabetes. Nutrients 2019; 11(9).

[22] Sala-Vila A, Fleming J, Kris-Etherton P, Ros E. Impact of α-linolenic acid, the vegetable ω-3 fatty acid, on cardiovascular disease and cognition. Adv Nutr 2022; 13(5): 1584-602.
[http://dx.doi.org/10.1093/advances/nmac016] [PMID: 35170723]

[23] Sinclair AJ, Guo XF, Abedin L. Dietary alpha-linolenic acid supports high retinal DHA levels. Nutrients 2022; 14(2): 301.
[http://dx.doi.org/10.3390/nu14020301] [PMID: 35057481]

[24] Zhao JV, Schooling CM. The role of linoleic acid in asthma and inflammatory markers: a Mendelian randomization study. Am J Clin Nutr 2019; 110(3): 685-90.
[http://dx.doi.org/10.1093/ajcn/nqz130] [PMID: 31287141]

[25] Dobrzyńska M, Przysławski J. The effect of camelina oil (α-linolenic acid) and canola oil (oleic acid)

on lipid profile, blood pressure, and anthropometric parameters in postmenopausal women. Arch Med Sci 2020; 17(6): 1566-74.
[http://dx.doi.org/10.5114/aoms.2020.94033] [PMID: 34900035]

[26] Gilron I, Robb S, Tu D, *et al.* Double-blind, randomized, placebo-controlled crossover trial of alpha-lipoic acid for the treatment of fibromyalgia pain: the IMPALA trial. Pain 2021; 162(2): 561-8.
[http://dx.doi.org/10.1097/j.pain.0000000000002028] [PMID: 32773602]

[27] Ricci R, Dedola C. Nutrients and the skin. BSAVA Manual of Canine and Feline Dermatology. BSAVA Library 2021; pp. 240-8.
[http://dx.doi.org/10.22233/9781910443811.31]

[28] Gogna S, Kaur J, Sharma K, *et al.* A systematic review on the role of alpha linolenic acid (ALA) in combating non-communicable diseases (NCDs). Nutrition and Food Science 2022. (ahead-of-print).

[29] Abebe W. Review of herbal medications with the potential to cause bleeding: dental implications, and risk prediction and prevention avenues. EPMA J 2019; 10(1): 51-64.
[http://dx.doi.org/10.1007/s13167-018-0158-2] [PMID: 30984314]

[30] Wu H, Xu L, Ballantyne CM. Dietary and pharmacological fatty acids and cardiovascular health. J Clin Endocrinol Metab 2020; 105(4): 1030-45.
[http://dx.doi.org/10.1210/clinem/dgz174] [PMID: 31678992]

[31] Veselinovic M, Vasiljevic D, Vucic V, *et al.* Clinical benefits of n-3 PUFA and ɤ-linolenic acid in patients with rheumatoid arthritis. Nutrients 2017; 9(4): 325.
[http://dx.doi.org/10.3390/nu9040325] [PMID: 28346333]

[32] Wen J, Khan I, Li A, *et al.* Alpha-linolenic acid given as an anti-inflammatory agent in a mouse model of colonic inflammation. Food Sci Nutr 2019; 7(12): 3873-82.
[http://dx.doi.org/10.1002/fsn3.1225] [PMID: 31890165]

[33] Yoon S, Gianturco SL, Pavlech LL, Storm KD, Yuen M V, Mattingly AN. Alpha Lipoic Acid: Summary Report. 2020.

[34] Balić A, Vlašić D, Žužul K, Marinović B, Bukvić Mokos Z. Omega-3 *Versus* omega-6 polyunsaturated fatty acids in the prevention and treatment of inflammatory skin diseases. Int J Mol Sci 2020; 21(3): 741.
[http://dx.doi.org/10.3390/ijms21030741] [PMID: 31979308]

[35] Sala-Vila A, Fleming J, Kris-Etherton P, Ros E. Impact of alpha-linolenic acid, the vegetable omega-3 fatty acid, on cardiovascular disease and cognition 2022.

[36] Wu J, Qiu M, Sun L, *et al.* α-Linolenic acid and risk of heart failure: a meta-analysis. Front Cardiovasc Med 2022; 8: 788452.
[http://dx.doi.org/10.3389/fcvm.2021.788452] [PMID: 35059448]

[37] Santos HO, Price JC, Bueno AA. Beyond fish oil supplementation: the effects of alternative plant sources of omega-3 polyunsaturated fatty acids upon lipid indexes and cardiometabolic biomarkers—an overview. Nutrients 2020; 12(10): 3159.
[http://dx.doi.org/10.3390/nu12103159]

[38] Li J, Pora BLR, Dong K, Hasjim J. Health benefits of docosahexaenoic acid and its bioavailability: A review. Food Sci Nutr 2021; 9(9): 5229-43.
[http://dx.doi.org/10.1002/fsn3.2299] [PMID: 34532031]

[39] Pei-Chen Chang J. Personalised medicine in child and Adolescent Psychiatry: Focus on omega-3 polyunsaturated fatty acids and ADHD. Brain, behavior, and immunity - health 2021; 16: 100310.

[40] Stark AH, Crawford MA, Reifen R. Update on alpha-linolenic acid. Nutr Rev 2008; 66(6): 326-32.
[http://dx.doi.org/10.1111/j.1753-4887.2008.00040.x] [PMID: 18522621]

[41] Wang L, Choi HS, Su Y, *et al.* The docosahexaenoic acid derivatives, diHEP-DPA and TH-DPA, synthesized *via* recombinant lipoxygenase, ameliorate disturbances in lipid metabolism and liver

inflammation in high fat diet-fed mice. Life Sci 2022; 291: 120219. [http://dx.doi.org/10.1016/j.lfs.2021.120219] [PMID: 35041834]

[42] Xu J, Ni B, Ma C, *et al.* Docosahexaenoic acid enhances hippocampal insulin sensitivity to promote cognitive function of aged rats on a high-fat diet. J Adv Res 2022. [PMID: 35618634]

[43] James G, Bohannan W, Adewunmi E, *et al.* Pharmacokinetics and metabolism in mouse retina of bis-allylic deuterated docosahexaenoic acid (D-DHA), a new dry AMD drug candidate. Exp Eye Res 2022; 222: 109193. [http://dx.doi.org/10.1016/j.exer.2022.109193] [PMID: 35870486]

[44] Ludden-Schlatter A, Lindegaard V, Branham KKR. In pregnant women, does LCPUFA supplementation reduce the risk of preterm or early preterm birth? Evidence-Based Practice 2022; 25(7): 35-6. [http://dx.doi.org/10.1097/EBP.0000000000001615]

[45] Miller SM, Zynda AJ, Sabatino MJ, Jo C, Ellis HB, Dimeff RJ. A pilot randomized controlled trial of docosahexaenoic acid for the treatment of sport-related concussion in adolescents. Clin Pediatr (Phila) 2022; 61(11): 785-94. [http://dx.doi.org/10.1177/00099228221101726] [PMID: 35722886]

[46] Bernasconi AA, Wilkin AM, Roke K, Ismail A. Development of a novel database to review and assess the clinical effects of EPA and DHA omega-3 fatty acids. Prostaglandins Leukot Essent Fatty Acids 2022; 183: 102458. [http://dx.doi.org/10.1016/j.plefa.2022.102458] [PMID: 35816925]

[47] Petermann AB, Reyna-Jeldes M, Ortega L, *et al.* Roles of the unsaturated fatty acid docosahexaenoic acid in the central nervous system: molecular and cellular insights. Int J Mol Sci 2022; 23(10): 5390. [http://dx.doi.org/10.3390/ijms23105390] [PMID: 35628201]

[48] Carbone BE, Abouleish M, Watters KE, *et al.* Synaptic connectivity and cortical maturation are promoted by the ω-3 fatty acid docosahexaenoic acid. Cereb Cortex 2020; 30(1): 226-40. [http://dx.doi.org/10.1093/cercor/bhz083] [PMID: 31034037]

[49] West EL, Majumder P, Naeem A, *et al.* Antioxidant and lipid supplementation improve the development of photoreceptor outer segments in pluripotent stem cell-derived retinal organoids. Stem Cell Reports 2022; 17(4): 775-88. [http://dx.doi.org/10.1016/j.stemcr.2022.02.019] [PMID: 35334217]

[50] Eynard AR, Repossi G. Role of ω3 polyunsaturated fatty acids in diabetic retinopathy: a morphological and metabolically cross talk among blood retina barriers damage, autoimmunity and chronic inflammation. Lipids Health Dis 2019; 18(1): 114. [http://dx.doi.org/10.1186/s12944-019-1049-9] [PMID: 30611256]

[51] Martins BP, Bandarra NM, Figueiredo-Braga M. The role of marine omega-3 in human neurodevelopment, including Autism Spectrum Disorders and Attention-Deficit/Hyperactivity Disorder – a review. Crit Rev Food Sci Nutr 2020; 60(9): 1431-46. [http://dx.doi.org/10.1080/10408398.2019.1573800] [PMID: 30880398]

[52] Bewicz-Binkowska D, Zgorzynska E, Dziedzic B, Walczewska A. Docosahexaenoic acid (DHA) inhibits fads2 expression in astrocytes but increases survival of neurons co-cultured with dha-enriched astrocytes. Int J Mol Cell Med 2019; 8(3): 232-40. [PMID: 32489952]

[53] Moriguchi T, Loewke J, Garrison M, Catalan JN, Salem N Jr. Reversal of docosahexaenoic acid deficiency in the rat brain, retina, liver, and serum. J Lipid Res 2001; 42(3): 419-27. [http://dx.doi.org/10.1016/S0022-2275(20)31666-7] [PMID: 11254754]

[54] Shati AA, El-Kott AF. Resolvin D1 protects against cadmium chloride-induced memory loss and hippocampal damage in rats: A comparison with docosahexaenoic acid. Hum Exp Toxicol 2021; 40(12_suppl) (Suppl.): S215-32.

[http://dx.doi.org/10.1177/09603271211038739] [PMID: 34405727]

[55] Sinclair AJ. Docosahexaenoic acid and the brain- what is its role? Asia Pac J Clin Nutr 2019; 28(4): 675-88.
[PMID: 31826363]

[56] Wen M, Zhao Y, Shi H, *et al.* Short-term supplementation of DHA as phospholipids rather than triglycerides improve cognitive deficits induced by maternal omega-3 PUFA deficiency during the late postnatal stage. Food Funct 2021; 12(2): 564-72.
[http://dx.doi.org/10.1039/D0FO02552F] [PMID: 33325958]

[57] Troesch B, Eggersdorfer M, Laviano A, *et al.* Expert opinion on benefits of long-chain omega-3 fatty acids (dha and epa) in aging and clinical nutrition. Nutrients 2020; 12(9): 2555.
[http://dx.doi.org/10.3390/nu12092555] [PMID: 32846900]

[58] Golanski J, Szymanska P, Rozalski M. Effects of omega-3 polyunsaturated fatty acids and their metabolites on haemostasis—current perspectives in cardiovascular disease. Int J Mol Sci 2021; 22(5): 2394.
[http://dx.doi.org/10.3390/ijms22052394] [PMID: 33673634]

[59] Carlson SE, Gajewski BJ, Valentine CJ, *et al.* Higher dose docosahexaenoic acid supplementation during pregnancy and early preterm birth: A randomised, double-blind, adaptive-design superiority trial. EClinicalMedicine 2021; 36: 100905.
[http://dx.doi.org/10.1016/j.eclinm.2021.100905] [PMID: 34308309]

[60] Van Dael P. Role of n-3 long-chain polyunsaturated fatty acids in human nutrition and health: review of recent studies and recommendations. Nutr Res Pract 2021; 15(2): 137-59.
[http://dx.doi.org/10.4162/nrp.2021.15.2.137] [PMID: 33841720]

[61] Liu C, Ralston NVC. Seafood and health: What you need to know? Advances in food and nutrition research. Elsevier 2021; pp. 275-318.

[62] Yu HR, Li LY, Xu CM, *et al.* Effect of dietary eicosapentaenoic acid (20:5n-3) on growth performance, fatty acid profile and lipid metabolism in coho salmon (Oncorhynchus kisutch) alevins. Aquacult Rep 2022; 23: 101084.
[http://dx.doi.org/10.1016/j.aqrep.2022.101084]

[63] Fukumoto K, Takemoto Y, Yoshikawa J, *et al.* Predictors of endothelial function improvement in patients with mild hypertriglyceridemia without evidence of coronary artery disease treated with purified eicosapentaenoic acid. Atherosclerosis 2020; 309: 27-32.
[http://dx.doi.org/10.1016/j.atherosclerosis.2020.07.013] [PMID: 32861211]

[64] Chapman MJ, Zamorano JL, Parhofer KG. Reducing residual cardiovascular risk in Europe: Therapeutic implications of European medicines agency approval of icosapent ethyl/eicosapentaenoic acid. Pharmacol Ther 2022; 237: 108172.
[http://dx.doi.org/10.1016/j.pharmthera.2022.108172] [PMID: 35304222]

[65] Toth PP, Chapman MJ, Parhofer KG, *et al.* Differentiating EPA from EPA/DHA in cardiovascular risk reduction. American Heart Journal Plus: Cardiology Research and Practice 2022; 100148.

[66] Gareri P. Omega-3 long-chain polyunsaturated fatty acids in the elderly: a review. OBM Geriat 2022; 6(2): 1-28.
[http://dx.doi.org/10.21926/obm.geriatr.2202198]

[67] Taneja NK, Singh A, Shivaprasad DP, Taneja P, Sachdev D. Nutraceuticals and natural-product derivatives for disease prevention. 2022.
[http://dx.doi.org/10.1002/9781119746843.ch21]

[68] Son SE, Koh JM, Im DS. Activation of free fatty acid receptor 4 (FFA4) ameliorates ovalbumin-induced allergic asthma by suppressing activation of dendritic and mast cells in mice. Int J Mol Sci 2022; 23(9): 5270.
[http://dx.doi.org/10.3390/ijms23095270] [PMID: 35563671]

[69] Bahreynian M, Feizi A, Daniali SS, Kelishadi R. Interaction between maternal dietary fat intake, breast milk omega-3 fatty acids and infant growth during the first year of life 2022.

[70] Salminen K. Nutrition and associated factors among older people in long-term care setting 2022.

[71] Lange KW, Nakamura Y, Reissmann A. Diet and food in attention-deficit hyperactivity disorder. Journal of Future Foods 2022; 2(2): 112-8.
[http://dx.doi.org/10.1016/j.jfutfo.2022.03.008]

[72] Shi P, Liao K, Xu J, Wang Y, Xu S, Yan X. Eicosapentaenoic acid mitigates palmitic acid-induced heat shock response, inflammation and repair processes in fish intestine. Fish Shellfish Immunol 2022; 124: 362-71.
[http://dx.doi.org/10.1016/j.fsi.2022.04.011] [PMID: 35421576]

[73] Gross BW, Gillio M, Rinehart CD, Lynch CA, Rogers FB. Omega-3 fatty acid supplementation and warfarin: a lethal combination in traumatic brain injury 2017.
[http://dx.doi.org/10.1097/JTN.0000000000000256]

[74] Block RC, Shearer GC, Holub A, *et al.* Aspirin and omega-3 fatty acid status interact in the prevention of cardiovascular diseases in framingham heart study. Prostaglandins Leukot Essent Fatty Acids 2021; 169: 102283.
[http://dx.doi.org/10.1016/j.plefa.2021.102283] [PMID: 33964664]

[75] Ventura HO, Milani RV, Lavie CJ, *et al.* Cyclosporine-induced hypertension. efficacy of omega-3 fatty acids in patients after cardiac transplantation. Circulation 1993; 88(5 Pt 2): II281-5.
[PMID: 8222166]

[76] Quispe R, Alfaddagh A, Kazzi B, *et al.* Controversies in the use of omega-3 fatty acids to prevent atherosclerosis. Curr Atheroscler Rep 2022; 24(7): 571-81.
[http://dx.doi.org/10.1007/s11883-022-01031-9] [PMID: 35499805]

[77] Mohammadi MM, Dehghan Nayeri N, Mashhadi M, Varaei S. Effect of omega-3 fatty acids on premenstrual syndrome: A systematic review and meta-analysis. J Obstet Gynaecol Res 2022; 48(6): 1293-305.
[http://dx.doi.org/10.1111/jog.15217] [PMID: 35266254]

[78] Myhre PL, Kalstad AA, Tveit SH, *et al.* Changes in eicosapentaenoic acid and docosahexaenoic acid and risk of cardiovascular events and atrial fibrillation: A secondary analysis of the OMEMI trial. J Intern Med 2022; 291(5): 637-47.
[http://dx.doi.org/10.1111/joim.13442] [PMID: 34982486]

[79] Chowdhury MH, Ghosh S, Kabir MR, Mamun MAA, Islam MS. Effect of supplementary omega-3 fatty acids on pregnant women with complications and pregnancy outcomes: review from literature. J Matern Fetal Neonatal Med 2022; 35(13): 2564-80.
[http://dx.doi.org/10.1080/14767058.2020.1786522] [PMID: 32643471]

[80] Garg PK, Guan W, Nomura S, *et al.* Associations of plasma omega-3 and omega-6 pufa levels with arterial elasticity: the multi-ethnic study of atherosclerosis. Eur J Clin Nutr 2022; 76(12): 1770-5.
[http://dx.doi.org/10.1038/s41430-022-01172-9] [PMID: 35680969]

[81] Yu F, Qi S, Ji Y, Wang X, Fang S, Cao R. Effects of omega-3 fatty acid on major cardiovascular outcomes: A systematic review and meta-analysis. Medicine (Baltimore) 2022; 101(30): e29556.
[http://dx.doi.org/10.1097/MD.0000000000029556] [PMID: 35905212]

[82] Bozzatello P, Brignolo E, De Grandi E, Bellino S. Supplementation with omega-3 fatty acids in psychiatric disorders: a review of literature data. J Clin Med 2016; 5(8): 67-93.
[http://dx.doi.org/10.3390/jcm5080067] [PMID: 27472373]

[83] Cuciniello R, Luongo D, Ferramosca A, *et al.* Conjugated linoleic acid downregulates Alzheimer's hallmarks in aluminum mouse model through an Nrf2-mediated adaptive response and increases brain glucose transporter levels. Free Radic Biol Med 2022; 191: 48-58.
[http://dx.doi.org/10.1016/j.freeradbiomed.2022.08.027] [PMID: 36028179]

[84] Burdge GC. α-linolenic acid interconversion is sufficient as a source of longer chain ω-3 polyunsaturated fatty acids in humans: An opinion. Lipids 2022; 57(6): 267-87. [http://dx.doi.org/10.1002/lipd.12355] [PMID: 35908848]

[85] den Hartigh L. Conjugated linoleic acid effects on cancer, obesity, and atherosclerosis: a review of pre-clinical and human trials with current perspectives. Nutrients 2019; 11(2): 370. [http://dx.doi.org/10.3390/nu11020370] [PMID: 30754681]

[86] Jinadasa B, Van Bockstaele F, Cvejic JH, Simal-Gandara J. Current trends and next generation of future edible oils. Future Foods. Elsevier 2022; pp. 203-31. [http://dx.doi.org/10.1016/B978-0-323-91001-9.00005-0]

[87] Jackson KH, Van Guilder GP, Tintle N, Tate B, McFadden J, Perry CA. Plasma fatty acid responses to a calorie-restricted, DASH-style diet with lean beef. Prostaglandins Leukot Essent Fatty Acids 2022; 179: 102413. [http://dx.doi.org/10.1016/j.plefa.2022.102413] [PMID: 35395436]

[88] Gautam PB, Gandhi K, Sharma R, Sharma N, Mann B. Conjugated linoleic acid: synthesis, physiological, and functional aspects. Functional Dairy Ingredients and Nutraceuticals. Apple Academic Press 2023; pp. 145-69.

[89] Veshkini A, Hammon HM, Vogel L, *et al.* Plasma proteomics reveals crosstalk between lipid metabolism and immunity in dairy cows receiving essential fatty acids and conjugated linoleic acid. Sci Rep 2022; 12(1): 5648. [http://dx.doi.org/10.1038/s41598-022-09437-w] [PMID: 35383209]

[90] Liang N, Emami S, Patten KT, *et al.* Chronic exposure to traffic-related air pollution reduces lipid mediators of linoleic acid and soluble epoxide hydrolase in serum of female rats. Environ Toxicol Pharmacol 2022; 93: 103875. [http://dx.doi.org/10.1016/j.etap.2022.103875] [PMID: 35550873]

[91] Cole RM, Angelotti A, Sparagna GC, Ni A, Belury MA. Linoleic acid-rich oil alters circulating cardiolipin species and fatty acid composition in adults: a randomized controlled trial. Mol Nutr Food Res 2022; 66(15): 2101132. [http://dx.doi.org/10.1002/mnfr.202101132] [PMID: 35596730]

[92] Feehan O, Magee PJ, Pourshahidi LK, *et al.* Associations of long chain polyunsaturated fatty acids with bone mineral density and bone turnover in postmenopausal women. Eur J Nutr 2022; 1-10. [PMID: 35908118]

[93] Zinn C, Lenferna De La Motte KA, Rush A, Johnson R. Assessing the nutrient status of low carbohydrate, high-fat (lchf) meal plans in children: a hypothetical case study design. Nutrients 2022; 14(8): 1598. [http://dx.doi.org/10.3390/nu14081598] [PMID: 35458160]

[94] Monnard C, Fleith M. Total fat and fatty acid intake among 1–7-year-old children from 33 countries: comparison with international recommendations. Nutrients 2021; 13(10): 3547. [http://dx.doi.org/10.3390/nu13103547] [PMID: 34684548]

[95] Jin R, Hao J, Yi Y, *et al.* Dietary fats high in linoleic acids impair antitumor t-cell responses by inducing e-fabp–mediated mitochondrial dysfunction. Cancer Res 2021; 81(20): 5296-310. [http://dx.doi.org/10.1158/0008-5472.CAN-21-0757] [PMID: 34400394]

[96] Wrzosek M, Zawadzka Z, Sawicka A, Bobrowska-Korczak B, Białek A. Impact of fatty acids on obesity-associated diseases and radical weight reduction. Obes Surg 2022; 32(2): 428-40. [http://dx.doi.org/10.1007/s11695-021-05789-w] [PMID: 34813039]

[97] Jasińska-Melon E, Mojska H, Przygoda B, Stoś K. *Trans* Fatty Acids Content in Whole-Day Diets Intended for Pregnant and Breastfeeding Women in Gynaecological and Obstetric Wards: Findings from the Study under the “Mum’s Diet” Pilot Program in Poland. Nutrients 2022; 14(16): 3360. [http://dx.doi.org/10.3390/nu14163360] [PMID: 36014867]

[98] Denton N. Waisted: The Biology of Body Fat. Oxford University Press 2022.

[99] Simon JA, Chen YH, Bent S. The relation of α-linolenic acid to the risk of prostate cancer: a systematic review and meta-analysis. Am J Clin Nutr 2009; 89(5): 1558S-64S. [http://dx.doi.org/10.3945/ajcn.2009.26736E] [PMID: 19321563]

[100] Cassanego G, Rodrigues P, De Freitas Bauermann L, Trevisan G. Evaluation of the analgesic effect of α-lipoic acid in treating pain disorders: A systematic review and meta-analysis of randomized controlled trials. Pharmacol Res 2022; 177: 106075. [http://dx.doi.org/10.1016/j.phrs.2022.106075] [PMID: 35026405]

[101] Roszkowska AM, Spinella R, Oliverio GW, *et al.* Effects of the topical use of the natural antioxidant alpha-lipoic acid on the ocular surface of diabetic patients with dry eye symptoms. Frontiers in Bioscience-Landmark 2022; 27(7): 202. [http://dx.doi.org/10.31083/j.fbl2707202] [PMID: 35866400]

[102] Li M, Kong Y, Lai Y, *et al.* The effects of dietary supplementation of α-lipoic acid on the growth performance, antioxidant capacity, immune response, and disease resistance of northern snakehead, Channa argus. Fish Shellfish Immunol 2022; 126: 57-72. [http://dx.doi.org/10.1016/j.fsi.2022.05.029] [PMID: 35598741]

CHAPTER 7

Prebiotics / Probiotics as Therapeutic Agents in the Healthcare System

Yamunna Paramaswaran[1], **Muthusamy Ramesh**[2], **Nallupillai Paramakrishnan**[3] and **Arunachalam Muthuraman**[4,*]

[1] *Faculty of Pharmacy, AIMST University, Jalan Bedong-Semeling, Bedong 08100, Kedah, Malaysia*

[2] *Department of Pharmaceutical Analysis and Quality Assurance, Institute of Pharmaceutical Sciences, Sandip Foundation, Nashik - 422213, India*

[3] *Department of Pharmacognosy, JSS College of Pharmacy, JSS Academy of Higher Education and Research, Mysuru - 570015, Karnataka, India*

[4] *Pharmacology, Toxicology, and Basic Health Sciences Unit, Faculty of Pharmacy, AIMST University, Jalan Bedong-Semeling, Bedong 08100, Kedah, Malaysia*

Abstract: Probiotics are live microorganisms found in foods or supplements that benefit the host, whereas prebiotics are non-digestible food ingredients that nourish beneficial gut bacteria. Typically, probiotics contain live microorganisms that help to maintain and improve the normal intestinal microflora, *i.e.*, "good" bacteria in the body. Prebiotics are mainly high-fiber-containing foods, and they act as food for human intestinal microflora. Both prebiotics and probiotics are useful for the healthy functions of human organ systems. The health benefits of these products are significantly shown in the regulatory mechanism at the cellular and molecular levels. The major physiological functions of these products are enhancing the metabolic alteration of good bacteria (microflora) and host cell secretion of mucus proteins. Besides, it also enhances calcium absorption, regulates mucosal barrier functions, and supports gut-endothelial barrier actions *via* the prevention of bad bacteria invasion and survival in the digestive system. The metabolite of probiotics also stimulates the host immune cell functions. Moreover, prebiotics act either directly or indirectly to support the microbiota for the development of healthy neurovascular, cardiovascular, renal, hepatic, and lung functions. However, the therapeutic actions and mechanisms of these products remain to be explored in various pathological conditions. Hence, this book chapter is focused on the exploration of prebiotics and probiotics in the management of various disorders in patients, besides foods and/or supplementary actions.

Keywords: Alpha-glucan, Galacto-oligosaccharides, Gut microbiota, Immune function, Inulin.

[*] **Corresponding author Arunachalam Muthuraman:** Pharmacology, Toxicology, and Basic Health Sciences Unit, Faculty of Pharmacy, AIMST University, Bedong 08100, Kedah, Malaysia.; E-mail: muthuraman.a@aimst.edu.my

Mukesh Singh Sikarwar, Arunachalam Muthuraman & Sohrab A. Shaikh (Eds.)

INTRODUCTION

The term "prebiotics" was first introduced by Glenn Gibson and Marcel Roberfroid in 1995. Prebiotics are substances obtained from certain types of carbohydrates, primarily non-digestible fiber, that serve as food for beneficial gut bacteria [1]. Further, these fibers are eaten by beneficial gut bacteria. Besides, the gut bacteria are collectively called gut flora or gut microbiota, which is essential for various important body functions [2]. The beneficial bacteria are good and help to protect the gut from harmful bacteria and fungi organisms [3]. In addition, these bacteria enhance immune functions; minimize the symptoms of depression, and help reduce obesity complications [4]. Some of the gut bacteria are formed from vitamin K and short-chain fatty acids [5]. Prebiotics are types of fiber present in vegetables, fruits, and legumes [6]. Some fibers are not digested by human enzymes and hormones, whereas good gut bacteria are easily digested for feed consumption [2]. The probiotic fiber-containing foods are beans, peas, oats, bananas, berries, asparagus, dandelion greens, garlic, leeks, and onions [7]. Gut bacteria convert the prebiotic fiber to short-chain fatty acids, *i.e.*, butyrate. Butyrate also regulates the natural movement of food in the gut compartment and boosts the blood flow into the colon tissue [8]. Further, a short-chain fatty acid also possesses anti-inflammatory and anti-cancer properties. Besides, these short-chain fatty acids are essential nutrients for colon cell linings and promote efficient gut-barrier functions *via* filtering the entry of harmful substances, bacteria, and viruses [9]. Overall, prebiotics are reduces gut inflammation, risk of cancer and improves healthy gastrointestinal functions [10].

Probiotics are live bacteria and provide various healthy body functions. Probiotics are beneficial bacteria found in various foods or supplements. The natural probiotic food is yogurt [11]. Beneficial bacteria (probiotics) are commonly found in fermented foods like sauerkraut, kimchi, kombucha tea, kefir, and pickled vegetables, where they are grown using naturally occurring sugars or fiber. Conversely, the pasteurization process is used to heat-treat foods, which kills all beneficial bacteria [12, 13]. Eating balanced amounts of prebiotics and probiotics helps to maintain healthy gut microbiota functions. Moreover, some foods have both beneficial bacteria and digestible fiber feed for gut-beneficial bacteria [14]. It is also known as symbiotic products like cheese, sauerkraut, and kefir [15]. The role of prebiotics and probiotics in the Healthcare system has been described in the following sections [16].

Physiological Functions of Prebiotics and Probiotics

Multiple types of microorganisms are present in the gut region. Normally, 10^{10} to 10^{12} live microorganisms per gram of tissue are present in the human colon [17].

These residual microorganisms are essential for the healthy functions of the stomach and small and large intestines [9]. Most of the microorganisms are anaerobic organisms and survive in the large intestine. It needs digestible fibers as food, and it is called prebiotics [11]. The imbalance of microbes will be developed with the influence of endogenous factors like mucin secretions [18]. Human dietary fibers, like non-digestible carbohydrates, are the chief source of microbial growth and energy development [19]. Prebiotics are influenced by gut microbial growth and functions; subsequently, they affect intestinal functions, such as the lack of human intestinal metabolism and integrity [20]. In addition, the suppression of gut pathogens (Bifidobacterium and Lactobacillus species) with lactic acid formation can modulate immune functions (antagonistic effects against pathogens) [21].

Normally, probiotics are carbohydrate fibers, and fermented products enhance the selective specific gut microbiota functions. Overall, prebiotics are categorized as carbohydrates (oligosaccharides) and non-carbohydrate products [22]. Various compounds like fructo-oligosaccharides, galacto-oligosaccharides, trans-galacto-oligosaccharides, alpha-glucan oligosaccharides, and inulin are the most common prebiotics [23]. The fermented products also act as prebiotics for gut microbiota for the production of short-chain fatty acids, lactic acid, butyric acid, and propionic acid [24]. All these compounds possess various beneficial effects on the body. Propionic acid helps the healthy functions of T-helper-2 cells in human airway tissue, macrophages, and dendritic cells of bone marrow. Fatty acids also reduce the colon's pH [24]. The peptidoglycan of fermentation products also acts as an immune stimulator for the prevention of pathogenic microorganisms-associated infections [18]. The beneficial effects of prebiotics are mainly due to the byproducts of microbial digestion, like butyrate, influencing the development of intestinal epithelial tissue, and fatty acids supporting blood circulation [25]. The primary properties of prebiotics are a) resistant to the stomach's acidic pH with lack of hydrolysis by digestive enzymes; b) unabsorbed in the gastrointestinal tract; c) fermented by intestinal microbiota; d) intestinal bacteria are selectively stimulated by this compound; e) improves the host's health. The details of prebiotics are explained in the following sections [18, 26].

Host Cell Functions of Prebiotics

Galacto-oligosaccharides are an extension product of lactose. It is categorized into two subgroups, *i.e.*, 1) excess galactose attachment in C3, C4, and C6; and 2) the trans-glycosylation of lactose [27]. These end products are a mixture of tri- to pentasaccharides with galactose, and they are also named trans-galacto-oligosaccharides. In infants, it potentially stimulates the Bifidobacteria and Lactobacilli [18]. Further, it also stimulates the Enterobacteria, Firmicutes, and

Bacteroidetes. The isomers of lactose, *i.e.*, lactulose, also act as prebiotics [28]. Other oligosaccharides, *i.e.*, sucrose extension-associated raffinose molecules, improve gut functions [29]. Starch and glucose-derived oligosaccharides like polydextrose are known to stimulate the Bifidobacteria [18]. Polydextrose consists of a glucan with various branches of glycosidic linkages. Some kinds of starch are resistant to digestion in the upper gut, promoting health *via* butyrate production [30]. Hence, it is considered a prebiotic. The groups of Firmicutes are degraded by *Ruminococcus bromii*, and *Bifidobacterium adolescentis* acts similarly to probiotic functions [31]. Furthermore, the oligosaccharide derivatives, like pectin (also called pectic oligosaccharides), also act as prebiotics. It has an extension of galacturonic acid or rhamnose, and is linked with arabinose, galactose, and xylose, and ferulic acid [18]. Fructan derivatives, consisting of inulin, fructo-oligosaccharide, and oligofructose, are stimulated by the lactic acid of gut bacteria, which enhances good bacterial health and host immune functions [32]. The non-carbohydrate oligosaccharides, like cocoa-derived flavanols, possess the criteria of prebiotic functions. It also promotes lactic acid formation from gut bacteria and enhances good bacterial growth and host immune functions [18].

Fructose-oligosaccharide exists in various plants, whereas the concentration of fructose-oligosaccharides is limited for the production of prebiotic effects. The synthesized fructose-oligosaccharide enriched the contents for probiotic actions [30]. It is produced by a chemical reaction method using glycosidase and glycosyl-transferase enzymes [33]. However, this method of production is hazardous and costly, and the yield is very low [34]. Another enzyme, *i.e.*, fructosyl-transferase, produces the prebiotic products from sucrose *via* transferring one to three fructose molecules [27]. This conversion needs fructosyl-transferase enzymes, which are present in various microorganisms like *Fusarium*, *Aspergillus*, *Aureobasidium*, *Penicillium*, and *Arthrobacter* species; *Zymomonas mobilis*, *Bacillus macerans*, *Candida, Kluyveromyces*, and *Saccharomyces cerevisiae*. It is an easy and cost-effective method of probiotic preparations. It is also able to make a safer way in the industrial scale-up process [27].

Galactose-oligosaccharide is produced by nucleophilic and electrophilic chemical displacement methods, and it is an uneconomical method in the industry [35]. The enzymatic method of approach for the production of galactose-oligosaccharides is made with galactosyl-transferase and galactosidase enzymes [36]. The stereoselective properties of galactosyl-transferase help to produce a large yield of galactose-oligosaccharide-type prebiotics [37]. However, the bio-catalysis for the galactosyl-transferase reaction is very costly due to the requirements of nucleotide sugars as a donor [18]. Moreover, the usage of globotriose and human milk oligosaccharides helps to reduce the cost of the previous product preparations.

Recently, the β-galactosidases have also been used for the preparation of galactose-oligosaccharide prebiotics [37]. β-galactosidases are present in various organisms like *Aspergillus oryzae*, *Sterigmatomyces elviae*, *Bifidobacteria*, and *Lactobacilli* [20]. Here, metal ions can be used as co-factors for β-galactosidases' actions, and it is economical [38].

Prebiotic Actions for Alteration of Gut Microbiota

The sources of energy (feed - prebiotics) for gut microbiota readily produce good products for healthy host gut functions *via* modulation of food composition and functions of microorganisms [39]. The changes of specific and selective gut microbiota, like *Escherichia coli* (E. Coli), with prebiotics enhance the blood flow in intestinal tissues [40]. Some of the host species, like *Actinobacteria*, *Firmicutes*, and *Bacteroidetes,* also use the prebiotics and fermented fructose-oligosaccharides, galactose-oligosaccharides, and xylooligosaccharides molecules [18]. In addition, the fermentation of starch and fructans by *Bifidobacterium* species also enhances the host microbiota growth and immune cell functions [39]. The alterations of gut pH (from 6.5 to 5.5) are also enhancing the propagation of gut microbiota along with Bacteroids, which leads to promoting the formation of butyrate. Butyrate is one of the essential fatty acids to improve gut function [39].

Prebiotics in the Healthcare System

Prebiotics provide multiple nutrients for the growth of gut microbiota. The degraded products of prebiotics, *i.e.*, short-chain fatty acids, enhance the blood circulation in the gastrointestinal tract as well as other distal organs [36]. The most important prebiotics, *i.e.*, fructooligosaccharides and galactooligosaccharides, are known to enhance the beneficial effects for maintaining human health and protection against various disorders. It also supports the functions of the immune system, central nervous system, and cardiovascular system [8].

The prebiotics immediately produce benefits for gastrointestinal disorders like irritable bowel syndrome, Crohn's disease, colorectal cancer, and necrotizing enterocolitis. Irritable bowel syndrome, like Crohn's disease, is characterized by chronic and severe abdominal pain and inflammation [24]. It can occur from any part of the gastrointestinal tract, *i.e.*, from the mouth to the anus. Moreover, the population of gut *Bifidobacteria* and *Faecalibacterium prausnitzii* minimizes the complication of irritable bowel syndrome and Crohn's disease *via* modulation of *Bacteroides* to *Firmicutes*-based probiotic products [41]. Clinically, the administration of an oligofructose dose of 20 grams per day, 5 grams of fructose-oligosaccharides per day for 6 weeks, and 3.5 grams of galactose-oligosaccharide per day for 12 weeks treats irritable bowel syndrome *via* enhancement of

Bifidobacteria actions [18]. Further, administration of 15 grams of fructose-oligosaccharides per day for 3 weeks enhances the *Bifidobacteria* population in the feces and is also evidenced to improve Crohn's disease [42]. Another study reported that 20 grams of oligofructose-enriched inulin per day for 4 weeks protects against the mild-to-moderate conditions of Crohn's disease [18].

In colorectal cancer conditions, the fermented products of prebiotics like butyrate protect against the risk of colorectal cancer *via* induction of apoptosis of cancer cells [43]. Clinically, the symbiotic therapy, *i.e.*, Lactobacillus rhamnosus and *Bifidobacterium Lactis* plus inulin, reduces the progression of colorectal cancer *via* improvement of vascular integrity and gut epithelial barrier functions [43]. The severe forms of necrotizing enterocolitis are also ameliorated by fructose-oligosaccharides and galactose-oligosaccharides types of prebiotics *via* enhancement of gut microbiota (*Bifidobacteria*) growth in preterm infants [18]. Further, the formation of prebiotics-based fatty acids improves feeding tolerance *via* enhancement of the gastric emptying process and bowel motility actions. However, better utilization of prebiotics still needs to be explored in the various clinical conditions [22].

In the immune system, prebiotics enhance immune functions by raising the gut-protective microbiota populations [19]. In addition, it reduces the populations of harmful bacteria like *Lactobacilli* and *Bifidobacteria*. Mannose oligosaccharide reduces the colony of *Salmonella* organisms *via* binding to type-1 fimbriae of *Salmonella* organisms, leading to blocking the adhesion of *Salmonella* to endothelial cells and also enhancing the expression of cytokine molecules [20]. In maternal conditions, prebiotics cross the placenta and affect the fetal immune cell functions. The administration of fructose-oligosaccharide in pregnancy modifies the microbiota and prevents skin inflammation *via* bifidogenic actions, whereas these bifidogenic effects are not transferred to the next generation [43]. However, the oligofructose and inulin mixture of prebiotics enhances the antibody responses against viral vaccines like influenza and measles, whereas the side effects of the influenza vaccine are minimized [44]. Further, it reduces diarrhea-associated fever and febrile seizures in infants; reduces the usage of antibiotics, and the duration of disease progression. $\beta(2\rightarrow1)$ fructans, a type of prebiotics, induce a healthy immune response with up-regulation of interleukin 4 in serum, and CD282+/TLR2+ myeloid receptor proteins in dendritic cells in healthy humans [24]. However, fructans are enhancing the secretion of salivary immunoglobulin A and the activation of immune cells [45]. The intake of fructose-oligosaccharide and galactose-oligosaccharide prebiotics reduces the risk of immune reactions in infants, such as atopic dermatitis, *via* downregulation of IL-6 expression and phagocytosis [24].

The nervous system also responds with the administration of prebiotics *via* the connection of the "gut-brain axis" system. Administration of prebiotics to piglets has reduced the gray matter instead of neural pruning, whereas the effects of prebiotics on the human brain have not been studied [39]. The actions of gut microbiota on the brain system occur *via* neural, endocrine, and immune actions. The intake of fructose-oligosaccharides and galactose-oligosaccharides stimulates the vagus nerve, leading to stimulation of the production of brain-derived neurotrophic factors, neurotransmitters, especially d-serine, and synaptic proteins like synaptophysin and N-methyl-D-aspartate [30]. In the neuroendocrine system, prebiotics regulate the hypothalamic-pituitary-adrenal axis *via* respective regulatory hormones like plasma peptide YY [30]. In addition, prebiotics enhance the microbiome growth-associated production of corticosterone and adrenocorticotropic hormone in mice [46]. The gut microbiota readily reacts with prebiotics and influences immune cells' mediated mood, learning, and memory, and psychiatric functions in neurological disorder patients [36]. The administration of polydextrose and galactose-oligosaccharide prebiotics reduces anxiety behavior in male piglets and enhances positive social interaction in rats [47]. In autism disorders, patients are shown higher levels of *Clostridium* and depletion of *Bifidobacterium* in feces [48]. The intake of prebiotics like wheat fiber is reducing autism disorders *via* reduction of the *Clostridium perfringens* population and raising the *Bifidobacteria* rates [49].

In the skin region, galactose-oligosaccharide prebiotics intake has shown beneficial effects *via* enhancement of water retention; improvement of the skin barrier function *via* expression of cell adhesion and matrix markers, *i.e.*, CD_{44} and collagen type-1; and prevention of immunoglobulin-associated erythema [27]. The administration of galactose-oligosaccharides with Bifidobacterium breve is reducing the toxicity of phenolic compounds like p-cresol in women [50]. Moreover, prebiotics lower the risk of cardiovascular disease *via* the reduction of inflammatory components. Clinically, the administration of inulin of 10 grams per day for three weeks reduces the blood triacylglycerides and liver lipogenesis [19]. In addition, the administration of fructose-oligosaccharides reduces the triacylglycerol level by around 7.5% in healthy individuals [37]. In contrast, some prebiotics like L-rhamnose possess lipogenic effects *via* the production of butyrate, acetate, and propionate molecules [51]. Another clinical trial refused this opinion. Hence, more extensive studies are needed to confirm the prebiotic role in cardiovascular disease. In bone disorders, disorders are mainly due to the lack of dietary absorption of calcium [8]. The 5 to 20-gram daily intakes of prebiotics like lactulose, trans-galactosylated oligosaccharides, and inulin with oligofructose significantly enhanced calcium absorption, whereas fructose- and galactose-oligosaccharides do not change calcium absorption [8].

Probiotic Actions for Gastrointestinal Functions

Probiotics are a mixture of live bacteria and/or yeasts. Normally, it is present in our bodies. Probiotics are present in various foods like yogurt, yeast, buttermilk, sourdough bread, cottage cheese, kombucha, tempeh, fermented pickles, fermented sauerkraut, kimchi, and miso soup [12]. Good bacteria are helping to eliminate the bad bacteria. In infectious conditions, bad bacteria are knocking on the door of impaired immune functions [49]. Probiotic microbes are a combination of bacteria, including fungi (yeasts), viruses, and protozoa. The characteristic features of probiotics are isolated from humans, survive in the intestine after ingestion, are proven for beneficial effects, and are safely consumed [52]. It possesses the following essential actions: anti-inflammation, regulation of T cells, immune-boosting actions *via* interaction of toll-like receptors and dendritic cells, and reduction of histone deacetylase-9 expression [52]. Besides, it also acts on the mouth, skin, lungs, urinary tract, and vagina. The probiotics associated with good bacteria are known to help the digestion of food, rid out the bad bacteria, support the synthesis of vitamins, make a healthy environment of intestinal endothelial linings, and improve the breakdown and absorption of medications [20]. The most common good bacteria in probiotic preparations are *Bifidobacterium* and *Lactobacillus* organisms. Besides, yeast, *i.e.*, Saccharomyces boulardii, is also employed in the preparation of probiotics. The usage of probiotics for medical conditions is discussed in the following section [53].

Probiotics in the Healthcare System

Probiotics are present in foods like yogurt with good bacteria, *i.e., Lactobacillus* and *Bifidobacterium*; and yeast, *i.e.*, Saccharomyces boulardii, which is occupied by various parts of the body, including the gut [39]. Medically, probiotics treat antibiotics and *Clostridioides difficile* infections associated with diarrhea [54]. Further, it reduces intestinal complications like cramps, constipation, inflammatory bowel disease, irritable bowel syndrome, urinary tract infections, gum disease, lactose intolerance, eczema *i.e.*, atopic dermatitis, upper respiratory infections, and sepsis in infants [55]. Fermented food products like pickles, kombucha, and kefir drinks enhance the availability of extra probiotics. Probiotic supplements are available in the form of foods, drinks, capsules, pills, powders, and liquids [53]. Sometimes, prebiotics like inulin, pectin, and resistant starches are mixed with probiotics and work as symbiotics to improve healthy gut effects [56]. However, rarely do probiotics affect the gastrointestinal tissue and cause mild stomach upset, bloating, flatulence, and diarrhea in the first attempt [53]. Probiotics are often administered to help prevent certain pre-existing infections and to mitigate the risk of new infections in vulnerable patient groups, such as those with a compromised immune system, critically ill patients, or individuals who have recently undergone surgery [57]. The major cautions of probiotic usage are a weakened immune system, developing resistance against antibiotics, and producing harmful byproducts of probiotic supplements [20]. Mostly, it is beneficial for healthy adults and kids. It reduces diarrhea, bloating, constipation, acid reflux symptoms, and eczema in children [58, 59]. There are certain mechanisms involved in the probiotic health effects, which produce the antagonistic action against the various microorganisms *via* secretion of anti-microbial substances, competitive adhesion to mucosa and epithelium, strengthening the gut-epithelial barrier function, and modulating the gut-immune system [60].

The intestinal non-pathogenic microorganism and a mucosal barrier are secrets of the anti-microbial peptides, immunoglobulin-A, and epithelial adhesion proteins, *i.e.*, E-cadherin and β-catenin [43]. Similarly, probiotic bacteria are also involved in the regulation of gut-endothelial barrier functions. The *Lactobacilli* potentially modulate the epithelial barrier function with the influence of the phosphorylation process of cell junctional adherence proteins *via* the raising of protein kinase C isoforms, *i.e.*, PKC-δ levels [61]. The administration of probiotics like *Lactobacillus casei* repairs gut-endothelial barrier damage, similar to the action of *Escherichia coli on the* mucosal barrier and mucosal integrity functions *via* expression and redistribution of tight junction proteins, *i.e.*, zonula occludens (ZO-2) and PKC [9, 61]. The peptides of *Lactobacillus rhamnosus* prevent the cytokine-associated cell apoptosis *via* activation of anti-apoptotic protein kinase B and inhibition of pro-apoptotic p38/mitogen-activated protein kinase activities [62]. Moreover, the *Lactobacillus* species are raising the expression of intestinal mucin in human intestinal cell lines *via* the *Lactobacillus* adhesion process [20]. Similarly, *Lactobacillus acidophilus* cell extracts also enhance the expression of mucin proteins (MUC-2) in HT29 cells. Hence, probiotics produce intestinal protection *via* mucous protein expression [63]. This adhesion property of probiotics modulates the intestinal immune system and antagonizes other harmful pathogen actions. Hence, intestinal barrier adhesion is one of the major events for the selection of new probiotic strains [20, 64].

Lactobacillus bacteria possess multiple surface determinants and readily interact with intestinal epithelial cells and mucus proteins. The intestinal epithelial cells are responsible for the secretion of complex glycoproteins, *i.e.*, mucin, and they prevent the adhesion of pathogens [36]. Another *Lactobacillus* species, *i.e.*, Lactobacillus reuteri, is directly targeted to mucus proteins, *i.e.*, Mucus-Binding Protein (MUB) [65]. This interaction between surface proteins of probiotics, mucous proteins with plasminogen, and enterocytes is observed in *Bifidobacterium lactis* and *Bifidobacterium bifidum,* respectively [19]. However, extensive studies are needed for the functional significance and interaction of mucous layer components, complex proteins, microbiota, and epithelial cells for clear underlying mechanisms in the development of innate and adaptive immune responses [22]. Probiotics also help in the production of anti-microbial substances like low molecular weight compounds (<1000 Da) such as organic acids. These anti-bacterial compounds are also named bacteriocins [66]. Such organic acids are acetic acid and lactic acid, which strongly inhibit Gram-negative bacteria growth *via* the destruction of cytoplasm components of the bacterial cell and lowering of bacterial intracellular pH levels [67, 68]. The bacteriocins of Gram-positive bacteria, *i.e.*, lactacin-B of *L. acidophilus*, plantaricin of *L. plantarum*, and nisin of *Lactococcus lactis,* possess a narrow spectrum of anti-bacterial activity for closely related bacteria [16]. Some of the bacteriocins are also known to produce strong antibacterial activity against food-borne pathogens. These bacteriocins inhibit cell wall synthesis, like nisin, making the complex to spore-forming pathogenic bacilli cell wall precursor, *i.e.*, lipid-II [66]. The specific anti-bacterial compounds like *bacteriocin* and *bifidocin-B* are produced by *B. bifidum* and exhibit the bactericidal action against the Gram-positive bacteria, *Salmonella enterica ser. typhimurium* [69]. Furthermore, intestinal *Bifidobacteria* and *Lactobacilli* bacteria produce conjugated linoleic acid, which possesses potential anti-carcinogenic effects [9]. In addition, conjugated linoleic acid of *L. plantarum* and *Bifidobacteria* produces the anti-obesity effect against diet-induced obesity in mice *via* modulation of fatty acid composition in the liver and adipose tissue [70]. Probiotics also make the de-conjugation of bile acids, which produces the strongest anti-microbial action compared to host bile salt compounds [53]. Moreover, some probiotic *Lactobacillus* strains like *Lactobacillus coryniformis* are producing bioactive metabolites (lactic acid, phenylacetic acid, benzoic acid, methylhydantoin, mevalonolactone, cyclo(L-Leu-L-Pro), and cyclo(L-Phe-L-Pro) which inhibit the growth of fungi and various species of bacteria [71]. Besides, the bread probiotics, *i.e.*, Fusarium culmorum and *Fusarium graminearum,* also produced the anti-fungal cyclic dipeptides, *i.e.*, cyclo (L-Phe-L-Pro) and cyclo(L-Phe-traps-4-OH-L-Pro), which inhibit the growth of food-borne filamentous fungi and yeasts [27, 72].

Probiotics also have a strong connection with the host immune system *via* interactions of the gut-immune system. It interacts with epithelial cells, dendritic cells, monocytes, macrophages, and lymphocytes [73, 74]. The probiotics release the specific antibody against the specific antigens *via* interaction of host B and T lymphocytes, leading to the production of the adaptive immune response [75]. However, innate immune responses are shared by a variety of pathogens *via* modulation of pathogen-associated molecular patterns, and pattern recognition receptors like toll-like receptors, extracellular C-type lectin receptors, and intracellular nucleotide-binding oligomerization domain-containing protein (NOD)-like receptors [73, 76]. The summaries of prebiotics and probiotics functions are illustrated in Fig. (**1**).

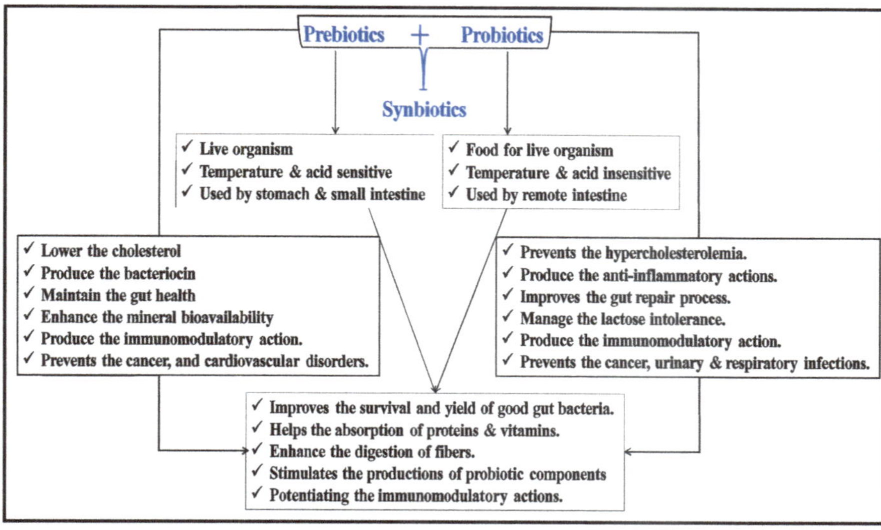

Fig. (1). The summaries of prebiotics and probiotics functions.

SUMMARY

Prebiotics and probiotics produce various health benefits *via* significant cellular and molecular mechanisms. Mostly, it enhances the metabolic alteration of good bacteria and host cell mucus proteins. It enhances calcium absorption and regulates mucosal functions, and supports gut-endothelial barrier actions for the prevention of bad bacteria invasion and survival. Further, metabolites of probiotics stimulate the host immune cells to establish the strongest action against pathogenic organisms like bacteria, viruses, and fungi. Further, prebiotic substances either directly or indirectly support the microbiota to make healthy neurovascular, cardiovascular, renal, hepatic, and lung functions. Pathological conditions improve the host cell's healthy functions *via* multiple molecular approaches. Especially, in cancer cells, prebiotics and probiotics interfere with the cell signaling process of cancer cells and induce the apoptosis process. In host cells, prebiotics, probiotics, and symbiotic products produce remarkable actions to prevent vascular diseases, obesity, and mental disorders *via* anti-inflammatory, cholesterol-lowering, and neuro-modulatory actions. Even the administration of prebiotics, probiotics, and symbiotics produces negative effects initially. The adaptation and safer usage of these products are always feasible. Even some of the therapeutic actions of these agents need to be addressed with suitable experimental studies and clinical trials. Further, long-term clinical trials and genomics-level assessments will support the strong confirmation of these products for health claims.

CASE STUDIES AND PRACTICE QUESTIONS

Case 1: *A 70-year-old male has a critical illness or immunosuppression. He has a risk of fungemia due to probiotic use containing Saccharomyces boulardii.*

Discussion Questions

a. Highlights the careful consideration of using the potential benefits of prebiotics/probiotics.
b. Discuss the immune function in this elderly patient in combating age-related changes.
c. List the prebiotics and probiotics.
d. Is it recommended to take probiotics and prebiotics together?
e. What is the difference between prebiotics, probiotics, and postbiotics?
f. What are the signs you need prebiotics?

Case 2: *A 65-year-old male patient hospitalized with impairment of bowel movements, malnutrition, and infections. He takes probiotics for 45 consecutive days and has shown to improve bowel movements.*

Discussion Questions

a. Highlights the bowel disorders and their symptoms in elderly patients.
b. Discuss the role of probiotics in the treatment of Inflammatory Bowel Disorders (IBD).
c. Describe the possible mechanisms and targets for the management of IBD.
d. Do probiotics bring down intestinal inflammation?
e. How to calm down the inflamed intestines?
f. Which one of the best methods is the fastest way to cure an inflamed gut?

Case 3: *A 46-year-old male patient has Chronic Kidney Disease (CKD). He is taking 3 g of short-chain fructo-oligosaccharides (SC-FOS) and 8 grams of mixed short- and long-chain inulin. After intake of prebiotics, there has been improvement in constipation and diarrhea, aid in calcium absorption, and improvement in immune function.*

Discussion Questions

a. Highlights the CKD pathogenesis.
b. Discuss the role of prebiotics in the treatment of CKD.
c. Describe the possible mechanisms and targets for the management of CKD.
d. Do prebiotics bring down renal inflammation?

e. How to calm down the inflamed renal tissue?
f. Describe the available supplement sources of prebiotics for the management of CKD patients.

Case 4: *A 52-year-old male patient has Parkinson's disease (PD). He also suffers from constipation. He recommended taking Short-Chain Fatty Acids (SCFAs).*

Discussion Questions

a. Highlights the PD pathogenesis and its symptoms.
b. How can constipation cause the leaky bowel conditions?
c. Discuss the role of prebiotics in the treatment of PD.
d. Describe the connection between the bowel and the brain functions.
e. How do prebiotics help to treat PD?
f. Describe the microbiome or bacterial compositions of the bowel with abnormal neurological function in Parkinson's disease.
g. How do SCFAs support the good bacteria in the gut of PD patients?

MCQs Questions

1. Which one of the following foods contains prebiotics, EXCEPT:
   A. Garlic
   B. Soybeans
   C. Wholegrains
   D. Glucose and galactose

2. Which one of the following molecules is absorbed by prebiotics?
   A. Iron
   B. Mucin
   C. Phytate
   D. Triacylglycerol

3. Which one of the following is NOT a property of probiotics?
   A. It is fermented by gut bacteria.
   B. It can be digested by salivary amylase.
   C. It can stimulate the growth of Lactobacillus.
   D. It can withstand relatively high temperatures.

4. Which one of the following is NOT a probiotic?
   A. *Escherichia coli*
   B. *Bifidobacterium lactis*
   C. *Lactobacillus plantarum*

D. *Streptococcus thermophilus*

5. Which one of the following is an example of a postbiotic, EXCEPT:
   A. Vitamin K
   B. Oligofructose
   C. Bifidobacteria
   D. Lactobacillus plantarum

Answers: 1) D; 2) A; 3) B; 4) A; 5) D

REFERENCES

[1] Kurian SJ, Baral T, Sekhar S, Rao M. Role of probiotics and prebiotics in digestion, metabolism, and immunity. Nutrition and Functional Foods in Boosting Digestion, Metabolism and Immune Health. Elsevier 2022; pp. 501-22.
[http://dx.doi.org/10.1016/B978-0-12-821232-5.00026-4]

[2] Bedu-Ferrari C, Biscarrat P, Langella P, Cherbuy C. Prebiotics and the human gut microbiota: from breakdown mechanisms to the impact on metabolic health. Nutrients 2022; 14(10): 2096.
[http://dx.doi.org/10.3390/nu14102096] [PMID: 35631237]

[3] Varela-Trinidad GU, Domínguez-Díaz C, Solórzano-Castanedo K, Íñiguez-Gutiérrez L, Hernández-Flores TJ, Fafutis-Morris M. Probiotics: protecting our health from the gut. Microorganisms 2022; 10(7): 1428.
[http://dx.doi.org/10.3390/microorganisms10071428] [PMID: 35889147]

[4] Dhamo K, Memushaj L, Shkreli R. Obesity prevention and treatment using probiotics and prebiotics. Journal of Biological Studies 2022; 5(1): 189-206.
[http://dx.doi.org/10.62400/jbs.v5i1.6625]

[5] Park J, Hosomi K, Kawashima H, *et al.* Dietary Vitamin B1 intake influences gut microbial community and the consequent production of short-chain fatty acids. Nutrients 2022; 14(10): 2078.
[http://dx.doi.org/10.3390/nu14102078] [PMID: 35631219]

[6] Syiemlieh I, Morya S. Dairy and non-dairy based probiotics: A review. Pharma Innov 2022; 11(6S): 2956-64.
[http://dx.doi.org/10.22271/tpi.2022.v11.i6Sak.13568]

[7] Cosme F, Inês A, Vilela A. Consumer's acceptability and health consciousness of probiotic and prebiotic of non-dairy products. Food Res Int 2022; 151: 110842.
[http://dx.doi.org/10.1016/j.foodres.2021.110842] [PMID: 34980381]

[8] Gatlin DM III. Prebiotics. Dietary Nutrients, Additives, and Fish Health. John Wiley and Sons, Ltd 2015; pp. 271-81.
[http://dx.doi.org/10.1002/9781119005568.ch13]

[9] Gibson GR, Probert HM, Loo JV, Rastall RA, Roberfroid MB. Dietary modulation of the human colonic microbiota: updating the concept of prebiotics. Nutr Res Rev 2004; 17(2): 259-75.
[http://dx.doi.org/10.1079/NRR200479] [PMID: 19079930]

[10] Tegegne BA, Kebede B. Probiotics, their prophylactic and therapeutic applications in human health development: A review of the literature. Heliyon 2022; 8(6): e09725.
[http://dx.doi.org/10.1016/j.heliyon.2022.e09725] [PMID: 35785237]

[11] Soccol CR, Medeiros ABP, Yamaguishi CT. The potential of probiotics. RE:view 2010; 22.

[12] Damián MR, Cortes-Perez NG, Quintana ET, *et al.* Functional foods, nutraceuticals and probiotics: a focus on human health. Microorganisms 2022; 10(5): 1065.

[http://dx.doi.org/10.3390/microorganisms10051065] [PMID: 35630507]

[13] Shams MH, Hashemzadeh F, Khorvash M, *et al.* Interaction of colostrum pasteurization with probiotics supplementation on health and performance of Holstein calves. Anim Feed Sci Technol 2022; 288: 115319. [http://dx.doi.org/10.1016/j.anifeedsci.2022.115319]

[14] Ye S, Shah BR, Li J, *et al.* A critical review on interplay between dietary fibers and gut microbiota. Trends Food Sci Technol 2022; 124: 237-49. [http://dx.doi.org/10.1016/j.tifs.2022.04.010]

[15] Leeuwendaal NK, Stanton C, O'Toole PW, Beresford TP. Fermented foods, health and the gut microbiome. Nutrients 2022; 14(7): 1527. [http://dx.doi.org/10.3390/nu14071527] [PMID: 35406140]

[16] Lauzon HL, Dimitroglou A, Merrifield DL, Ringø E, Davies SJ. Probiotics and prebiotics: concepts, definitions and history. Aquaculture Nutrition. John Wiley and Sons, Ltd 2014; pp. 169-84. [http://dx.doi.org/10.1002/9781118897263.ch7]

[17] Hu X, Yang F. Analysis of the therapeutic effect of changyanning on intestinal flora in inflammatory bowel disease 2022. [http://dx.doi.org/10.1155/2022/3757763]

[18] Tungland BC, Meyer D. Nondigestible oligo- and polysaccharides (dietary fiber): their physiology and role in human health and food. Compr Rev Food Sci Food Saf 2002; 1(3): 90-109. [http://dx.doi.org/10.1111/j.1541-4337.2002.tb00009.x] [PMID: 33451232]

[19] Heidt PJ. Probiotics: bacteria and bacterial fragments as immunomodulatory agents 2002.

[20] Fioramonti J, Theodorou V, Bueno L. Probiotics: what are they? What are their effects on gut physiology? Best Pract Res Clin Gastroenterol 2003; 17(5): 711-24. [http://dx.doi.org/10.1016/S1521-6918(03)00075-1] [PMID: 14507583]

[21] Burakova I, Smirnova Y, Gryaznova M, *et al.* The effect of short-term consumption of lactic acid bacteria on the gut microbiota in obese people. Nutrients 2022; 14(16): 3384. [http://dx.doi.org/10.3390/nu14163384] [PMID: 36014890]

[22] Tannock GW. Probiotics: Time for a dose of realism: 11.

[23] Davani-Davari D, Negahdaripour M, Karimzadeh I, *et al.* Prebiotics: definition, types, sources, mechanisms, and clinical applications. Foods 2019; 8(3): 92. [http://dx.doi.org/10.3390/foods8030092] [PMID: 30857316]

[24] Afrc RF. Probiotics in man and animals. J Appl Bacteriol 1989; 66(5): 365-78. [http://dx.doi.org/10.1111/j.1365-2672.1989.tb05105.x] [PMID: 2666378]

[25] O'Riordan KJ, Collins MK, Moloney GM, *et al.* Short chain fatty acids: Microbial metabolites for gut-brain axis signalling. Mol Cell Endocrinol 2022; 546: 111572. [http://dx.doi.org/10.1016/j.mce.2022.111572] [PMID: 35066114]

[26] Pranoto Y. Starch and its derivatives as potential source of prebiotics 2022. [http://dx.doi.org/10.1002/9781119702160.ch16]

[27] Vilà B, Esteve-Garcia E, Brufau J. Probiotic micro-organisms: 100 years of innovation and efficacy; modes of action. Worlds Poult Sci J 2010; 66(3): 369-80. [http://dx.doi.org/10.1017/S0043933910000474]

[28] Wang M, Wang L, Lyu X, Hua X, Goddard JM, Yang R. Lactulose production from lactose isomerization by chemo-catalysts and enzymes: Current status and future perspectives. Biotechnol Adv 2022; 60: 108021. [http://dx.doi.org/10.1016/j.biotechadv.2022.108021] [PMID: 35901861]

[29] Elango D, Rajendran K, Van der Laan L, *et al.* Raffinose family oligosaccharides: friend or foe for human and plant health? Front Plant Sci 2022; 13: 829118.

[http://dx.doi.org/10.3389/fpls.2022.829118] [PMID: 35251100]

[30] Petschow B, Doré J, Hibberd P, *et al.* Probiotics, prebiotics, and the host microbiome: the science of translation. Ann N Y Acad Sci 2013; 1306(1): 1-17.
[http://dx.doi.org/10.1111/nyas.12303] [PMID: 24266656]

[31] Sun Y, Zhang S, Nie Q, *et al.* Gut firmicutes: Relationship with dietary fiber and role in host homeostasis. Crit Rev Food Sci Nutr 2022; 1-16.
[PMID: 35822206]

[32] Tawfick MM, Xie H, Zhao C, Shao P, Farag MA. Inulin fructans in diet: Role in gut homeostasis, immunity, health outcomes and potential therapeutics. Int J Biol Macromol 2022; 208: 948-61.
[http://dx.doi.org/10.1016/j.ijbiomac.2022.03.218] [PMID: 35381290]

[33] Xia W, Sheng L, Mu W, *et al.* Enzymatic preparation of gentiooligosaccharides by a thermophilic and thermostable andbeta;-glucosidase at a high substrate concentration. Vol. 11. Foods 2022.

[34] Ham SY, Kim HS, Cha E, Lim T, Byun Y, Park HD. Raffinose inhibits streptococcus mutans biofilm formation by targeting glucosyltransferase. Microbiol Spectr 2022; 10(3): e02076-21.
[http://dx.doi.org/10.1128/spectrum.02076-21] [PMID: 35575506]

[35] Kasdekar N, Walke G, Deshpande K, Hotha S. Glycosyl vinylogous carbonates as glycosyl donors by metal-free activation. J Org Chem 2022; 87(9): 5472-84.
[http://dx.doi.org/10.1021/acs.joc.1c02427] [PMID: 35414184]

[36] Roberfroid M. Functional food concept and its application to prebiotics. Dig Liver Dis 2002; 34 (Suppl. 2): S105-10.
[http://dx.doi.org/10.1016/S1590-8658(02)80176-1] [PMID: 12408452]

[37] Martins GN, Ureta MM, Tymczyszyn EE, Castilho PC, Gomez-Zavaglia A. Technological aspects of the production of fructo and galacto-oligosaccharides. enzymatic synthesis and hydrolysis. Front Nutr 2019; 6: 78.
[http://dx.doi.org/10.3389/fnut.2019.00078] [PMID: 31214595]

[38] Khan M, Husain Q. Effect of metal ions present in milk on the structure and functional integrity of native and polyaniline chitosan nanocomposites bound β-galactosidase: A multi-spectroscopic approach. Food Chem 2019; 279: 312-20.
[http://dx.doi.org/10.1016/j.foodchem.2018.12.022] [PMID: 30611496]

[39] Monteagudo-Mera A, Rastall RA, Gibson GR, Charalampopoulos D, Chatzifragkou A. Adhesion mechanisms mediated by probiotics and prebiotics and their potential impact on human health. Appl Microbiol Biotechnol 2019; 103(16): 6463-72.
[http://dx.doi.org/10.1007/s00253-019-09978-7] [PMID: 31267231]

[40] Panther EJ, Dodd W, Clark A, Lucke-Wold B. Gastrointestinal microbiome and neurologic injury. Biomedicines 2022; 10(2): 500.
[http://dx.doi.org/10.3390/biomedicines10020500] [PMID: 35203709]

[41] Chong PP, Chin VK, Looi CY, Wong WF, Madhavan P, Yong VC. The microbiome and irritable bowel syndrome – a review on the pathophysiology, current research and future therapy. Front Microbiol 2019; 10: 1136.
[http://dx.doi.org/10.3389/fmicb.2019.01136] [PMID: 31244784]

[42] Guarino M, Altomare A, Emerenziani S, *et al.* Mechanisms of action of prebiotics and their effects on gastro-intestinal disorders in adults. Nutrients 2020; 12(4): 1037.
[http://dx.doi.org/10.3390/nu12041037] [PMID: 32283802]

[43] Delzenne NM, Williams CM. Prebiotics and lipid metabolism. Curr Opin Lipidol 2002; 13(1): 61-7.
[http://dx.doi.org/10.1097/00041433-200202000-00009] [PMID: 11790964]

[44] Rodrigues CMC, Plotkin SA. Impact of vaccines; health, economic and social perspectives. Front Microbiol 2020; 11: 1526.
[http://dx.doi.org/10.3389/fmicb.2020.01526] [PMID: 32760367]

[45] Dobrange E, Peshev D, Loedolff B, Van den Ende W. Fructans as immunomodulatory and antiviral agents: the case of *Echinacea.* Biomolecules 2019; 9(10): 615. [http://dx.doi.org/10.3390/biom9100615] [PMID: 31623122]

[46] Vagnerová K, Vodička M, Hermanová P, *et al.* Interactions between gut microbiota and acute restraint stress in peripheral structures of the hypothalamic–pituitary–adrenal axis and the intestine of male mice. Front Immunol 2019; 10: 2655. [http://dx.doi.org/10.3389/fimmu.2019.02655] [PMID: 31798585]

[47] Arnold JW, Roach J, Fabela S, *et al.* The pleiotropic effects of prebiotic galacto-oligosaccharides on the aging gut. Microbiome 2021; 9(1): 31. [http://dx.doi.org/10.1186/s40168-020-00980-0] [PMID: 33509277]

[48] Martirosian G, Ekiel A, Aptekorz M, *et al.* Fecal lactoferrin and Clostridium spp. in stools of autistic children. Anaerobe 2011; 17(1): 43-5. Available from: https://www.sciencedirect.com/science/article/pii/S1075 996410001721 [http://dx.doi.org/10.1016/j.anaerobe.2010.12.003] [PMID: 21167951]

[49] Peredo-Lovillo A, Romero-Luna HE, Jiménez-Fernández M. Health promoting microbial metabolites produced by gut microbiota after prebiotics metabolism. Food Res Int 2020; 136: 109473. [http://dx.doi.org/10.1016/j.foodres.2020.109473] [PMID: 32846558]

[50] Kaur AP, Bhardwaj S, Dhanjal DS, *et al.* Plant prebiotics and their role in the amelioration of diseases. Biomolecules 2021; 11(3): 440. [http://dx.doi.org/10.3390/biom11030440] [PMID: 33809763]

[51] Portincasa P, Bonfrate L, Vacca M, *et al.* Gut microbiota and short chain fatty acids: implications in glucose homeostasis. Int J Mol Sci 2022; 23(3): 1105. [http://dx.doi.org/10.3390/ijms23031105] [PMID: 35163038]

[52] Chiu YH, Lin SL, Tsai JJ, Lin MY. Probiotic actions on diseases: implications for therapeutic treatments. Food Funct 2014; 5(4): 625-34. [http://dx.doi.org/10.1039/c3fo60600g] [PMID: 24549263]

[53] Correia MITD, Liboredo JC, Consoli MLD. The role of probiotics in gastrointestinal surgery. Nutrition 2012; 28(3): 230-4. [http://dx.doi.org/10.1016/j.nut.2011.10.013] [PMID: 22305005]

[54] Pal R, Athamneh AIM, Deshpande R, *et al.* Probiotics: insights and new opportunities for Clostridioides difficile intervention. Crit Rev Microbiol 2022; 1-21. [PMID: 35574602]

[55] Verdu EF. Probiotics effects on gastrointestinal function: beyond the gut? Neurogastroenterol Motil 2009; 21(5): 477-80. [http://dx.doi.org/10.1111/j.1365-2982.2009.01297.x] [PMID: 19432946]

[56] Kinross J. Probiotics and synbiotics reduce infective complications from colorectal surgery Techniques in Coloproctology. Springer 2022; pp. 1-3.

[57] Schucht J, Marshall WA, Brown C, Caminiti N, Rosenthal M. Surgical nutrition and post-surgical management. Nutrition, Weight, and Digestive Health 2022; pp. 139-54.

[58] Vadala BS, Kumar P, Dwivedi MK. Probiotics in mitigation of food allergies and lactose intolerance. Probiotics in the Prevention and Management of Human Diseases. Elsevier 2022; pp. 213-21. [http://dx.doi.org/10.1016/B978-0-12-823733-5.00022-2]

[59] Depoorter L, Vandenplas Y. Probiotics in pediatrics. Probiotics 2022; pp. 425-50. [http://dx.doi.org/10.1016/B978-0-323-85170-1.00014-2]

[60] Pandey K, Modi A. Implications of probiotics and prebiotics on immune functions. Prebiotics, Probiotics and Nutraceuticals. Springer 2022; pp. 187-201. [http://dx.doi.org/10.1007/978-981-16-8990-1_10]

[61] Huo J, Wu Z, Sun W, *et al.* Protective effects of natural polysaccharides on intestinal barrier injury: A review. J Agric Food Chem 2022; 70(3): 711-35.
[http://dx.doi.org/10.1021/acs.jafc.1c05966] [PMID: 35078319]

[62] Soliman MG, Mansour HA, Hassan WA, Shawky E. Impact of oral probiotics in amelioration of immunological and inflammatory responses on experimentally induced acute diverticulitis. Probiotics Antimicrob Proteins 2022; 1-11.
[PMID: 35838945]

[63] Breugelmans T, Oosterlinck B, Arras W, *et al.* The role of mucins in gastrointestinal barrier function during health and disease. Lancet Gastroenterol Hepatol 2022; 7(5): 455-71.
[http://dx.doi.org/10.1016/S2468-1253(21)00431-3] [PMID: 35397245]

[64] di Vito R, Conte C, Traina G. A multi-strain probiotic formulation improves intestinal barrier function by the modulation of tight and adherent junction proteins. Cells 2022; 11(16): 2617.
[http://dx.doi.org/10.3390/cells11162617] [PMID: 36010692]

[65] Yu Y, Zong M, Lao L, Wen J, Pan D, Wu Z. Adhesion properties of cell surface proteins in Lactobacillus strains in the GIT environment. Food Funct 2022; 13(6): 3098-109.
[http://dx.doi.org/10.1039/D1FO04328E] [PMID: 35226005]

[66] Mercado V, Olmos J. Bacteriocin production by bacillus species: isolation, characterization, and application. Probiotics Antimicrob Proteins 2022; 14(6): 1151-69.
[http://dx.doi.org/10.1007/s12602-022-09966-w] [PMID: 35881232]

[67] Han S, Lu Y, Xie J, *et al.* Probiotic gastrointestinal transit and colonization after oral administration: a long journey. Front Cell Infect Microbiol 2021; 11: 609722.
[http://dx.doi.org/10.3389/fcimb.2021.609722] [PMID: 33791234]

[68] Castro-López C, Romero-Luna HE, García HS, Vallejo-Cordoba B, González-Córdova AF, Hernández-Mendoza A. Key stress response mechanisms of probiotics during their journey through the digestive system: a review. Probiotics Antimicrob Proteins 2022; 1-21.
[PMID: 36001271]

[69] Verma DK, Thakur M, Singh S, *et al.* Bacteriocins as antimicrobial and preservative agents in food: Biosynthesis, separation and application. Food Biosci 2022; 46: 101594.
[http://dx.doi.org/10.1016/j.fbio.2022.101594]

[70] Mei Y, Chen H, Yang B, Zhao J, Zhang H, Chen W. Research progress on conjugated linoleic acid bio-conversion in Bifidobacterium. Int J Food Microbiol 2022; 369: 109593.
[http://dx.doi.org/10.1016/j.ijfoodmicro.2022.109593] [PMID: 35287032]

[71] Salman M, Javed MR, Ali H, *et al.* Bioprotection of zea mays l. from aflatoxigenic aspergillus flavus by loigolactobacillus coryniformis bch-4. PLoS One 2022; 17(8): e0271269.
[http://dx.doi.org/10.1371/journal.pone.0271269] [PMID: 35917314]

[72] Wang Y, Wu J, Lv M, *et al.* Metabolism characteristics of lactic acid bacteria and the expanding applications in food industry. Front Bioeng Biotechnol 2021; 9: 612285.
[http://dx.doi.org/10.3389/fbioe.2021.612285] [PMID: 34055755]

[73] Kaur H, Ali SA. Probiotics and gut microbiota: mechanistic insights into gut immune homeostasis through TLR pathway regulation. Food Funct 2022; 13(14): 7423-47.
[http://dx.doi.org/10.1039/D2FO00911K] [PMID: 35766374]

[74] Tóth M, Muzsai S, Regulski K, *et al.* The phagocytosis of *Lacticaseibacillus casei* and its immunomodulatory properties on human monocyte-derived dendritic cells depend on the expression of lc-p75, a bacterial peptidoglycan hydrolase. Int J Mol Sci 2022; 23(14): 7620.
[http://dx.doi.org/10.3390/ijms23147620] [PMID: 35886967]

[75] Chen J, Liang H, Lu J, He Y, Lai R. Probiotics improve postoperative adaptive immunity in colorectal cancer patients: a systematic review and meta-analysis. Nutr Cancer 2022; 74(8): 2975-82.
[http://dx.doi.org/10.1080/01635581.2022.2056619] [PMID: 35341415]

[76] Li M, Zhang R, Li J, Li J. The role of c-type lectin receptor signaling in the intestinal microbiota-inflammation-cancer axis. Front Immunol 2022; 13: 894445.
[http://dx.doi.org/10.3389/fimmu.2022.894445] [PMID: 35619716]

CHAPTER 8

Phytochemicals as Nutraceuticals

Mukesh Singh Sikarwar[1,*] and **Vaibhav Kumar Rathi**[2]

[1] *Amity Institute of Pharmacy, Amity University, Gwalior, Madhya Pradesh, India*

[2] *Department of Pharmacy, Quantum University, Roorkee (Haridwar), Uttarakhand, India*

Abstract: Phytochemicals serve as essential components in nutraceuticals derived from plants and in functional food products. Plants are designed to generate phytochemicals as protective responses when faced with environmental stressors. The complexity of these phytochemicals suggests they possess significant potential for various physiological actions. A significant number of secondary metabolites generated by plants find applications in the field of medicine. Nutraceuticals are products sourced from food that offer both nutritional and medicinal benefits, typically taken in forms similar to pharmaceuticals, such as capsules, pills, or tablets. Functional foods are typically consumed like regular foods, which clearly differentiates them from nutraceuticals. Nutraceuticals differ from functional foods in that they are not classified as food. Instead, they consist of extracts or dosage forms derived from food, aimed at enhancing health outcomes. Phytochemicals like alkaloids, glycosides, carotenoids, phenolics, sulfides, flavonoids, phytoestrogens, and many other phytochemicals are used as nutraceuticals. Recently, the traditional system of medicines started launching nutraceuticals, for example, Ayurveda nutraceutical products range from beauty products to Non-Communicable Disease (NCD) management like diabetes, hypertension, and cancer management. Nutraceuticals reduce oxidative stress by quenching the free radicals in NCD, hence have the value of appropriate therapeutic nutritional interventions. This chapter is an attempt to compile the background, source, chemistry, and clinical studies of different classes of phytochemicals having the potential of nutraceuticals.

Keywords: Chemical structure, Clinical trials, Nutraceutical, Phytochemical.

INTRODUCTION

Phytochemicals are the microchemicals that are produced inside the cells of plants, and secondary metabolites are the phytochemicals that are produced due to defense mechanisms in plants and various other reasons, including environmental

* **Corresponding author Mukesh Singh Sikarwar:** Amity Institute of Pharmacy, Amity University, Gwalior, Madhya Pradesh, India; E-mail: mukeshsikarwar@gmail.com

Mukesh Singh Sikarwar, Arunachalam Muthuraman & Sohrab A. Shaikh (Eds.)

stress and adverse environments for the survival of the plant. Secondary metabolites produced from these plants could be utilized as nutraceuticals. To be a nutraceutical plant, it should have medicinal value apart from its nutritional value [1]. Phytochemicals as a nutraceutical could be classified based on chemical class and their action. Nutraceutical products for eye care, skin care, hair care, energy boosters, antihypertensives, anti-obesity, antidiabetic, hormone regulators, stimulants, anti-ageing, and rejuvenators are widely available in the market [2]. In this chapter, some of the important nutraceuticals are discussed.

CAROTENOIDS: A AND Β-CAROTENE, LYCOPENE, XANTHOPHYLLS, LEUTIN

Carotenoids are largely present in photosynthetic plants and nonphotosynthetic tissues within the unique cells called xanthophores. Different hues of meals, including fruits and vegetables, are attributable to the presence of carotenoids. The trans form of carotenoids isomerizes to the cis form during the digestion of food. Carotenoids mainly exist in fruits and vegetables, and their composition is determined by climate variables and geographic areas. α and β-Carotene, lycopene, xanthophylls, and leutin are some of the main carotenoids frequently exploited as nutraceuticals. Carotenoids are more abundant in the peel than pulp of the fruits and are efficient synergistically in polyherbal form. Certain carotenoids, like zeaxanthin and lutein, have a tremendous role in the protection of macula lutea against photooxidative damage and reduce the risk of age-related macular degeneration [3, 4]. Lycopene and beta carotenes provide protection by their antioxidant potential.

Carotenoids and terpenoids are made up of isoprene units, with each unit having five carbons; therefore, carotenoids can be classified in the chemical class of terpenoids. Carotenoids are mostly tetraterpenoids and are made up of 40 carbon skeletons with a conjugated polyene chain. Condensation of isoprenyl units could synthesize the carotenes (hydrocarbons) or xanthophylls (hydrocarbons containing oxygen). Various colors in fruits and vegetables are due to carotenoid pigments, and these colors are due to the absorption of light by different chain lengths. Carotenoids are isolated from natural resources and synthesized in the laboratory [5]. More than 600 naturally occurring carotenoids are known; however, very few are commercialized. Humans do not have the mechanism to synthesize the carotenoids *de novo*; hence, carotenoids are a required part of the diet and supplements since they perform a huge number of essential biological tasks. Carotenoids are mainly stored in the liver and adipose tissues. However, at greater concentrations, it could accumulate in the adrenal gland, lungs, corpus luteum, and testes. Human plasma and tissue were also found to have an increased number of carotenoids such as phtoene and phytofluene, a colorless substance [6].

α-Carotene

α-carotene is found in dark green foods such as green beans, spinach, and broccoli [7]. After central cleavage, α-carotene converts to one molecule of physiologically active retinol. The conversion effectiveness of β-carotene to vitamin A (retinol) is theoretically higher than that of α-carotene (Fig. **1**). Alpha carotene includes only one retinyl group, whereas beta carotene contains two. Alpha carotene is an equally significant carotene since it has potential antioxidants, anti-cancer, and immunomodulatory properties. Although α-carotene contains provitamin A activity, clinical trials on it are limited due to its connection with β-carotene and the difficulty of isolating it. Carrots have significant levels of α-carotene, which have been linked to increased blood concentrations [8]. It is also found in certain types of squash and pumpkin [9]. One study demonstrated that α-carotene is more effective than β-carotene in reducing the proliferation of human malignant tumour cells [10].

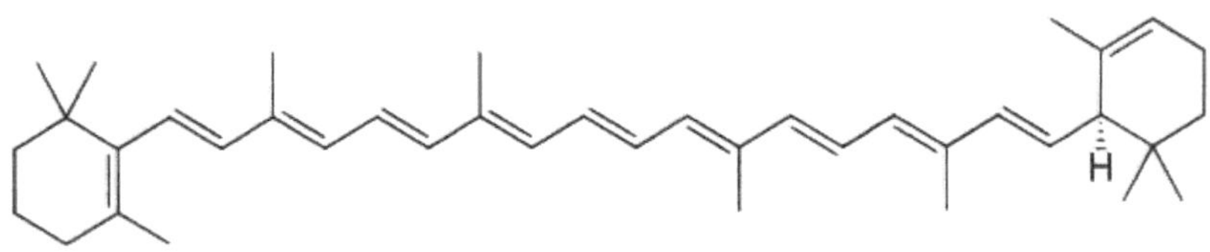

Fig. (1). Chemical structure of α-carotene.

α-carotene has a β-ionone ring at one end and an α-ionone ring at the other end. A study found that greater amounts of α-carotene, all-trans-beta-carotene, and total lycopene were linked to improved cardiac autonomic function. The CVD-stratified research revealed that increasing blood concentrations of alpha-carotene had positive effects on cardiac autonomic dysfunction [11].

β-Carotene

The term β-carotene comes from the Greek word "beta" (β) and the Latin word carota, which means carrot. Beta carotene is a prominent component of the carotenoid family that occurs naturally as a pigment in plants. β-carotene 15, 15′-monooxygenase produces two retinol molecules in the presence of oxygen, making it a significant precursor of vitamin A found in fruits and vegetables [12]. β-carotene is a provitamin that converts into vitamin A through metabolism (Fig. **2**). Apricots, asparagus, carrots, broccoli, Chinese cabbage, grapefruits, beetroot, cantaloupe, pumpkin, sweet potato, pink grapefruit, tomatoes, watermelon, mango, papaya, peaches, prunes, oranges, lettuce, peas, spinach, chilli powder, and paprika are the most common natural sources. β-Carotene has the greatest provitamin A activity, and deficiency can cause xerophthalmia, blindness, and early death [13]. Because of its antioxidant qualities, this nutraceutical has the potential to aid people suffering from chronic diseases such as diabetes, cancer, and cardiovascular disease [14]. Beta carotene can degrade owing to heat, light, and other environmental factors; hence, efforts are being made to increase its stability by encapsulation or innovative drug delivery systems [15]. Compared to alpha and epsilon carotene, beta carotene exhibits the highest antioxidant activity among the carotenes [16]. Beta-carotene is primarily responsible for the provitamin function of seaweed. A β-Carotene-15,150-dioxygenase can break it, which eventually leads to the creation of compound retinal [17]. The recommended daily intake of β-Carotene is around 15 mg [18].

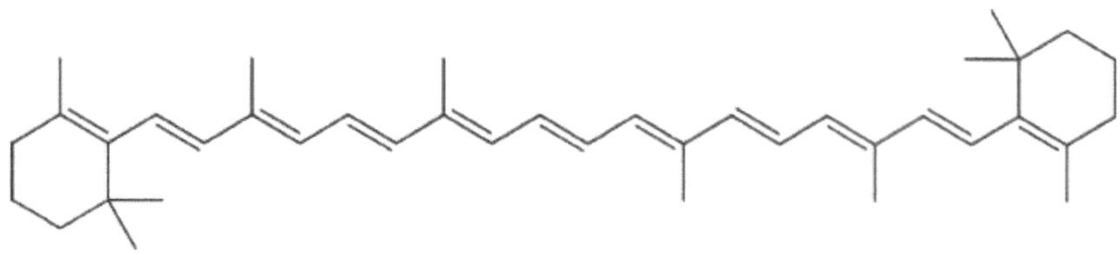

Fig. (2). Chemical structure of β-carotene.

There is no intrinsic vitamin A found in Algae, yet it includes provitamins such as β-carotene. Red seaweed *Gracilaria changgi, Kappaphycus alvarezzi,* and brown algae kombu were discovered to have high values of β-carotene with vitamin A activity. Moderate quantities of vitamin A were identified in wakame, arame, sea grapes, and sea lettuce [19 - 22]. Synthetic form of β-Carotene has acquired around 98% of the β-carotene market and only the remaining fraction, equivalent to 2-3%, is derived from bio-resources, such as fruits and vegetables, algae, fungus, and bacteria [23]. β-Carotene ′ oxygenase-1 and β-carotene 9′,10′ oxygenase-2, also known as BCO1 and BCO2, respectively, are the two known carotenoid cleavage enzymes in humans [24]. While high-pressure treatment tends to retain or even enhance the quantity of carotenoids, boiling in hot water causes both lycopene and β-carotene to partially degrade and isomerise [25].

Although high doses of β-carotene and vitamin E can be prooxidant, β-carotene is not teratogenic [9]. However, the ATBC study found that β-carotene (20 mg/d) increased the incidence of common colds in people who were engaging in strenuous exercise and the risk of pneumonia in smokers who were 21 years of age or older [26, 27]. According to a study, when β carotene [30 mg/d] was given as a supplement to subjects with colonic polyps or colon cancers for three months, the CD4 count increased only in cancer patients whose CD4 percentage was lower than that of patients with polyps and controls. However, only AIDS patients with more than 10 cells/microliter had higher CD4+ cell counts after taking 60 mg/d of β-carotene. β-carotene (60 mg/d, 3 months) raised NK but not CD4 in HIV patients [28 - 30]. In a study, 50 mg/kg β-carotene for 21 days increased the concentrations of IgA and total quantity of Antibody-Secreting Cells (ASC) in the jejunum [31]. In 1996, Gollnick *et al.* reported on the photoprotection properties of beta-carotene [32]. The β-carotene that may help immune cells function better was found and investigated by Hughes *et al.* [33].

β-Carotene is used medicinally to treat erythropoietic protoporphyria, a photosensitivity disorder, at a very high dose of 180 mg/day. Long-term bioassays in experimental animals showed that β-Carotene had no mutagenic or carcinogenic effects and did not show toxicity at high doses [34]. Clinical studies and epidemiological research have indicated that β-carotene may increase immune response and lower the incidence of cataracts, age-related macular degeneration, cardiovascular disease, and several forms of cancer [35 - 37]. In Kenya, children aged 5 to 13 years exhibited slightly greater blood retinol and β-carotene concentrations after ingesting β-carotene-fortified cassava [38]. β-carotene supplementation improved the plasma antioxidant capacity of older women in a randomized double-blind placebo-controlled study [39].

Carrot root includes α- and β-carotene, both largely in crystal forms, which are not easily solubilized by the digestive process. β-Carotene nutraceuticals have substantially better bioavailability than β-carotene that is produced from the diet. Micozzi *et al.* revealed that a 30 mg/day dose of all-trans β-carotene induced more than a fivefold rise in plasma β-carotene compared to 29 mg/day of β-carotene obtained from carrots [40]. β-carotene is a tetraterpene with chemical formula $C_{40}H_{56}$ and molecular weight 536.88. Depending on formulations, it comprises all trans (Z) isomers of β-carotene with various amounts of cis-isomer. It can be found as red to brownish-red to violet crystals or crystalline powder [41].

Lycopene

One of the most prominent carotenoids in nature is lycopene. The pigment lycopene gives tomatoes their red hue. Lycopersicon esculentum is the tomato's scientific name. In 1873, lycopene was originally isolated from the Tamus communis (black bryony); however, Schunck later called it lycopene in 1903 [42]. Approximately 80% of dietary lycopene is gained from tomatoes [43]. Lycopene sources include watermelon, pink grapefruit, papaya, and guava. Lycopene is available in the form of supplements or tomato extracts as well. Lycopene (C40H56) is a non-provitamin A lipophilic phytochemical (Fig. **3**). It is relatively robust to mild heat processing when the fat is missing, yet prolonged heat might induce deterioration. Lycopene is more stable in the matrix of tomato, compared to isolated, purified equivalents [44 - 49].

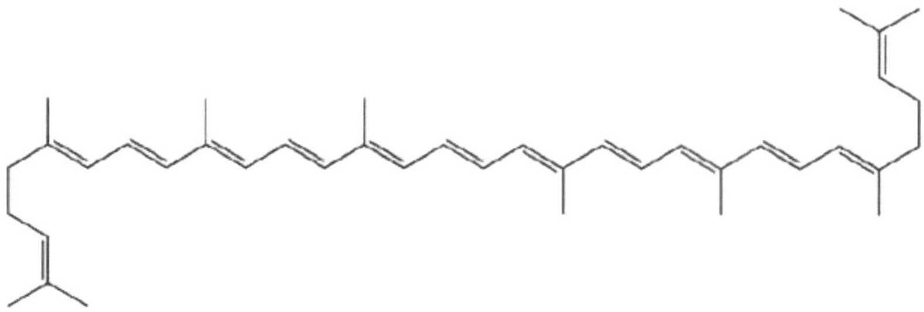

Fig. (3). Chemical structure of lycopene.

Homogenized tomatoes give higher bioavailable lycopene. It may be owing to mechanical disruption, which plays a crucial role in bioaccessibility [50]. Better absorption of lycopene from tomatoes is better when it's heat-treated but not fried [51, 52]. Some research showed that lycopene-rich fruits and vegetables have cancer-protective action *via* shielding against oxidative and other damage to DNA in humans [53]. Lycopene's unsaturated nature is a powerful antioxidant and a singlet oxygen quencher [54]. One of the pilot investigations revealed the possible significance of tomato extract containing lycopene in the treatment of prostate cancer [55]. Another clinical trial indicated the benefits of supplementation with lycopene in patients with localized prostate cancer reported the favourable effects in prostate cancer [56]. Clinical investigation in men and women with healthy weight data suggested that postprandial lipemia-induced oxidative stress and related inflammatory response are decreased by ingesting tomato products after a meal. A study demonstrating the preventive effect is decreasing cardiovascular disease risk, since there is a significant association between oxidation and inflammation in vascular tissues [57].

According to human research, taking tomato juice supplements on a regular basis reduced waist circumference, cholesterol, and inflammatory adipokine levels in young, healthy women. The study also showed that it may help obese people lose weight [58]. The 30-day Lycopene dietary intervention affected CRP levels in female heart failure patients, according to results from a pilot study [59]. Eating meals high in lycopene before being exposed to UV radiation has been shown to reduce the erythema response, indicating that tomato consumption affects the skin's reaction to these harmful stimuli [60]. This may be because lutein and lycopene-enriched tomato nutrient complex inhibited UVA-1 and UVA/B-induced elevation of heme-oxygenase 1, intercellular adhesion molecule 1, and matrix metallopeptidase 1 mRNA, which are indicators of oxidative stress, photodermatoses, and photoaging. A double-blind, placebo-controlled, and crossover study proposed photoprotection by oral supplementation with β-carotene and lycopene [61].

In a mouse research, lycopene was shown to have protective effects on the heart against histological abnormalities caused by atrazine (ATR) and to have substantial chemoprotective potential against ATR-induced cardiac damage by reducing the inflammatory response [62]. An investigation into the antioxidant capacity of lycopene in fatty liver degeneration showed that it had therapeutic benefits on hepatic and blood lipids, lowering TNF-α, raising HDL, and lowering malondialdehyde [63]. The effect of lycopene on the glycaemic state and antioxidant capacity in patients with type 2 diabetes was examined in a case-control study involving 87 patients and 122 healthy individuals. According to a study, lycopene may reduce oxidative stress and improve the pathophysiology of people with type 2 diabetes. It also has a higher peripheral antioxidant capacity and improves glycaemic control [64].

Xanthophylls

Tetraterpenes, or carotenoids, are molecules with a log chain of hydrocarbons (40 C atoms) called carotenes and molecules with one or more oxygen atoms in their structure called xanthophylls. Despite being generally non-polar compounds with the exception of lutein, xanthophylls are more polar than carotenes due to changes in the locations of oxygen atoms in their structures, such as keto, carboxy, methoxy, and epoxy [65]. Fucoxanthin, lutein, astaxanthin, zeaxanthin, and β-cryptoxanthin are the most prominent xanthophylls. Fucoxanthin is a common marine carotenoid that makes up around 10% of the whole production (Fig. **4**). It is found in diatoms (Bacillariophyta), *Laminaria japonica, Undaria pinnatifida, Sargassum fusiformis, Sargassum horneri, and the Fucus genus*, including *Fucus serratus* and *Fucus vesiculosus* [66]. A potent antioxidant with ten times the antioxidant activity of other carotenoids, astaxanthin is a red pigment [67]. Because xanthophylls are insoluble in water, they share properties with lipids and, as a result, have analogous transport pathways in the body's aqueous environment [68]. The two most prominent xanthophylls that build up in the brain and eye are lutein and zeaxanthin, which give the macula lutea in the eye its yellow tint. Green leafy vegetables and β-cryptoxanthin found in peppers, papayas, and pumpkins are dietary sources of lutein and zeaxanthin. Seashells, fish, and some types of mushrooms are marine sources of astaxanthin and canthaxanthin [68, 69].

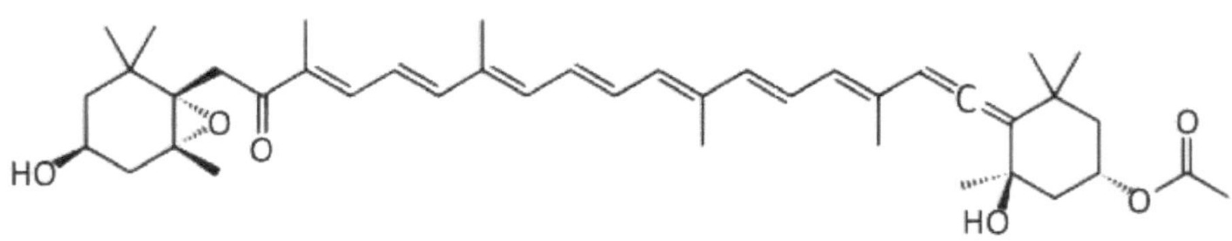

Fig. (4). Chemical structure of fucoxanthin.

Researchers say that because lutein and zeaxanthin build up in the brain and their plasma concentrations in healthy older individuals are connected to cognitive function, they are crucial for cognitive health [70]. High intakes of lutein and zeaxanthin were associated with a 22% reduced risk of cataract extraction compared to those in the lowest quintile, according to prospective research comparing carotenoid and vitamin A intakes with risk of cataract extraction in US women [71]. Photosynthetic microorganisms and plant parts generate lutein and zeaxanthin, particularly in stressful or high-light situations [72]. Animals cannot manufacture xanthophylls like zeaxanthin and lutein, and epidemiological research has indicated a negative association between xanthophylls and illnesses, including age-related eye disease, some forms of cancer, and others [73]. Consumption of Astaxanthin in combination with fish oil increased the lipid-lowering effects and increased phagocytic activity compared to the consumption of astaxanthin alone [74]. The chemical structure of astaxanthin is illustrated in Fig. (**5**).

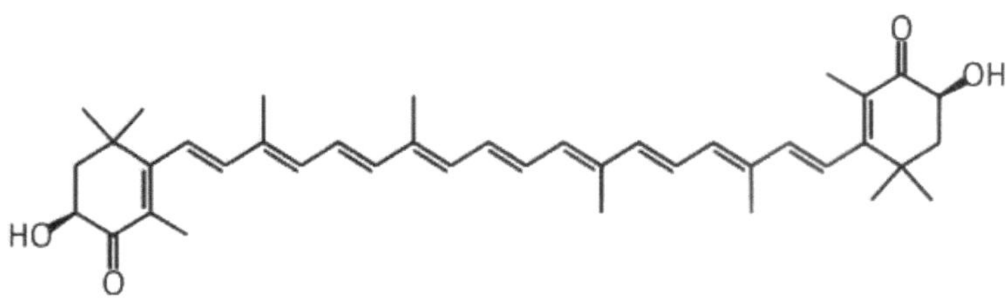

Fig. (5). Chemical structure of astaxanthin.

Lutein

Mangoes, maize, sweet potatoes, carrots, squash, tomatoes, and dark, leafy greens like bok choy, kale, and collards are also rich sources of these carotenoids. Lutein dipalmitate, commonly referred to as helenin, is found in the plant *Helenium autumnale* and is used to treat visual abnormalities. In plants, lutein and zeaxanthin are present as mono-or diesters of fatty acids and exist in non-esterified forms. Fruits and vegetables high in lutein include broccoli, pepper, grapes, carrot, maize, spinach, kiwi fruit, orange, kale, squash, orange juice, and zucchini. The marigold flower (*Tagetes erecta*) extract provides a crystalline lutein product that comprises 86% by weight of the carotenoids lutein and zeaxanthin [75]. Zeaxanthin and meso-zeaxanthin, two of lutein's stereoisomers, are found in the human retina. The concentration of lutein yellow xanthophyll carotenoid in the eyes is 78, which is roughly 500 times higher than its concentration in other body tissues. It is concentrated in the macula of the eye and shields the retinal pigment epithelial cells from blue light damage and the macula from oxidative stress [76 - 78]. Lutein and zeaxanthin in concentrations of ~6–10 mg/d may be important for eye health.

Chemically, the lutein is formed of cyclic structures at both ends of its conjugated chain and 40 carbon atoms. With the exception of the position of the double bond in one ring, which provides lutein a molecule with three chiral centres as opposed to zeaxanthin's two, their chemical structures are equivalent [79]. Because of its chemical nature, lutein helps maintain retinal function and prevent a number of eye disorders. By providing a better reaction with serum oxygen, lutein's two hydroxyl groups make it more polar and hydrophilic than carotene and effectively scavenge Reactive Oxygen Species (ROS), including superoxide anion (O^{2-}), perhydroxyl radical (HO2·), and hydroxyl radical (OH·), thereby reducing cellular damage caused by radical actions [80]. By lowering early inflammatory responses and UV-induced hyperproliferative rebound following oral lutein and zeaxanthin intake, the effects of UVB irradiation are minimized [81].

In research evaluating the primary carotenoids in human plasma, it was demonstrated that in CAD patients, lutein and zeaxanthin were the only two that exhibited an inverse connection with IL-6, a biomarker of inflammation for CAD [82]. By evaluating macular pigment optical density and retinal sensitivity, a clinical study of lutein and zeaxanthin supplementation was carried out to establish the influence of carotenoids in different phenotypes of early Age-related Macular Degeneration (AMD). The results demonstrated a substantial increase in macular pigment optical density in the reticular pseudodrusen [83]. The impact of lipoprotein profiles, apoE, and serum cytokines on the population with atherosclerosis was studied. Research has revealed that lutein supplementation decreases inflammatory cytokines and modulates blood lipids, a critical sign of early atherosclerosis [84]. Lutein is a natural food colorant and has health-promoting properties that make lutein a high-value nutraceutical ingredient (Table **1**) [85].

Table 1. Lutein supplementation for eye diseases.

Eye Disease	Supplement	Study Design	Key Findings	References
Atrophic Age-Related Macular Degeneration (AMD)	Lutein with or without other antioxidants	Double-blind, randomized, placebo-controlled trial	Supplementation with lutein alone or in combination with other nutrients led to improvements in visual function.	[86]
Atrophic AMD	Lutein and Antioxidants	Randomized controlled trial with 12-month follow-up	Supplementation with lutein was found to enhance Macular Pigment Optical Density (MPOD).	[87]

(Table 1) cont.....

Eye Disease	Supplement	Study Design	Key Findings	References
AMD	Lutein	Randomized Controlled Trial	MPOD levels increased significantly following lutein supplementation.	[88]
Early-stage AMD	Lutein	Double-blind, placebo-controlled, randomized trial across two centers	Lutein was effective in increasing MPOD in patients with early-stage AMD.	[89]
Intermediate AMD (CAREDS)	Lutein and Zeaxanthin	Observational study from the Women's Health Initiative	Women under 75 showed protection against intermediate AMD when supplemented with lutein and zeaxanthin.	[90]
Nonproliferative Diabetic Retinopathy	Lutein	Randomized, double-blind, placebo-controlled study	Improvements were noted in contrast sensitivity at lower spatial frequencies.	[91]
Diabetic Retinopathy	Lycopene with Lutein/Zeaxanthin	Community-based cross-sectional study	Antioxidant levels were found to be lower in individuals with diabetic retinopathy than in those without.	[92]
Retina Health in Preterm Infants	Lutein	Randomized Controlled Trial	Lutein supplementation demonstrated a protective effect on retinal health and development in preterm infants.	[93]
Myopia	Lutein	Cross-sectional, population-based study	Higher plasma lutein levels were associated with a reduced risk of developing myopia.	[94]
MPOD in Healthy Individuals	Lutein	Randomized clinical study	Among healthy Japanese participants without high myopia, lutein was more effective than zeaxanthin in enhancing MPOD within the fovea.	[95]
Age-related Nuclear Cataract	Lutein/Zeaxanthin	Clinical study	Elevated plasma levels of these carotenoids were linked to a reduced risk of developing nuclear cataracts, suggesting a protective role with aging.	[96]

PHENOLIC: TOCOPHEROLS, TOCOTRIENOLS, RESVERATROL

Phenolic compounds are a family of phytochemicals defined by the presence of one or more hydroxyl (-OH) groups connected to aromatic rings. These substances, notably polyphenols, are widely dispersed throughout diverse sections of plants, including leaves, stems, flowers, fruits, bark, roots, and rhizomes. In the plant world, phenolic chemicals contribute to key processes such as growth, development, and defense mechanisms. They also alter the sensory aspects of meals, including their color, fragrance, and flavor. Numerous scientific investigations have emphasized the numerous biological actions of phenolic compounds, which include anti-inflammatory, antioxidant, antibacterial, antiviral, antidiabetic, and anticancer characteristics. Common groups of phenolic substances include flavonoids, phenolic acids, lignans, and stilbenes (Table **2**).

Table 2. Various classes of phenolic compounds.

S.N.	Class	Number of Carbons	Basic Skeleton	Plant Source
1.	Simple phenols, benzoquinones	6	C_6	*Juglans nigra*
2.	Phenolic acids	7	C_6–C_1	*strawberries, raspberries, blueberries*
3.	Phenylacetic acid	8	C_6–C_2	*Gardenia jasminoides*
4.	Hydroxycinnamic acid, coumarin, isocoumarin	9	C_6–C_3	*Coffee beans, Cinnamomum cassia*
5.	Naphthoquinone	10	C_6–C_4	*Juglans nigra*
6.	Xanthone	13	C_6–C_1–C_6	*Garcinia mangostan*
7.	Stilbene	14	C_6–C_2–C_6	*Vitis vinifera*
8.	Flavonoids, isoflavonoids	15	C_6–C_3–C_6	*Glycine max*
9.	Lignans, neolignans	18	$(C_6$–$C_3)_2$	*Flaxseeds (Linum usitatissimum)*
10.	Biflavonoids	30	$(C_6$–C_3–$C_6)_2$	*Ginkgo biloba*
11.	Condensed tannins, Catecholmelanine, and Lignins	n	$(C_6$–$C_3)n$ $(C_6)n$ $(C_6$–C_3–$C_6)n$	*Pinus roxburghii* *Mucuna pruriens* *Acacia catechu* [97]

Tocopherols

Vitamin E, or tocopherols, is a class of fat-soluble compounds that are essential for protecting cells from damage caused by free radicals. Leafy green vegetables, nuts, seeds, and vegetable oils are the usual sources of tocopherols. Tocopherols in cells are mostly found in fat stores and lipid-rich regions of the cell, such as mitochondrial membranes. Vegetable oils, certain oilseeds, and nuts are the main sources of tocopherols in vegetables [98]. Vitamin E is a class of lipid-soluble α, β, γ, and δ-tocopherols. Only photosynthetic species, including cyanobacteria, algae, plants, fungi, corals, sponges, and tunicates, are capable of synthesizing tocopherols (Figs. **6** - **8**).

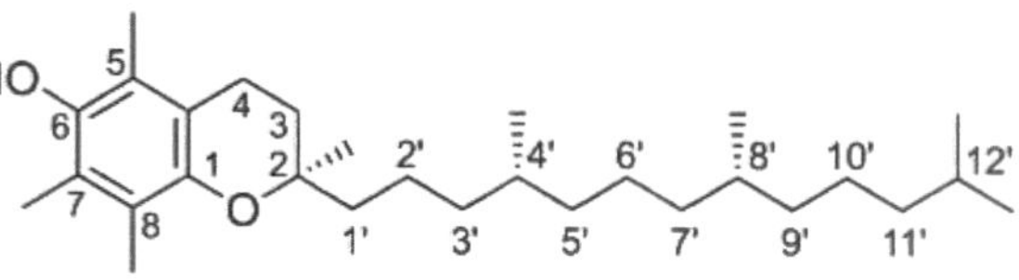

Fig. (6). Chemical structure of α-tocopherols.

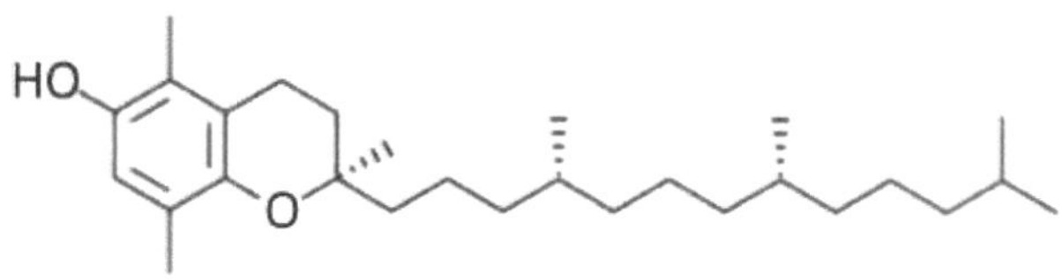

Fig. (7). Chemical structure of β-tocopherols.

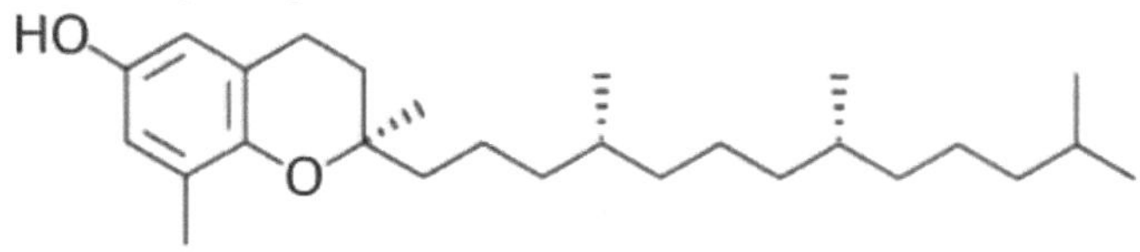

Fig. (8). Chemical structure of δ-tocopherols.

Tocopherols are monophenols, which occur as alpha, beta, delta, and gamma tocopherols and vary in chemical structure from one another by the number and position of methyl groups. There are eight stereoisomers for every tocopherol because of the presence of three chiral centers. Alpha-tocopherol is the prevalent tocopherol mainly found in food oils, as demonstrated by almond, peanut, olive, and sunflower oils. The gamma-tocopherol is found in certain food oils like corn, camelina, canola, linseed, walnut oils, and soybean [99]. Tocopherols, as nutraceuticals, have drawn interest due to their possible health advantages. Studies have shown that it has antioxidant properties [100] and improves cardiovascular health [101], immune function [102], eye [103], brain [104], and skin health [103].

Tocotrienols

Tocotrienols are a subgroup of vitamin E sharing similar chemical structures with tocopherols. However, tocotrienols have an unsaturated side chain, which distinguishes them from tocopherols (Fig. **9**). Tocotrienols contain a chromanol ring and a phytyl tail. The hydroxyl group (OH) is at position 2, and a methyl group (CH3) is at position 5 in the chromanol ring. The phytyl tail is made up of a 16-carbon isoprenoid chain. The tocotrienols show unsaturation by having three double bonds (triene) in the phytyl tail, unlike tocopherols, which have a saturated phytyl tail. Tocotrienols are four types of alpha, beta, gamma, and delta tocotrienols. Similar to tocopherols, tocotrienols are also hydrophobic molecules, soluble in oils and fats but insoluble in water.

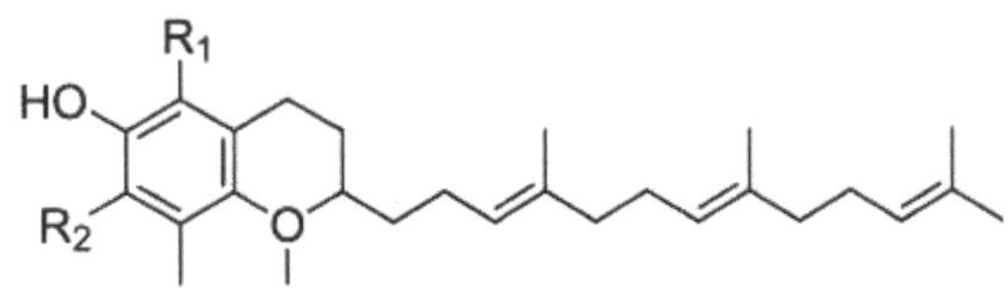

R1	R2	Nomenclature
CH_3	CH_3	α
CH_3	H	β
H	CH_3	γ
H	H	δ

Fig. (9). Chemical structure of tocotrienols.

Tocotrienols have gained attention for their potential health benefits, such as antioxidant, cardioprotective, neuroprotective effects, anti-cancer properties, and skin, liver, and metabolic health (Table **3**).

Table 3. Tocotrienol clinical trials for different diseases.

Study Design	Dose	Clinical Activity	Duration	Outcome	References
Randomized, double-blind, placebo-controlled pilot	300 mg twice daily	Fatty liver disease	12 weeks	Aminotransferase levels and inflammatory and oxidative stress markers were improved in patients with NAFLD.	[105]
Randomized, double-blinded study	200 mg twice a day	type 2 diabetes	8 weeks	significantly reduced serum creatinine levels, representing a useful addition to the current treatment for diabetic nephropathy.	[106]
Randomized, double-blind, and placebo-controlled	200 mg/day twice	CVD	2 years	Tocotrienols were found to attenuate the progression of white matter lesions.	[107]

(Table 3) cont.....

Study Design	Dose	Clinical Activity	Duration	Outcome	References
Double-blinded, placebo-controlled pilot	200 mg/day Twice	Breast cancer	5 years	No correlation was found between adjuvant tocotrienol therapy and breast cancer survival rate in women with early breast cancer.	[108]
Randomized, placebo-controlled, double-blind	400 mg/day	Metabolic syndrome	16 weeks	Tocotrienol supplementation exerted potential beneficial effects on cytokines and lipid profiles in adults with metabolic syndrome.	[109]
Double-blinded, placebo-controlled, randomized	430 mg/day 860 mg/day	Postmenopausal women with osteopenia	12 weeks	At a dose of 600 mg per day for 12 weeks, Tocotrienol seems to be harmless in postmenopausal osteopenic women.	[110]

Resveratrol

Red grape skin, peanuts, blueberries, Japanese knotweed (*Polygonum cuspidatum*), and numerous other berries are natural sources of resveratrol. A stilbenoid molecule with two phenol rings connected by an ethylene bridge is resveratrol (3,5,4′-trihydroxy-trans-stilbene). This molecule, a phytoalexin of the polyphenol class, is generated by a variety of plants in response to stress brought on by damage or stressed pathogenic bacteria or fungi. About 92 novel resveratrol compounds have been found from a range of families, including the Dipterocarpaceae, Paeoniaceae, Vitaceae, Leguminosae, Gnetaceae, Cyperaceae, Polygonaceae, Gramineae, and Poaceae families. These compounds contain 39 dimers, 23 trimers, 13 tetramers, 6 resveratrol monomers, 6 hexamers, 4 pentamers, and 1 octamer. The two isomeric forms of resveratrol (trans-3,5,4--trihydroxystilbene), cis- and trans-resveratrol, are depicted in the chemical structure (Fig. **10**). Resveratrol's trans form and effects are responsible for its diverse biological activities, which generally involve cellular responses including differentiation, apoptosis, cell cycle arrest, and anti-proliferation of cancer cells [111]. Traditional medicine exploited pterostilbene, a naturally occurring methoxylated resveratrol analogue from *Pterocarpus santalinus* (red sandalwood), to treat diabetes [112].

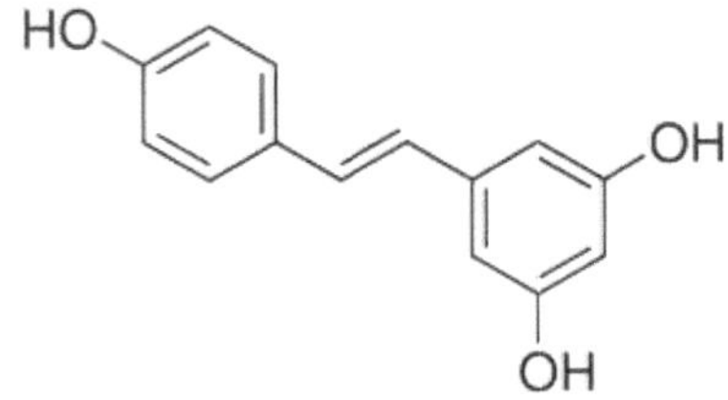

Fig. (10). Chemical structure of resveratrol.

Resveratrol's biological activities include free radical scavenging: research has indicated that trans-resveratrol may have the ability to scavenge OOH and, most likely, OOR radicals [113]. Anticancer Activity: Resveratrol has been shown in several *in vitro* and *in vivo* investigations to inhibit all stages of carcinogenesis, including initiation, promotion, and progression [114]. By controlling a distinct group of transcription factors, upstream kinases, and their regulators, resveratrol targets intracellular signalling pathway components such as pro-inflammatory mediators, tumour angiogenic and metastatic switches, and regulators of cell survival and death [115]. *Cardioprotective Effects:* Resveratrol improved left ventricular function, decreased cardiac hypertrophy, interstitial fibrosis, contractile dysfunction, and remodelling, and plasma BNP (B-type natriuretic peptide) levels in heart failure [116]. *Neuroprotective Effects:* Resveratrol enhanced mitochondrial biogenesis and functioning *via* the AMPK/PGC1α/SIRT1 (sirtuin 1)/vitagenes pathway [117]. *Anti-Inflammatory Activity:* Resveratrol inhibits NF-κB, tumour necrosis factor-α, and interleukin-6 serum levels, macrophage inflammatory protein-2 and cyclooxygenase-2 activity levels, ROS generation, and caspase-3/9 in rabbit models to prevent inflammation produced by acute pharyngitis [118]. *Antimicrobial Activity:* Resveratrol may help cure infectious illnesses caused by Staphylococcus aureus and pneumonia caused by S. aureus [119].

Clinical Studies

Obesity: Timmers *et al.* also found that obese males who received 150 mg of resveratrol daily for 30 days had improved cellular and systemic metabolic indicators, such as increased muscle mitochondrial respiration and decreased blood levels of lipids and glucose. *Non-alcoholic fatty liver disease:* Studies have indicated that giving resveratrol to people with NAFLD at a lower dose for a shorter period of time can be helpful. After taking 300 mg of resveratrol daily for three months, the patients' ALT and AST levels decreased, their lipid metabolism improved, and their glucose and inflammatory levels decreased [120]. *Diabetes:* According to research, taking resveratrol daily for three months improved glycaemic management by lowering HbA1c levels, systolic blood pressure, Total Cholesterol (TC), and total protein [121]. *Neurological diseases:* Resveratrol has been demonstrated to influence the activities of metabolic regulators AMPK, SIRT1, and PGC-1α, which have been implicated in the development of neurological illnesses [122]. *Cancer:* Research suggests that by altering the epigenetics of genes linked to breast cancer, resveratrol may be a chemopreventive medication for the disease; this finding will be confirmed in upcoming clinical studies [123].

SULFIDES: DIALLYL SULFIDES, ALLYL TRISULFIDE

Sulfides are a wide group of sulfur-containing compounds that are bonded to one or more other elements. They may be categorized on the basis of their bonding and structure. For instance, Binary sulfides, mixed sulfides, organic sulfides, metal sulfide complexes, and biological sulfides. Phytochemicals that are sulfur-bearing, like the allyl sulfides, occur in garlic and onions and are widely used for their possible health benefits, such as antioxidant, anti-inflammatory, and antimicrobial effects. Until the sulphur compounds in alliaceous vegetables are broken down, crushed, or chewed in an enzyme-substrate process, they are not bioactive. Alliin is changed into allicin in this process of cellular tissue breakdown, and the enzyme alliinase then swiftly changes it into diallyl sulphide, diallyl disulphide, or diallyl trisulphide [124].

Diallyl Sulfides

Two allyl groups (-CH2-CH=CH2) are linked to a central sulphur atom in this family of organic compounds. Diallyl disulfide (DADS), which has the chemical formula (C3H5)2S2, is the most well-known member of this group (Fig. **11**). Diallyl trisulfide (DATS) and diallyl sulphide (DAS) are additional components. Garlic, onions, shallots, and leeks are among the plants of the Allium genus that naturally contain diallyl sulphides. DAS has been proven in multiple studies to specifically inhibit CYP2E1 in a range of cell types, therefore lowering cellular toxicities generated by HIV proteins, diabetes, alcohol, and pharmaceuticals. Diallyl sulphides are poorly soluble in water and have high boiling temperatures. They taste and smell strong. Diallyl sulphides have been explored for possible health advantages. They have been revealed to have antioxidant, antibacterial, and anti-inflammatory effects. Diallyl sulphides preferentially inhibit cytochrome P450 2E1 (CYP2E1), which is important for the liver's metabolism of numerous xenobiotics, such as alcohol and opioids. When alcohol and pharmaceuticals are metabolised by CYP2E1, reactive oxygen species and reactive metabolites are generated. These substances affect the membranes of proteins, lipids, and DNA, which eventually destroys the liver. DAS has been proven in multiple studies to specifically inhibit CYP2E1 in a range of cell types, therefore lowering cellular toxicities generated by HIV proteins, diabetes, alcohol, and pharmaceuticals.

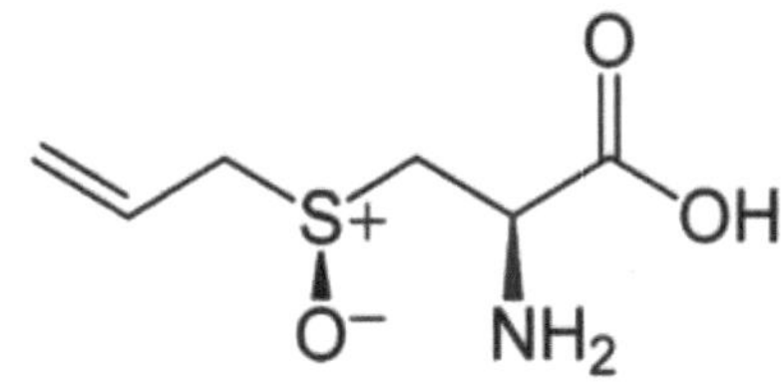

Fig. (11). Chemical structure of alliin.

Biological Activities

According to research, diallyl disulfide may be able to alleviate neuropathic pain in rats administered CCI by stimulating the H2S-BDNF-Nrf2 signaling pathway [126]. Cardiovascular health: Dialyl sulphides can lessen the risk of heart disease by increasing blood flow, decreasing blood pressure, and lowering cholesterol. Anticancer activity: Diallyl sulphides have anti-cancer characteristics and can inhibit some cancer cell types from multiplying. Diallyl sulphides may have advantages such as immune system activation and lower sensitivity to infections [125 - 127]. Diallyl sulphides have neuroprotective characteristics that may help lessen the risk of neurodegenerative illnesses, including Parkinson's and Alzheimer's disease.

Allyl Trisulfide

Allyl trisulfide (ATS) is an organic compound having the formula (C3H5)2S3, belonging to the family of allyl sulfides, although with an extra sulfur atom in its molecule. It is often present in garlic and contributes to the unique scent and flavor of garlic. Diallyl trisulfide is an organic trisulfide where both of the hydrogens are substituted with allyl groups (Fig. **12**). Diallyl trisulfide (DATS) or Allitridin. It contains antifungal, antitumour and antioxidant action, an estrogen receptor antagonist, an antineoplastic agent, a vasodilator agent, an antioxidant, an anti-inflammatory agent, a pesticide, an antiprotozoal drug, a platelet aggregation inhibitor and an antilipemic medicine [128 - 130].

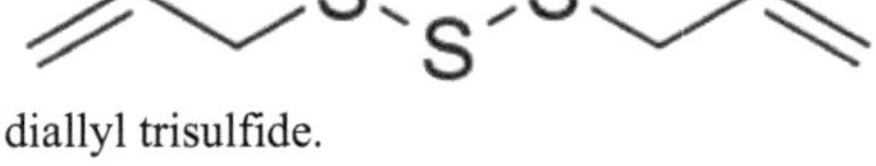

Fig. (12). Chemical structure of diallyl trisulfide.

In raw garlic, diallyl trisulfide is formed when the enzyme alliinase acts on allicin, and then allicin decomposes into various sulfur-containing compounds, including diallyl trisulfide, upon crushing or chopping garlic cloves (Table **4**).

Table 4. Anticancer effects of Diallyl sulfides and Allyl trisulfide.

S.N.	Active Constituents	Biological Activity	Mode of Action	References
1.	Diallyl trisulfide from garlic	Anticancer effect	When diallyl trisulfide attaches itself to certain cysteine residues in β-tubulin, it forms Sallylmercaptocystein, which stops the cell cycle and triggers caspase-3 to trigger apoptosis.	[131]
2.	Diallyl trisulfide (DATS)	PC-3 Human Prostate Cancer	The elevation of pro-apoptotic proteins Bak and Bax was linked to the growth inhibition of PC-3 xenografts caused by DATS. Vascular endothelial growth factor receptor-2 protein was down-regulated by DATS, which inhibited PC-3 cell motility in culture.	[132]
3.	Diallyl disulfide and diallyl trisulfide isolated from *Allium sativum* L.	Paclitaxel-resistant triple-negative breast cancer cells	Diallyl disulfide and diallyl trisulfide activated caspase 3 and 9 to cause apoptosis and blocked the cell cycle, which prevented PTX-resistant cells from proliferating.	[133]
4.	Diallyl sulfide (DAS), diallyl disulfide (DADS), and diallyl trisulfide (DATS)	Human colon cancer colo 205 cells	Certain signal proteins, including PI3K, Ras, MEKK3, MKK7, ERK1/2, JNK1/2, and p38, are inhibited by DAS, DADS, and DATS. The MMP-2, MMP-7, and MMP-9 enzymes are inhibited as a result. They also inhibit COX-2 and NF-κB, which reduces cell proliferation.	[134]
5.	Diallyl trisulfide (DATS) from garlic	Pancreatic Cancer Cells	DATS treatment in AsPC-1 pancreatic cancer cells reduced Gli1 transcription factor mRNA and protein levels. It increased the protein levels of the Sonic Hedgehog pathway's initiating ligand and Patched receptor. Additionally, DATS suppressed ectopic Gli1 expression.	[135]
6.	Processed Diallyl trisulfide (DATS)	HNSCC Tumor Growth and Cancer Stemness	DATS caused notable G2/M cell cycle arrest in AsPC-1 cells, elevating cyclin B1, Cip1/p21, and Ser-10 phospho-histone H3 levels. NAC pretreatment diminished mitotic arrest, indicating that Reactive Oxygen Species (ROS) play a role.	[136]
7.	Diallyl Trisulfide from garlic	Human Colon Cancer Cells	Diallyl trisulfide (DATS) binds to specific cysteine residues on tubulin, forming S-allylmercaptocysteine, which halts the cell cycle and induces apoptosis through caspase-3 activation.	[137]

(Table 4) cont.....

S.N.	Active Constituents	Biological Activity	Mode of Action	References
8.	Diallyl trisulfide (DATS) is found in garlic	Triple-Negative Breast Cancer (TNBC)	Suppressing MMP2/9 by Blocking NF-κB and ERK/MAPK Signaling Pathways.	[138]
9.	Diallyl sulfide (DAS), diallyl disulfide (DADS), and diallyl trisulfide (DATS) from Garlic	Skin Cancer	Diallyl trisulfide (DATS) increased intracellular reactive oxygen species (ROS), triggered cytosolic Ca2+ mobilization, and decreased mitochondrial membrane potential (ΔΨm). Western blot analysis confirmed the expression of molecules linked to G2/M arrest and apoptosis, aligning with cell cycle and viability results.	[139]
10	Diallyl trisulfide (DATS)	Colorectal cancer cells	DATS boosted ROS production in primary colorectal cancer cells, activating the mitochondria-mediated apoptotic pathway. This was marked by increased cytochrome c, Apaf-1, AIF, caspase-3, and caspase-9 levels. A decreased ΔΨm and elevated Bax/Bcl-2 ratio further drove caspase-9 and -3 activation.	[140]

FLAVONOIDS: RUTIN, NARINGIN, QUERCETIN, ANTHOCYANIDINS, CATECHINS, AND FLAVONES

The term “flavonoids” or “bioflavonoids” comes from the Latin flavus, which refers to their inherent yellow hue. Secondary metabolites called flavonoids have an aromatic ring joined to a phenolic -OH group. Flavonoids, which give plants their colour, aroma, and flavour, are abundant in the vacuoles of their cells, fruits, and seeds [141]. The C6-C3-C6 structure of all flavonoids is made up of two benzene rings, A and B, which are connected by an oxygen-containing heterocyclic pyrene ring (C) (Fig. **13**). The core heterocyclic ring's saturation level serves as the basis for the general classification of flavonoids into two types. For example, anthocyanidins, flavones, flavonols, and isoflavones exhibit C2=C3 unsaturation, whereas saturated flavonoids are represented by flavanones, dihydroflavonols, and flavan-3-ols [142]. Band II (240–285), which corresponds to the A ring benzoyl system, and band I (300–400 nm), which corresponds to the B ring cinnamonoyl system, are the two main maxima of absorption found in flavonoids. Because of their structural resemblance to oestrogens, such as oestradiol, isoflavones, which have a B ring linked to position three of the C ring, are also known as phytoestrogens. While the B ring is attached in position 4 of neoflavonoids, those with the B ring attached in position 2 can be divided into several subgroups according to the structural properties of the C ring. For instance, catechins, anthocyanins, chalcones, flavones, flavonols, flavanones, and flavanonols [143]. Flavones have a double bond between the second and third locations of the C ring and a ketone functional group at the fourth position. The presence of a hydroxyl at the third position in the C ring, which can be further glycosylated, sets flavonols apart from flavones. In dihydroflavones or flavanones, the double bond at positions two and three is saturated, but not in flavones. Flavanonols are derivatives of 3-hydroxy flavanone. Chalcones are flavonoids with an open C ring [144, 145]. Flavonoids' high metabolism, quick excretion, and restricted absorption make them minimally bioavailable. However, of all the flavonoid subclasses, isoflavones appear to be the most accessible, whereas galloylated catechins and anthocyanins are extremely poorly absorbed [146].

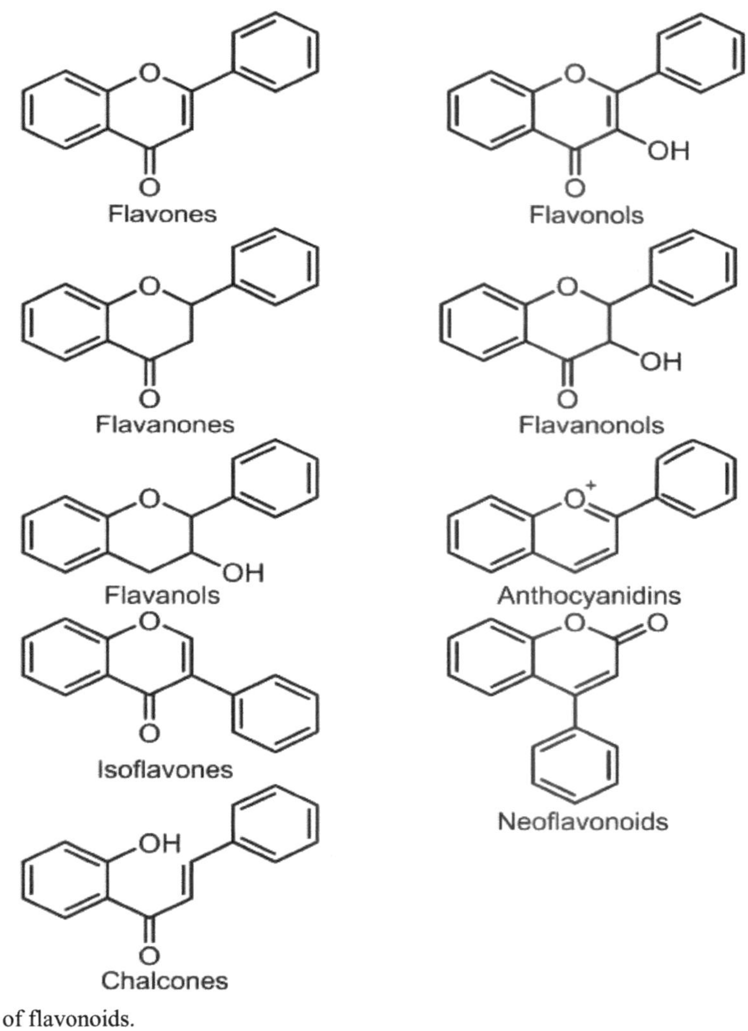

Fig. (13). Types of flavonoids.

Quercetin, kaempferol, icariin, myricetin, naringin, daidzein, luteolin, genistein, hesperidin, apigenin, and a few more flavonoids are some important flavonoids. The two biosynthetic routes that produce flavonoids in plants are the polyketide, which produces blocks for polymeric C2 units, and the phenylpropanoid, which produces the phenylpropanoid skeleton (C6-C3). Nowadays, flavonoids are an essential part of pharmacological, cosmetic, therapeutic, and nutraceutical applications [147].

Rutin

Rutin is a flavonol flavonoid that is mostly found in plants (3, 3′, 4′, 5, 7-pentahydroxyflavone-3-rhamnoglucoside (Fig. **14**). Other names for it include quercetin-3-rutinoside and rutoside. Prevention of neuroinflammation, support of neural crest cell survival, anticonvulsant, anti-Alzheimer, and treatment for hyperkinetic movement disorder are among the pharmacological actions of rutin. Other actions include antidepressant, analgesic, and antinociceptive, antiarthritic, antidiabetic, anti-hypercholesterolemic, antiplatelet aggregatory, antiulcer, antiasthmatic, and anticancer [148].

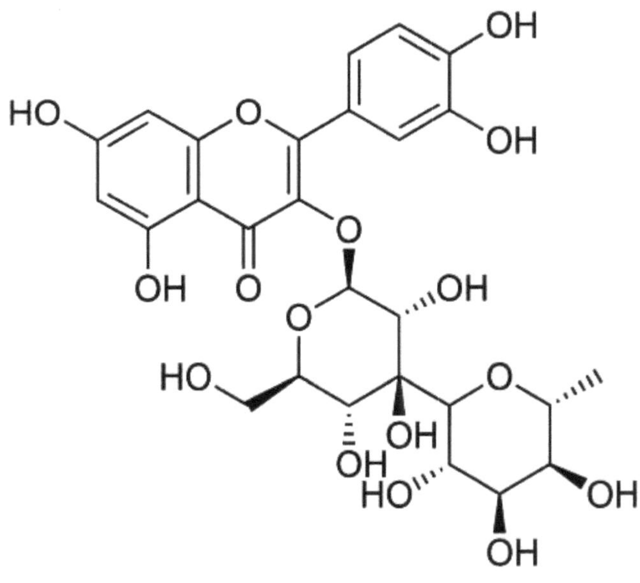

Fig. (14). Chemical structure of rutin.

'Rutin' is derived from the Ruta graveolens plant, which is mostly composed of rutin. The chemical structure of rutin consists of the flavonolic aglycone quercetin and the disaccharide rutinose.

- The hydroxyl group at position five, the double bond, and the double-bonded oxygen in the oxane ring are essential for the flavonoid activity of rutin.
- The neuroprotective properties of rutin are attributed to the 4-Oxo group and 2,3 double bonds in the C ring.
- Compared to aglycone quercetin, C-3 position glycosylated quercetin exhibits less potent free radical scavenging action [148].

For its anticancer properties, rutin is linked to the regulation of signalling pathways such as NF-κB, PI3K/Akt/mTOR, Nrf2, ERK, JNK, and p38 MAPK. Rutin has been shown to disrupt intracellular signalling molecules, including TNF-α, Bax, ILs, Beclin, VEGF, Bcl-2, and caspases, in a number of *in vitro* and *in vivo* tests [149]. Rutin protects fibroblasts against redox imbalances caused by UVA and UVB rays at the level of gene and protein expression. Additionally, it has antiapoptotic properties and prevents phospholipid metabolism alterations, which lowers endocannabinoid levels [150]. Potential uses for rutin-loaded nanophytosomes included adding water-insoluble nutraceuticals to food items [151]. When linoleate rutin is derivatised, a bioconjugate is created that may be used as an active component in preserving cellular integrity, homeostasis, and healing or as a flavonoid prodrug with a favourable toxicological profile. With improved biological qualities, rutin linoleate may find use in pharmaceutical nutraceutics to prevent skin, liver, and cardiovascular diseases [152].

According to research, when rutin is given orally to rats and rabbits, the metabolites 3, 4-dihydroxyphenylacetic acid, 3-methoxy-4-hydroxyphenylacetic acid, and 3-hydroxyphenylacetic acid are found in the urine. In a different investigation, plasma levels of quercetin were only 3.5 μmol/L when healthy people were fed 50 mg of either rutin or quercetin. Additionally, microbial metabolites from human urine were shown to contain up to 50% of a 75 mg rutin dosage that was consumed [153]. When 500 mg of rutin supplement was compared to an identical amount of glucose placebo in a 6-week randomised single-blind placebo-controlled experiment, the plasma levels of flavonoids such as quercetin, kaempferol, and isorhamnetin were shown to be considerably higher [154]. The effectiveness of a rutin-enriched extract in treating mild to moderate ulcerative colitis was investigated in a Chinese clinical study. Results show that it was just as successful as mesalazine in improving ulcerative colitis-related clinical and endoscopic findings while also lowering blood levels of inflammatory markers such as TNF-α, IL-1 beta, and IL-8 [155].

In a clinical experiment, 50 volunteers with mild to severe ulcerative colitis were given 500 mg of rutin and 500 mg of ascorbic acid twice daily or a placebo for six weeks to examine the benefits of the combination. According to the results, there was a large decrease in the blood levels of oxidative stress and inflammatory indicators such as malondialdehyde, nitric oxide, prostaglandin E2, TNF-α, and IL-10, along with a significant improvement in the clinical and endoscopic parameters linked to ulcerative colitis [156]. When rutin supplements were compared to a placebo, the effects on blood pressure markers, serum antioxidant enzymes, and quality of life in patients with type 2 diabetes mellitus were found to be significantly lower for systolic, diastolic, pulse, mean arterial pressure, and heart rate, while superoxide dismutase, catalase, and glutathione peroxidase and quality of life parameters were significantly higher than baseline (All $p < 0.05$) [157].

Naringin

Naringin (4′,5,7-trihydroxyflavanone-7-rhamnoglucoside) and its aglycone, naringenin, are flavanones that are mostly found in citrus fruits such as lemon, orange, mandarin, and grapefruit. Two rhamnose units joined at the C7 and three rings, two of which are benzene rings, joined by a chain of three carbon atoms make up Naringin's structure (Fig. **15**).

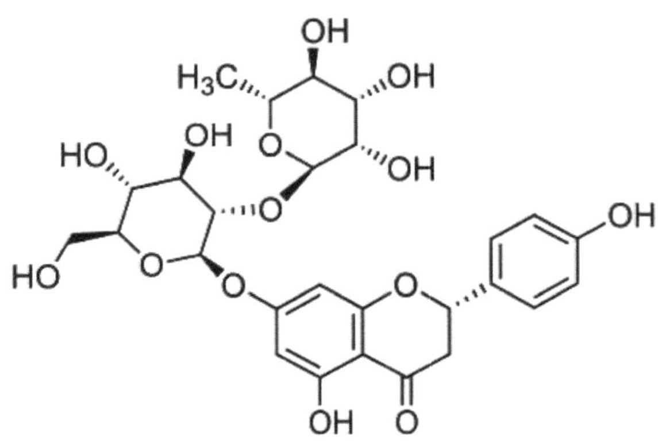

Fig. (15). Chemical structure of naringin.

A pyran ring, two aromatic rings, and fifteen carbon atoms make up the fundamental chemical composition of naringin. The seventh carbon of the aglycone derivative naringenin is attached to the disaccharides rhamnose and glucose, where rhamnose is the terminal sugar. Naringin's chemical structure, which includes the amount and precise location of hydroxyl groups on the two aromatic rings, the presence of sugar moieties, and other characteristics, is responsible for all of its health benefits, including microbiome modulation, anti-inflammatory, anti-osteoporotic, and radical scavenging (reactive oxygen species). Numerous nanotechnology-based drug delivery strategies have enhanced the bioavailability and pharmacokinetics of naringin, ultimately providing protection against deterioration and unintentional contact over extended periods of circulation [158].

Naringin had an anti-inflammatory effect by inhibiting the generation of PGE2, NO, IL-6, and TNF-α in LPS-induced RAW cells. Naringin also decreased arthritis, joint stiffness, and the synthesis of inflammatory mediators and proinflammatory cytokines. In the Monosodium Iodoacetate (MIA)-induced osteoarthritis paradigm, naringin is limited to the subchondral bone and cartilage tissues. One medicinal drug that successfully cures osteoarthritis and its related symptoms is naringin [159]. Naringenin is a member of the flavanone subclass and has a variety of pharmacological characteristics and nutraceutical benefits; nevertheless, it has pharmacokinetic problems, such as low dissolution rate and poor absorption [160].

In animal studies, the aglycone of the flavanone naringin has been demonstrated to alleviate obesity, dyslipidemia, and insulin resistance. These flavonoids primarily function by down-regulating genes linked to lipid metabolism and up-regulating AMPK and PPARα [161]. Because naringenin inhibits alpha-glucosidase and alpha (α)-amylase, it has been demonstrated to have anti-diabetic effects [162]. Numerous cardiovascular-protective properties, including lipid-lowering, insulin-sensitizing, anti-oxidative, anti-inflammatory, and antihypertensive effects, were revealed by naringenin. Naringin improved endothelial function, raised nitric oxide generation, reduced the risk of cerebral thrombosis, and slowed the age-related rise in systolic blood pressure in stroke-prone spontaneously hypertensive rats [163].

In a double-blind crossover study, twelve patients with stage I hypertension were given 500 mL/day of either a fruit juice with 593 μM naringin or a lower-dose juice (143 μM naringin) for five weeks. While there was no discernible difference in the two groups' systolic blood pressure drop, the high-dose naringin group's diastolic blood pressure decreased more [164]. The lipoprotein profile and plasmatic lipids of dyslipidemic individuals improved after six months of therapy with a commercial bergamot-derived extract (containing around 95 μM naringin/capsule) [165]. In clinical research, LDL cholesterol levels decreased, and the activity of several antioxidant enzymes, including catalase and superoxide dismutase, increased after taking 400 mg of naringin per capsule every day for eight weeks [166]. The impact of 240 mL of orange flavanone drinks (about 15 mg naringenin) was assessed utilising Flow-Mediated Dilatation (FMD) of the brachial artery at 0 to 7 hours in a clinical study including healthy males between the ages of 30 and 65. The activity of a certain flavanone's metabolites on nitric oxide was probably the reason for the decrease in postprandial endothelial dysfunction [167]. By lowering liver lipid peroxidation, increasing liver antioxidant content, and inhibiting NF-kB activation, naringenin treatment has been shown in clinical studies to help protect against oxidative stress and inflammation linked to Non-alcoholic Fatty Liver Disease (NAFLD). It also reduces the expression of hepatic pro-inflammatory genes like tumour necrosis factor-α (TNF-α), interleukin-6 (IL-6), and IL-1β [168].

Naringenin doses between 150 and 900 mg are safe for healthy individuals, and serum concentrations match the dosage. Taking 300 mg of naringenin twice a day is likely to have a physiological impact because it works effectively in primary human adipocytes (8 μM) [169]. In male Wistar rats, studies were conducted to assess the protective effects of naringin and naringenin against paclitaxel-induced cardiotoxicity and nephrotoxicity. After medication treatment, naringin and/or naringenin dramatically reduced the kidney and heart's histological changes and lesion scores. Furthermore, the treatments corrected the negative effects on antioxidant defences and cardiac and renal lipid peroxidation by increasing GSH, SOD, and GPx. The restoration of antioxidant defences and defence against oxidative stress has been linked to naringin and naringenin [170]. By modifying a variety of signalling pathways, including nuclear factor erythroid 2-related factor/NAD(P)H quinone oxidoreductase 1, antioxidant capacity, decreased necroptosis, and overexpression of neuroprotective ciliary neurotrophic factor, the natural citrus flavonoid naringenin co-administration markedly reduced cognitive dysfunction with an apparent neuroprotective effect [171].

Quercetin

Quercetin is a well-known dietary antioxidant and a member of the flavonoid family. Innumerable nutritional supplements and meals, including fruit, vegetables, tea, and wine, contain it, and it is said to have positive health effects. Quercetin's potential health benefits may be related to its capacity to scavenge highly reactive molecules like Peroxynitrite and the hydroxyl radical [171]. Many foods and drinks, including flowers, bark, stems, roots, wine, vegetables, tea, and fruits, including apples, dill, berries, cilantro, and onions, contain quercetin, also known as 3,5,7,3′,4′pentahydroxyflavone (Fig. **16**). Three benzene rings and five hydroxyl groups make up its chemical makeup. It has been established that quercetin's antioxidant properties are significantly influenced by the hydroxyl moieties at rings A and B, 3, 5, 7, 3′, and 4′, the double bond between the second and third carbons, and the carbonyl function on the fourth carbon (Table **5**) [172].

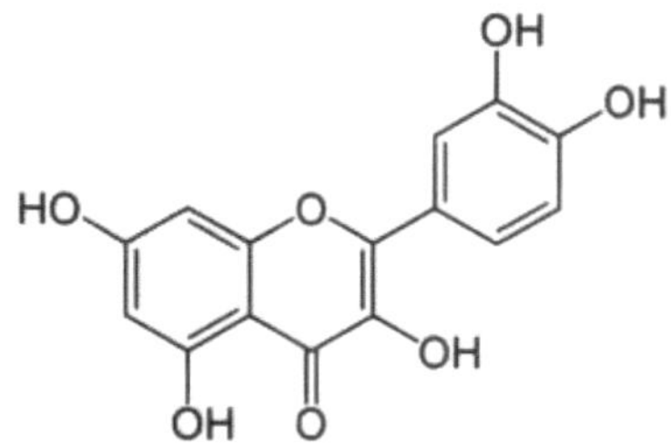

Fig. (16). Chemical structure of quercetin.

Table 5. Health benefits and mechanism of quercetin.

Activity	Mechanism
Neuroprotection	Reactive oxygen scavenging.
Diabetes	Thus, lowering cell proliferation and the labyrinthine interhemal membrane's (LIM) thickness helps avoid gestational diabetes mellitus.
Cardio protection	Lowers oxidative stress and inflammatory proteins in the heart and inhibits apoptosis.
Bone formation	Inhibits the action of osteoclasts.
Tuberculosis	Affects isocitrate lyase, an enzyme that is required for M. tuberculosis to adhere to host cells.
Cancer	Inhibits cell proliferation.
Hyperuricemia	Increases the excretion of renal urate and scavenges free radicals [173].

For 10 weeks, 72 women participated in a double-blind, randomised clinical experiment. The individuals were given 500 milligrams of quercetin daily. Triglycerides (TG), total cholesterol, and low-density lipoprotein cholesterol did not substantially decrease with quercetin, but it did considerably lower interleukin-6 (IL-6), High-density Lipoprotein Cholesterol (HDL-C), systolic blood pressure (SBP), and tumour necrosis factor-α (TNF-α) [174]. In a double-blind crossover trial, 49 healthy participants were given 150 mg of either quercetin or a placebo for eight weeks, separated by three weeks of washout. Quercetin decreased waist circumference, postprandial SBP, postprandial triacylglycerol, and raised HDL and TNFα [175]. Patients with diabetic renal disease received an oral combination of 1000 mg of quercetin and 100 mg of dasatinib; the test showed a reduction in the load of senescent cells in adipose tissue in just 11 days, which in turn reduced the release of inflammation and dysfunctional components [176].

For a 12-week experiment, eighty-four patients were divided into two groups: 42 were given a 500 mg daily quercetin pill, and 42 were given a 500 mg daily starch placebo. Because it increased transferrin and lowered iron, ferritin, transferrin saturation, and high-sensitivity C-reactive protein, quercetin is an effective treatment for improving iron status in thalassemia. Furthermore, quercetin was shown to have no effect on inflammation, as evidenced by its lack of discernible effects on tumour necrosis factor-α (TNF-α) and total iron binding capacity [177]. Fifty female RA patients were randomly assigned to a placebo group and a quercetin (500 mg/day) group for eight weeks in a double-blind, placebo-controlled, randomised controlled clinical study. High-sensitivity tumour necrosis factor-α (hs-TNF-α) was dramatically reduced by quercetin, which also reduced morning discomfort, pain after exercise, and Early Morning Stiffness (EMS) [178].

In a randomised clinical study, 84 PCOS-afflicted women participated. One gram of quercetin was given to the treatment group every day for 12 weeks, whereas a placebo was given to the control group. It was shown that quercetin supplements increased the AMPK level by 12.3% and the expression of the ADIPOR1 and ADIPOR2 transcripts compared to the control group [179]. To determine the effect of quercetin on the postprandial hyperglycemia of individuals with Type 2 Diabetes Mellitus (T2DM), a crossover, blinded, and randomised trial was carried out. In individuals with type 2 diabetes, 400 mg of quercetin was proven to be an effective strategy to reduce postprandial hyperglycemia [180]. After consuming 500 mg of quercetin daily for eight weeks, patients who suffered myocardial infarction showed a substantial rise in TAC and a drop in TNF-α levels. Furthermore, there was an improvement in the quality of life's insecurity component [181]. Through its ability to regulate certain hormones and secondary metabolites, quercetin and kaempferol effectively protect plants against stress. The pharmacokinetic study's applicability to human health was assessed. According to the literature evaluation, they prevent the formation of atherosclerotic plaques by lowering LDL oxidation and platelet aggregation. Additionally, they guard against harm to the heart cells' mitochondria, lowering the chance of cardiovascular problems [182].

Anthocyanidins

The sugar-free versions of anthocyanins are called aglycones, or anthocyanidins. Natural pigments called anthocyanins give plant materials their vivid hues and sensory appeal. Cyanidins are polyphenolic natural compounds that are members of the flavonoid class. Fruits like berries, grapes, and cherries contain coloured polyphenolic chemicals called anthocyanins, which are produced by the phenylpropanoid pathway and have a variety of structural patterns. Plant flavonoid pigments called anthocyanins ($C_{15}H_{11}O+$) are produced *via* the phenylpropanoid pathway. They are anthocyanidin aglycones that are joined to sugar molecules. The chromophore structure of anthocyanidins is made up of two benzene rings joined by a heterocyclic oxygen ring. Different compounds are produced by differences in the hydroxylation, methylation, and glycosylation patterns. Anthocyanins offer a number of health advantages, including lifespan, cellular health, protection against oxidative stress, enhanced endothelial function, lowered blood pressure, and decreased inflammation. It regulates glucose metabolism, improves insulin sensitivity, helps manage diabetes and obesity, and improves skin health by boosting collagen synthesis and shielding the skin from UV rays. Examples of anthocyanidins include delphinidin, petunidin, cyanidin, malvidin, peonidin, and pelargonidin. Consuming foods like berries and grapes that contain cyanidin and delphinidin may have a number of health advantages [183].

The most prevalent and plentiful anthocyanins are those that undergo an O-glycosylation at the flavonoid skeleton's C-3 (C ring) to produce -O-β-glucoside derivatives. In the structure of anthocyanin, a glycosidic linkage is found between a monosaccharide or disaccharide; further, a second sugar residue is found attached to the aglycon. The basic skeleton is made up of a pyran and a phenolic ring joined together, with an additional phenolic ring attached at position 2 of the pyran. Glycosylation of the A-C bicycle at the 3, 5, and 7 positions provides scope for a great variety of possible structural and functional molecules, and two sites on the B-ring, at the 3′ and 5′ positions, provide scope for more than one substituent [184].

Anthocyanidins possess a basic structure termed the flavylium cation, consisting of a 3,5,7-trihydroxy-2-phenylbenzopyrane skeleton (Fig. **17**). This is the general core structure of anthocyanins. The majority of natural anthocyanins are attached to sugar molecules, generally at positions C3, C5, and C7. Such sugars are glucose, galactose, xylose, arabinose, rutinose, and rhamnose. The six principal anthocyanidins are cyanidin, delphinidin, pelargonidin, peonidin, petunidin, and malvidin. They vary in the amount and location of hydroxyl and methoxyl groups on their rings, which determine their color, stability, and how well they can be absorbed by the body.

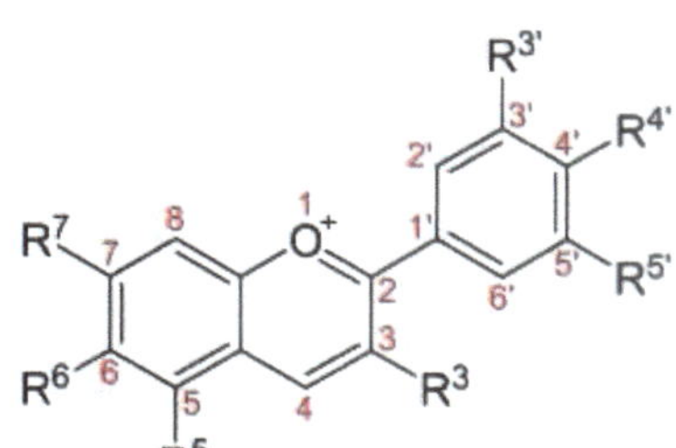

Fig. (17). Chemical structure of anthocyanidin.

Water-soluble antioxidant pigments are called anthocyanidins. The main nutritional sources of anthocyanins include red fruits (such as berries and grapes), purple maize, wine, cereals, and vegetables like cabbage. In addition, blueberry anthocyanidins have anti-inflammatory, anti-mutagenic, rhodophylactic, antioxidant, and DNA-protective properties [185]. Malvidin-3-glucoside was absorbed in plasma and urine after 3 and 6 hours of consuming red wine and red grape juice, according to research, with bioavailability being around twice as high following red grape juice intake as following red wine consumption [186]. Within six hours of consuming 300 millilitres of red wine, six healthy volunteers' urine anthocyanin levels (218 mg anthocyanins) peaked, according to another study [187]. According to a study, it may be advantageous to consume 11g of elderberry concentrate, which contains 17.2% w/w of anthocyanins, on an empty stomach. According to research, healthy participants who ate 500g of strawberries every day for a month had a substantial decrease in triglycerides, total cholesterol, and low-density lipoprotein cholesterol, but no change in high-density lipoprotein cholesterol. Consuming strawberries also raised vitamin C and plasma total antioxidant capacity, with all parameters reverting to baseline following the washout period. The fruits were discovered to have significant levels of anthocyanins and vitamin C [188].

Anthocyanins and Ginkgo Biloba Extract (GBE) have been shown to be beneficial for a variety of vascular disorders. Based on the vascular hypothesis of the process of glaucomatous optic nerve injury, this experiment was carried out to evaluate the impact of GBE and anthocyanins on visual function in patients with Normal Tension Glaucoma (NTG). The study's findings suggest that in certain NTG instances, anthocyanins and GBE may help improve visual function [189]. Bilberry extract, a plant-derived antioxidant that is high in anthocyanins, has been used as a common ocular health supplement all over the world. By injecting lipopolysaccharide, researchers created a mouse model of Endotoxin-induced Uveitis (EIU) that exhibits both uveitis and retinal inflammation. According to a study, bilberry extract high in anthocyanins protects vision during retinal inflammation [190]. About 38 individuals with open-angle glaucoma using antiglaucoma drops participated in a double-masked, randomised, placebo-controlled study to investigate the impact of black currant anthocyanins (BCACs) on the course of the condition. Research showed that when BCACs were administered, ocular blood flows improved throughout the course of the 24-month observation period as compared to individuals who received a placebo [191].

Patients with metabolic syndrome who consumed meals containing 320 mg of anthocyanins for four weeks had a decrease of 13% in fasting blood glucose, 25% in triglycerides, 33% in LDL-C, and 28% in hs-CRP levels, according to a clinical trial [192]. It was shown that anthocyanin supplementation (320 mg/day) decreased the expression of pro-inflammatory genes and NF-κB pathways, such as TNF-α, IL-6, IL-1A, PCAM-1, and COX-2, in both the MetS and control groups [193]. According to the study, yoghurt enriched with riceberry rice anthocyanins significantly increased the plasma ferric reducing capacity, trolox equivalent antioxidant capacity, and oxygen radical absorption capacity in healthy volunteers while also lowering plasma MDA [194]. The effect of anthocyanin-rich supplements on the cognitive function of middle-aged and older people in good cognitive health was investigated. According to research, anthocyanin-rich supplements may help older persons retain their neuro-activities and cognitive processing speed, improving their everyday functioning and quality of life [195].

Berries are rich in anthocyanins, and research indicates that eating a diet rich in polyphenols may improve health by lowering oxidative stress. The purpose of this study was to examine the effects of a standardised extract of the maqui berry (Aristotelia chilensis) on lipid peroxidation products in healthy overweight smokers. Studies have shown that dietary regimens using maqui berry extract can improve oxidative status (Ox-LDL and F2-isoprostanes) in persons who smoke, are overweight, and are otherwise healthy [196]. Researchers examined the effects of a test meal including lutein, astaxanthin, and anthocyanin on the ocular function of Japanese individuals in good health who had suffered from eye fatigue from using visual display terminals. Forty-four patients in total were randomly assigned to either the active or placebo groups. Two active or placebo pills were given daily for six weeks. According to a study, eating the test meal for six weeks prevented the accommodative function from declining as a result of visual display terminal operation [197].

Catechins

A naturally occurring polyphenol component, catechin is a member of the flavonoid family, specifically the flavan-3-ol subclass. It is found in a variety of foods, including green tea, black grapes, strawberries, and chocolate. Four pairings of stereoisomers most prominently seen in green tea are epigallocatechin (EGC) and gallocatechin (GC), epicatechin and epicatechin, epicatechin gallate and epicatechin gallate (ECG), and epigallocatechin gallate (EGCG) and gallocatechin gallate [198]. Catechu, the boiling extract or tannic juice of Mimosa catechu (Acacia catechu), is the name of the catechin chemical family. Catechin has a dihydropyran heterocycle (the C-ring) with a hydroxyl group on carbon 3 in addition to two benzene rings (the A- and B-rings). The B ring is comparable to a catechol moiety, whereas the A ring is comparable to a resorcinol moiety. The molecule has two chiral centers on carbons two and three. It has four diastereoisomers as a result. Two of the isomers are called epicatechin because of their cis configuration, while the other two are called catechin because of their trans configuration. The constituents of the proanthocyanidins, a kind of condensed tannin, are epicatechin and catechin (Fig. **18**).

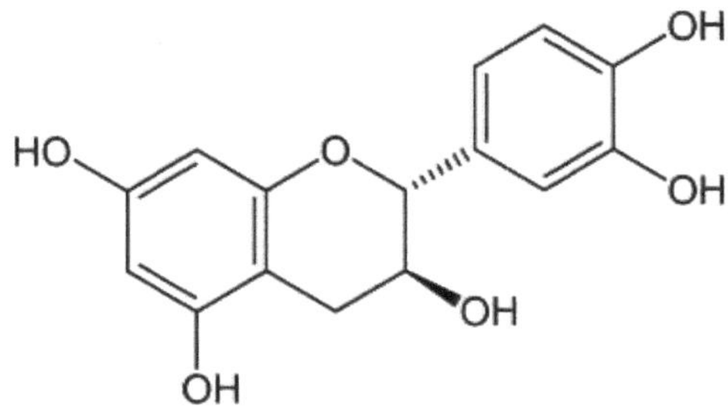

Fig. (18). Chemical structure of catechin.

Catechins offer many health benefits by neutralizing free radicals and shielding the skin against damage brought on by UV radiation and environmental pollution. They induce collagen synthesis and prevent the synthesis of enzymes (termed matrix metalloproteinases) that dissolve the structure of the skin. Of all catechins, EGCG and ECG are particularly potent antioxidants due to a unique chemical moiety termed gallate. This renders them more effective in neutralizing free radicals than general antioxidants such as vitamin C (ascorbic acid), vitamin E (tocopherol), and Trolox [199]. It is challenging to extract catechins for two reasons: either they are found in plant tissue that is bound to proteins or sugars, or they can form polymerised derivatives with different levels of solubility, and their chemical structures and interactions with other food ingredients are not entirely understood. Second, it is challenging to create an appropriate extraction procedure since they are extremely vulnerable to oxidation, light, high temperatures, and alkaline environments [200].

Catechin, a flavonoid derived from *Camellia sinensis*, is known for its potent antioxidant properties and potential therapeutic benefits in treating cancer, diabetes, and infections. Catechin could inhibit the activation of the PI3K/Akt pathway in gastric cancer cells. The active component of green tea, catechin, has a powerful anti-tumor effect [201]. Catechin possesses numerous beneficial biological activities, such as combating viruses, bacteria, and toxic molecules known as free radicals, so it may be applied as a nutraceutical (a food item with medicinal benefits). It is also of potential use in combating cancer, cardiovascular protection, inhibiting inflammation, and maintaining brain function. Furthermore, catechin reduces fat deposition in arteries, guards against DNA damage, binds to cell walls to protect them, and inhibits the formation of toxic microbes on such walls [202 - 204].

Randomised Clinical Trials (RCTs) investigating the effects of green tea, catechin, and other green tea supplements on liver enzyme levels were thoroughly reviewed and analysed in this work. According to the study, the effect of green tea on liver enzymes varies depending on an individual's health, with a slight increase in healthy people and a moderate decrease in NAFLD patients [205]. The meta-analysis included 31 studies with 3321 participants overall. In people of normal weight as well as those who are overweight or obese, a study found that consuming green tea reduces LDL cholesterol and TC but not HDL cholesterol or triglycerides [206]. The study looked at how a Green Tea Extract (GTE) supplement containing 1315 mg of catechins (843 mg of EGCG) affected risk factors for breast cancer. It used a randomised, double-blind, placebo-controlled study. The results showed that GTE considerably reduced levels of 'bad' LDL cholesterol and Total Cholesterol (TC), especially in those with high cholesterol at the beginning of the research [207]. In a 12-week clinical study, 60 healthy Japanese men and women between the ages of 30 and 75 were given green tea containing α-glucosyl hesperidin (GT-gH). The supplement included 146 mg of EGCG and 178 mg of α-glucosyl hesperidin. According to the study, GT-gH inhibited weight growth and had stronger anti-obesity benefits in people under 50 [208].

Flavones

A relatively broad subclass of the phenolic group of specialised metabolites found in plants is flavonoids. With the B ring on C-2 and a C-2/C-3 double bond, flavones are a fairly big group (Fig. **19**). With almost 2,500 recognised members and their glycosides, flavones are a relatively big group. By providing defence against UV rays and oxidative stress, improving interspecies relationships, and aiding in plant development through lignification and anthocyanin colouration, flavones play a significant role in plants' adaptation to terrestrial settings. Animals can benefit greatly from flavones because of their high chemical variety, which is made possible by modifications to the chemical backbone, including hydroxylation, O-/C-glycosylation, O-methylation, and acylation. Since flavones are typical byproducts of the benzopyran class, they are essential oxygen heterocycles found in fruits and vegetables. The chemical backbone of flavone ($C_{15}H_{10}O_2$) is 2-phenylchromen-4-one (2-phenyl-1-benzopyran-4-one). Each of the three functional groups found in flavones-hydroxy, carbonyl, and conjugated double bond—has a distinct reactivity.

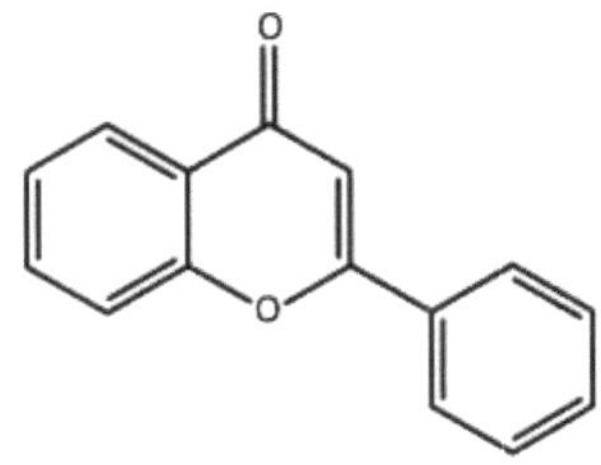

Fig. (19). Chemical structure of flavones.

Flavones that dissolve in water and ethanol have a colourless to yellow crystalline form. However, when in an alkali solution, they turn yellow. Many fruits and vegetables, including broccoli, celery, carrots, parsley, onion leaves, cabbage, peppers, most flowers, apple skins, wheat sprouts, tea, and citrus fruits, contain flavones, including apigenin, luteolin, and tricetin [209], by adding a double bond between the C-2 and C-3 sites, an enzyme known as flavone synthase catalyses the transformation of flavanones into flavones. The ability of flavone synthases to catalyse the conversion of comparable substrates (flavanones) into the same products (flavones) using two distinct enzyme types and a somewhat different mechanism makes them special. 2-hydroxyflavanones, which are produced from flavanones by F2H CYP enzymes, are used as substrates by several flavones, particularly those with C-glycosylation [210]. Natural compounds called flavones have health-promoting qualities. They have antiviral, liver-protective, blood-clo--preventing, anti-inflammatory, anti-allergic, antioxidant, and anti-cancer properties. Apigenin, luteolin, tangeritin, chrysin, and 6-hydroxy flavone are a few examples of prevalent flavones. Depending on the quantity and location of hydroxyl (-OH) or methoxy (-OCH_3) groups, their chemical structures differ [211].

Flavones have two substituents on the C-ring: a 2,3-double bond and a 4-carbonyl. To elucidate the antidepressant mechanism of action of luteolin, seventeen network pharmacology preclinical investigations and molecular docking analysis were conducted. Numerous processes, including dopamine transport, synaptic protection, anti-oxidative stress, anti-apoptosis, anti-inflammation, anti-endoplasmic reticulum stress, modulation of the hypothalamic-pituitary-adrenal axis, and 5-HT metabolism, contribute to luteolin's antidepressant effects [212]. A pilot study was conducted on outpatients who had a documented history of COVID-19 and post-infection olfactory loss that continued for over 90 days following negative SARS-CoV-2 testing. The combination of oral PEA and luteolin supplementation and olfactory rehabilitation considerably expedited the recovery of olfactory function, especially in those with chronic olfactory impairment [213].

The study aims to examine the anticancer effects of tricetin (TCN) on two human liver cancer cell lines, Hep G2 and PLC/PRF/5. The work demonstrates that ROS generation induces TCN-induced cell death in liver cancer cells, suggesting that both internal and extrinsic apoptotic pathways contribute to this potential cancer chemopreventive medication [214]. In this study, researchers looked at how tricetin, a flavone molecule, could protect against acute pancreatitis. The results showed that cerulein, a cholecystokinin-like peptide, could not harm mouse pancreatic cells when tricetin was present. Additionally, tricetin inhibited the activation of PARP-1, an enzyme that responds to oxidative DNA damage, and the levels of the inflammatory markers IL-1β, IL-6, and TNF-α in the pancreas [215].

PHYTOESTROGENS: ISOFLAVONES, DAIDZEIN, GENISTEIN, LIGNANS

Phytoestrogens are non-steroidal estrogen-like substances found in all plants, with legumes having the highest concentrations.

Isoflavones

Isoflavones, possessing a steric configuration identical to steroidal estrogens, interact with the human estrogen receptor, thus enabling them to produce diverse estrogenic or anti-estrogenic activities. Isoflavones resemble 17-β-estradiol in chemical structure, which could serve as agonists or antagonists of estrogen depending on endocrine levels of estrogen, but isoflavone actions are quite complicated due to numerous variables like chemical structures and mechanisms (Fig. **20**) [216]. Isoflavones are flavonoids that have a slightly different structure from flavones. In isoflavones, the phenyl group is bonded at the 3-position rather than the 2-position on the chromone ring. They are typically present in Fabaceae family plants (such as soybeans and legumes). Some of the most recognized isoflavone phytoestrogens are genistein, daidzein, glycitein, biochanin A, and formononetin. These molecules have structures that enable them to act like estrogen in the body.

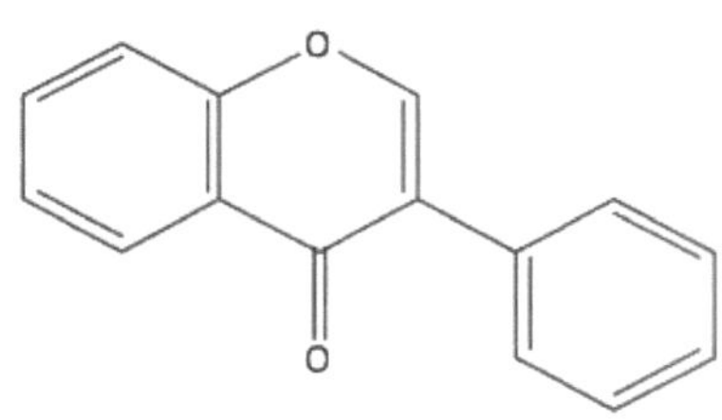

Fig. (20). Chemical structure of isoflavones.

Genistin, daidzin, and glycitin are the three main isoflavones found in the glycoside form in soybeans. Legumes, such as soybeans, red clover, white clover, and lucerne, are important sources of isoflavones for farm animals' diets. The breakdown of isoflavones in their glycoside state during digestion results in the removal of the sugar component, forming active compounds called aglycones, namely genistein, daidzein, and glycitein. These isoflavones can be found in unprocessed soy products, including miso, tofu, and soymilk. After consumption, isoflavone aglycones are absorbed from the top part of the small intestine and reach their peak in the bloodstream within an hour. Plant isoflavonoids have an important role in interactions with microorganisms. By triggering nodulation genes, isoflavonoids help legumes and rhizobia (bacteria that fix nitrogen) form symbiotic associations. Phytoalexins, which can comprise isoflavones, isoflavanones, pterocarpans, isoflavans, and coumestans, are another type of isoflavonoids that serve as natural defences [217].

Being chemoprotective, isoflavones can serve as an alternative treatment for a variety of hormonal conditions, including osteoporosis, menopausal symptoms, cardiovascular disease, and breast and prostate cancer. Enhancing intake of soy products, proteins, or isoflavones has been shown to improve indicators of bone resorption and formation or decrease bone mass loss in postmenopausal women [218]. According to research, eating meals high in soy isoflavones decreased the chance of mortality by 29% and the risk of recurrence by 32% in women with breast cancer [219]. Consuming isoflavones was linked to a decreased risk of prostate cancer development, according to a meta-analysis of eight studies [220]. F2-isoprostane and other lipid peroxidation indicators were shown to be lower in a two-week soy protein containing 56 mg of isoflavones than in a protein containing only 2 mg of isoflavones [221].

Daidzein

Daidzein is a naturally occurring compound in soybeans and legumes, which falls under the category of isoflavones, and it is shikimate pathway-derived. Daidzein, 7-hydroxy-3-(4-hydroxyphenyl)-4H-chromen-4-one, is a naturally occurring non-steroidal phytoestrogenic compound that acts on the estrogen receptor (Fig. **21**).

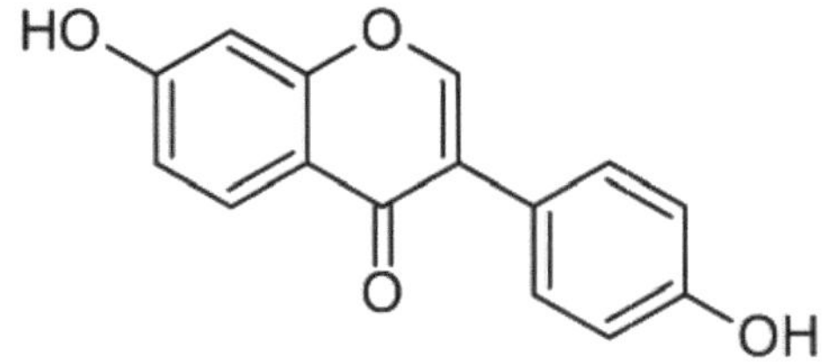

Fig. (21). Chemical structure of daidzein.

Daidzein is also known as an aglycone. Because of its limited solubility in water, it is dissolved in alcohol or an alcohol/water combination for medicinal applications. According to studies, daidzein promotes osteoblast development and suppresses osteoclasts' ability to resorb bone [222]. A neuroprotective substance called daizein affects a number of neurological processes, such as behaviour, cognition, growth, development, and reproduction, by interacting with different signalling molecules and receptors. Because of its association with the cerebrovascular system, it also exhibits actions against a variety of neuropathological diseases [223]. Certain bacteria in the colon and lower small intestine produce equol from the isoflavone daidzin or daidzein. The asymmetric carbon atom at position C3 gives this non-planar, phenolic molecule its unique three-dimensional shape. R(-)-equol and S(-)-equol are the two mirror-image structures (enantiomers) that result from this; however, only S(-)-equol is naturally generated by gut flora [224].

Numerous ailments, including menopausal symptoms, cardiovascular and bone disorders, cancer, mental illness, obesity, type 2 diabetes, renal disease, and ageing skin, can be prevented and treated with equol, according to recent clinical studies and reviews. Additionally, because of its antioxidant properties, daidzein may help protect the reproductive system from harmful environmental influences and prevent ovarian cancer and oxidative stress-related reproductive problems [225]. An isoflavone phytoestrogen called daidzein is frequently used as a nutraceutical to treat conditions including inflammation, cancer, and osteoporosis. Daidzein has a number of positive health benefits, including anti-inflammatory, antioxidant, and anti-bleeding (antihemolytic) properties. Additionally, daizein protects against breast cancer, osteoporosis, diabetes, and heart disease. Daidzein's oestrogenic mimetic action makes it an attractive natural health component because all of these disorders are frequently linked to oestrogen status [226].

GENISTEIN

Genistein is an isoflavone in the flowering plant Dyer's Genista tinctoria L. and is found commonly in plants of the Fabaceae family. It mimics estrogen and is a member of the aglycone form of isoflavones, which are the biologically active forms (Fig. **22**). Isoflavones in nature predominantly occur in glycosylated forms (attached to sugars) and are processed or digested to become active aglycones. In mammals, isoflavones may act like estrogen either as an agonist or an antagonist of its action. They may bind to natural hormones such as estradiol (E2 or 17β-estradiol) by either augmenting their activity or inhibiting estrogen receptors, at times inducing alterations that decrease receptor activity. The estrogenic activity of genistein is derived from its chemical structure, specifically the hydroxyl groups at carbon positions 4 and 7 of its phenol rings. These are structurally analogous to estradiol's functional groups, so that genistein is able to bind to both α and β types of estrogen receptors. Its endocrine effects are primarily attributable to its primary metabolite, (−)-(S)-equol, a strong phytoestrogen yielded by gut microflora.

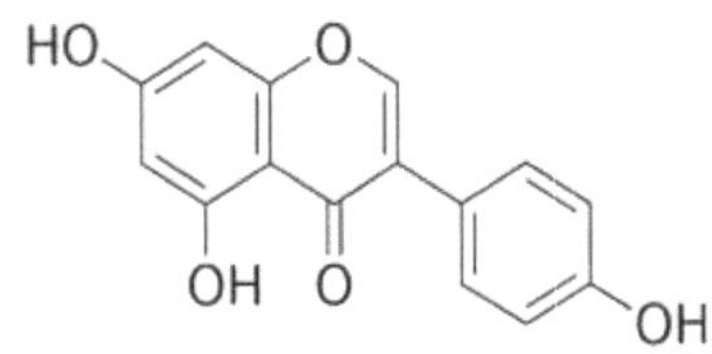

Fig. (22). Chemical structure of genistein.

A study found an inverse relationship between plasma isoflavones like daidzein and genistein and fibroadenoma risk, suggesting that higher soy intake may lower the risk of fibroadenomas and breast cancer [227]. According to research, women who are unable to get progestin treatment for endometrial hyperplasia may benefit from genistein aglycone. Treatment with genistein reduces endometrial thickness, improves ER-β1 staining, and results in bleeding regression, indicating that it may be used as a progestin substitute [228]. According to research, genistein can lower the expression of biomarkers linked to the development and prognosis of prostate cancer, including genes linked to the cell cycle like p27Kip1 and androgen-related biomarkers like KLK4 [229]. Due to its protein kinase inhibitory properties, genistein administration has been shown to increase superoxide production in patients with kidney neoplasms following cisplatin therapy [230]. The Akt and NF-κB pathways, which are linked to the growth, spread, and resistance to chemotherapy of cancer cells and are frequently overactive in pancreatic cancer, can be inhibited by genistein. A genistein-based molecule in one research showed a good pharmacokinetic profile and was non-toxic, suggesting that it might be safely studied further in pancreatic cancer patients [231].

According to a study conducted on 389 postmenopausal women, homocysteine levels, a risk factor for coronary artery disease that is independent of other variables, and cardiovascular risk factors were positively impacted by genistein aglycone, calcium, vitamin D3, and a balanced diet [232]. Taking 54 mg of genistein daily for a year, as opposed to a placebo, significantly decreased the incidence of diabetes in a clinical study with 120 postmenopausal women with metabolic syndrome [233]. According to a clinical study on the effects of phytoestrogens like genistein on postmenopausal women's lipid metabolism, these substances raised HDL and apolipoprotein A-1 while lowering LDL and apolipoprotein B [234].

Lignan

The word "Lignan was originally proposed by Haworth to a series of dimeric phenylpropanoids in which two C6-C3 are joined by their central carbon (C8). The majority of natural lignans are oxidized at C9 and C9′ and form a wide variety of structurally diverse lignans depending on oxygen incorporation into the skeleton and patterns of cyclization [235] (Fig. **23**).

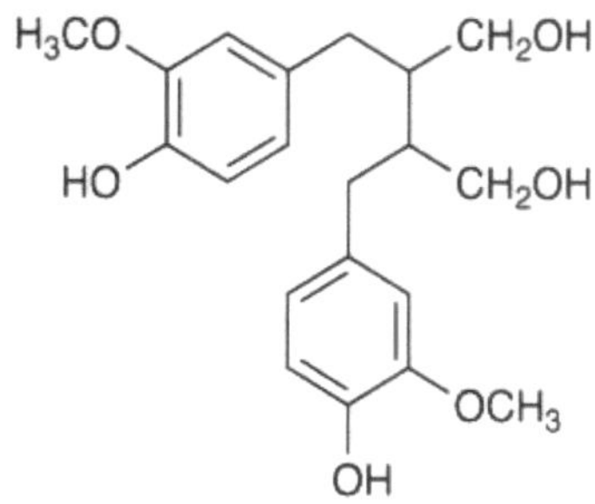

Fig. (23). Chemical structure of lignin.

Whole grains and seeds such as flax, sesame, rye, oats, wheat, millet, barley, and buckwheat, as well as nuts and legumes, naturally contain lignans, which are plant nutrients. Aryltetralin (*e.g.*, podophyllotoxins), arylnaphthalene (*e.g.*, justcidins), furan (*e.g.*, belischmins), furofuran (*e.g.*, epimagnolin) derivatives, dibenzylbutane (*e.g.*, enterodiol), dibenzylbutyrolactone (*e.g.*, enterolactone), dibenzylbutyrolactol (*e.g.*, gnetucleistol F), and dibenzocyclooctadiene (*e.g.*, gomisins) are the eight main subtypes of lignans. Depending on whether they include an oxygen atom at the C9 (or 9′) position, several of these lignans can be further classified. Additionally, hybrid lignans are unique molecules that combine the structures of lignans with those of other plant compounds that have both lignan-like chemical structures and biological activities, such as coumarins (coumarinolignans), xanthones (xantholignans), flavonoids (flavolignans), and stilbenes (stilbenolignans). Additionally, lignans can be used to treat microbial infections, diabetes, cardiovascular illnesses, and as antioxidants to treat other significant or mild inflammatory reactions.

Additionally, lignans have been shown to have anti-tumor properties and to be cancer-protective at the early stages of carcinogenesis. The gold standard of top-ranked lignans, podophyllotoxins, shows cytotoxic action and topoisomerase-II inhibitory potentials. They also spawned several therapeutically useful medications, including etoposide, teniposide, Etopophos, NK611, and GL331 [236]. Both primary and secondary preventive settings have been used to examine the effects of lignan-rich flaxseed in preventing prostate cancer. Prostate epithelial proliferation and serum total PSA were shown to have significantly decreased

[237]. A meta-analysis that comprised five intervention studies using flaxseed lignan supplements revealed a decrease in plasma total and low-density lipoprotein cholesterol, as well as positive associations with C-reactive protein [238].

Long-term lignan consumption has been associated with a decreased incidence of total Coronary Heart Disease (CHD) in both men and women, according to a study [239]. This may be because lignan and fibre intake work in concert. This clinical case study describes how a 31-year-old PCOS woman's hormone levels were affected by taking 30 grams of flaxseed per day. This case study's clinically significant decrease in androgen levels and corresponding decrease in hirsutism highlight the need for more research on the effects of flaxseed supplementation on hormone levels and PCOS clinical symptoms [240]. Long-term lignan consumption was linked to a decreased incidence of type 2 diabetes, according to cohort research, primarily among obese people and premenopausal women [241].

OATS, WHEAT BRAN, RICE BRAN, SEAFOODS, COFFEE, AND TEA AS FUNCTIONAL FOODS

When included in a regular diet in the proper amounts, functional foods and phytochemicals have gained popularity because of their health advantages. Operational Natural or processed foods that include biologically active substances that offer health advantages in addition to nutritional value are known as functional foods. The majority of functional foods, including fruits, vegetables, cereals, nuts, seeds, herbs, spices, and drinks, include phytochemicals, which are important organic substances. Numerous biological actions, including neuroprotective, anti-diabetic, antioxidant, anti-cancer, and anti-inflammatory properties, are possessed by these substances. Phytochemicals fall into a wide range of groups, including nitrogen-containing compounds, polyphenols, alkaloids, terpenoids, and organosulfur compounds. One serving of fruits or vegetables (around 120 grams) may contain up to 100 distinct phytochemicals, out of the more than 900 different phytochemicals that have been identified in food. Research now shows that animal foods like milk, fermented milk products, and cold-water fish also contain important bioactive compounds like probiotics, conjugated linolenic acid, long-chain omega-3, -6, and -9 polyunsaturated fatty acids, and bioactive peptides. Previously, it was thought that these functional ingredients were primarily found in plant-based foods, especially whole grains, fruits, and vegetables [242]. Japan first proposed the concept of functional food in the early 1980s. The first functional foods law was put into effect in Japan during that decade and was known as FOSHU, or “Foods for Specified Health Use”. Meals that may regulate biological processes and aid in disease prevention were initially referred to as functional meals.

To increase the flexibility of the approval procedure, Japan additionally accepts Qualified FOSHU, Standardised FOSHU, and Reduction of Disease Risk FOSHU in addition to conventional FOSHU (Food with Specified Health Use). Foods that exhibit certain health advantages but lack the scientific proof or a clear mechanism to meet the complete FOSHU requirement are considered qualified FOSHU. Foods with well-established approval criteria and scientific proof make up standardised FOSHU; Items are approved if they meet the required criteria for reduction of disease risk. Foods containing components with demonstrated nutritional and scientific benefits have been proven to reduce the risk of specific illnesses and may qualify for approval under the FOSHU system. Apart from these categories, conventional functional foods that are made of natural or whole-food ingredients are also said to provide health advantages due to their antioxidants, vitamins, minerals, and good fatty acids. Anthocyanins, for example, are found in blueberries and have anti-inflammatory and antioxidant properties. Isoflavones found in soybeans have been associated with a decreased risk of heart disease and some types of cancer. Because of their antioxidant properties, tomatoes may lower the risk of cancer due to their high lycopene concentration. Both green tea (containing catechins) and garlic (containing allicin) are well-known for their anti-inflammatory and anti-cancer properties, making them excellent examples of functional foods that are high in phytochemicals [243].

Oat

Because of its high nutritional content, oats (*Avena sativa* L.), a unique cereal crop, are highly valued for use in medicine, cosmetics, animal feed, and human nourishment. Carbohydrates, dietary soluble fibre, balanced protein, lipids, different phenolic compounds, vitamins, and minerals are all abundant in this cereal. Avenanthramides, p-hydroxybenoic acid, vanillic acid, tricin, ferulic acid, caffeic acid, protocatechuic acid, sinapic acid, apigenin, luteolin, kaempferol, and quercetin are only a few of the many phenolic chemicals found in oats. Oats are a nutrient-dense cereal with a high soluble fibre content that has several physiological advantages, including reducing hyperglycemia, hyperinsulinemia, and hypercholesterolaemia. Soluble fibres like (1→3, 1→4)-β-D-glucan or β-glucan are responsible for the majority of the physiological effects of oat soluble fibre, which is caused by the increased viscosity. As a modulator of the glycaemic, insulin, and cholesterol responses to diet, β-glucan, a useful component of oats, has been linked to health benefits [244]. Oats are also linked to several health benefits, including a decreased risk of cancer, gastrointestinal disorders, cardiovascular disease, and type 2 diabetes mellitus.

The nutritional value and health-conscious appeal of fermented oats have led to their growing popularity. With potential health benefits including anti-inflammatory and antioxidant qualities, they offer a more comprehensive phytochemical and nutritional profile that may reduce the risk of chronic diseases. Carbohydrates like sugars and starches are hydrolysed by bacteria, fungi, or yeast during fermentation, which improves their absorption of vitamins, minerals, and other nutrients and makes them easier to digest [245]. A diet high in fibre, such as oats, helps improve gut flora. Oats include plant proteins, unsaturated fatty acids, and antioxidant phytochemicals, making them a useful dietary element with prebiotic potential. The gut microbiota is influenced by oat consumption, and associations have been shown between oat consumption and the abundance of *Bifidobacterium, Faecalibacterium prausnitzii, Lactobacillus, Roseburia*, and *Akkermansia muciniphila*. In 210 individuals with moderate hypercholesterolaemia, Chinese research found that consuming 80g of oats daily for 45 days decreased their levels of total and non-high-density lipoproteins [246].

Wheat Bran

One of the most significant cereal crops in the world, wheat (*Triticum aestivum*), is primarily used for animal feed and human sustenance. An estimated 90 million tonnes of Wheat Bran (WB), a significant by-product of milling wheat, are generated each year. Wheat bran is an inexpensive and abundant source of vitamins, minerals, dietary fibre, and other bioactive substances such as phytosterols, alkylresorcinols, phenolic acids, and arabinoxylans. The germ, bran, and endosperm are the three main parts of a wheat grain; the bran forms the outer layer. Comprising xylans, lignin, cellulose, galactan, and fructans, the bran component comprises around 53% fibre. Wheat bran is valued for its anti-inflammatory and antioxidant properties in addition to its culinary and non-food applications. Because of its high phytochemical and dietary fibre content, clinical trials and epidemiological studies have demonstrated that regular consumption of high-fiber foods, like wheat bran, can significantly reduce the risk of chronic diseases like colon cancer, diabetes, obesity, and cardiovascular disease [247]. By controlling the host's gut flora, dietary fibres derived from rice and wheat bran are beneficial to human health. During fermentation, dietary fibres can promote the production of several beneficial metabolites, primarily short-chain fatty acids, which are closely linked to protecting against a number of illnesses [248].

Hard red winter wheat, wheat bran, white flour, and bread made from wheat flour were all examined in the study. In comparison to whole wheat, refined flour, and bread, wheat bran was shown to contain considerably higher levels of dietary fibre (42.8%), fat (4.25%), ash (5.79%), and important minerals and B vitamins. Arabinoxylan, a non-starch β-(1,4)-linked polysaccharide with a xylose backbone that is replaced by arabinose residues at C(O)-2 and/or C(O)-3, is a major component of bran. Additionally, the C(O)-5 position of the arabinose units can be esterified to produce phenolic acids, ferulic acid, and p-coumaric acid. In addition to being a significant source of antioxidant phenolic compounds like ferulic acid and alkylresorcinols, the latter of which is the most common, wheat bran is especially rich in B vitamins such as thiamin, niacin, vitamin B6, and folate. Several processing techniques, including heat, alkaline, enzymatic, ultrasonic, and fermentation treatment, have been studied to increase the release and bioavailability of ferulic acid. Most importantly, when consumed as a cereal fibre that contains β-glucan, arabinoxylan itself has been associated with lowering blood glucose levels in people with type 2 diabetes [249, 250]. LDL-cholesterol reduction associated with barley and oat β-glucan in clinical trials [251].

Rice Bran

For almost half of the world's population, rice (*Oryza sativa* L.) is a staple meal, and for 25% of people, it is essential to their daily sustenance. Ten percent of the weight of raw rice is made up of rice bran, a mill by-product that is rich in vitamins, minerals, vital fatty acids, and dietary fibre. The remaining portion of rice bran is used to produce oil, with the remaining 90% being used as feed for cattle and fowl. The majority of the nutrients are found in it, including carbs (34–62%), lipids (15–20%), protein (11–15%), crude fibre (7–11%), and ash (7–10%). It is mostly composed of aleurone, pericarp, subaleurone layer, and germ [252]. Fatty acids, including palmitate, linoleate, and oleate, make up the majority of rice bran, which is an excellent source of rice lipids and bioactive chemicals. Additionally, rice bran contains 4-hydroxy-3-methoxycinnamic acid, which has photoprotective and antioxidative qualities. Ricebran contains dietary fibres such as α-glucan, pectin, and gum, as well as bioactive substances like γ-oryzanol, tocotrienol, tocopherol, and α-sitosterol. The main antioxidant, γ-oryzanol, has ten times the activity of tocopherol. Depending on the kind of rice cultivar, these phytochemical levels vary [253]. Due to its high fat content and the powerful enzyme lipase, which breaks down the oil and renders it rancid and unfit for consumption, rice bran has a relatively limited shelf life. Antioxidant substances such as polyphenols, vitamin E, tocotrienols, and carotenoids, which are abundant in rice bran, help shield DNA and other bodily tissues from oxidative damage. Rice bran, which is high in dietary fibre and has medicinal potential, may be used to make highly sought-after functional or value-added meals [254]. When given as 6% of a diet for eight weeks, rice bran-whether ethanol-extracted or enzyme-treated-has been shown to improve blood pressure, lipid profiles, and glucose metabolism. In stroke-prone spontaneously hypertensive rats, supplementing with adenosine, an active component of functional bran, has been shown to ameliorate metabolic syndrome [253]. Supplementing with Ferulic Acid (FA), an active component of functional bran, has been shown to raise lipid profiles and blood pressure [255].

Strong antioxidants called anthocyanins are abundant in rice bran from coloured rice cultivars. Trichin, apigenin, cyanidin rutinoside, cyanidin glucoside, epicatechins, eriodictyol, luteolin, isohamnetin, hesperetin, hermnetin, and peonidin glucoside are examples of monomeric, dimeric, and polymeric anthocyanins. The two main anthocyanins present in rice bran are peonidin-3-O-glucoside and cyanidin-3-O-glucoside. The antioxidant activity of rice bran is further enhanced by the presence of flavones and flavonols, such as flavan-3-ols and flavan-1-ols [256]. Through the inhibition of serum ACE activity, the enhancement of glucose impairment, insulin sensitivity, leptin impairment, and serum adiponectin level, as well as the modulation of transcription factors and gene expression, fermented rice bran significantly reduced the rise in blood pressure (Table **6**) [257].

Table 6. Clinical studies on rice bran bioactivities.

S.No	Functional Food Source	Dose and Duration	Reported Biological Effects	Reference
1	Rice bran with or without 2% plant sterols	Combined with a 25% energy-restricted diet for 8 weeks in overweight and obese adults	Helped in weight management and lowering cholesterol levels.	[258]
2	Rice bran extract containing acylated steryl glucosides	30–50 mg/day for 12 weeks in obese Japanese men	Reduced body weight and cholesterol.	[259]
3	Brown rice bran extract enriched with acylated steryl glucosides	50 mg for 6 months in postmenopausal Vietnamese women	Contributed to weight loss, cholesterol reduction, and anti-inflammatory effects.	[260]
4	Rice bran powder	70 g/day along with a low-calorie diet for 12 weeks in overweight and obese individuals	Exhibited anti-inflammatory properties.	[261]
5	Stabilized rice bran	20 g daily for 12 weeks in patients with type 2 diabetes	Showed antidiabetic and lipid-lowering benefits.	[262

Sea Food

Because seafood is high in ω-3 fatty acids, carotenoids, chitosan, enzymes, dietary fibres, phenolic compounds, and proteins, it is frequently utilised to create functional and nutraceutical meals [263]. Omega-3 fatty acids, chitosan, carotenoids, enzymes, protein hydrolysates, algal phenolics, and carbohydrates are examples of functional food components that are essential for promoting health, lowering the risk of disease, and lowering healthcare costs. They include fish oil (mainly omega-3-polyunsaturated fatty acids), seal blubber oil, algal oil, shark liver oil and squalene, shark cartilage, chitin, chitosan, and their monomers and oligomers, enzymes, peptides, and related compounds, vitamins (A, especially its precursor β-carotene, D, and E), seaweed (macroalgae) and its constituents, protein hydrolysates, and other products. These marine-based nutraceuticals have recently attracted the attention of the pharmaceutical and health food industries. Additionally, the primary metabolites of marine mussels from the genera Mytilus and Perna have been shown to be useful for the production of pharmaceuticals, functional foods, and food additives [264].

Enzymes treated with Fish Protein Hydrolysates (FPH) may be employed as cardioprotective agents in functional foods or medications, while sardine muscle antihypertensive proteins, such as angiotensin I-converting enzyme inhibitors (ACE), have the potential to be used as antihypertensive medicines. Fish skin and flesh extracts include antioxidants with significant superoxide-scavenging activity that can be used as functional foods and medications to defend against physiologically harmful reactive oxygen species [265]. The health advantages of seafood are associated with a high consumption of n-3 PUFAs, such as EPA and DHA. These fatty acids are abundant in fish oil, which is promoted as a functional food for better health. According to a meta-analysis, those who ate fish once a week had a 15% reduced risk of dying from CVD than people who didn't eat any fish [266].

Coffee and Tea

Coffee is one of the most popular drinks around the world and is frequently taken with food. Coffee has various bioactive compounds like caffeine, trigonelline, pyrogallic acid, quinolinic acid, tannic acid, and nicotinic acid. Coffee is also a significant source of minerals and provides about 8% of the recommended daily intake of calcium and contributes to magnesium availability. Caffeine, coffee's major stimulant, has been found to improve mental attention, cognitive function, alertness, and diminish fatigue while slowing the onset of sleep. It has been shown that coffee and tea infusions can increase plasma antioxidant capacity, with coffee's action primarily due to enhanced concentrations of uric acid and phenolic compounds. Coffee and tea are both high in antioxidants and phenolic compounds; however, the roasting involved in coffee production could diminish some of these healthy compounds. Nevertheless, roasting still produces Maillard Reaction Products (MRPs), which could increase the antioxidant content of the final beverage. Daily coffee consumption has been associated with reduced susceptibility to Low-Density Lipoprotein (LDL) oxidation, possibly lowering malondialdehyde levels and LDL-cholesterol. Also, caffeine and its metabolites, *i.e.*, theobromine and xanthine, have dual activities both as antioxidants and pro-oxidants. Habitual coffee consumption has been found to have beneficial effects on mood and mental well-being (epidemiological and clinical studies) and to be associated with improved neurological outcomes (*e.g.*, lesser risk of Parkinson's disease), metabolic syndrome management (*e.g.*, diabetes and gallstones), and liver and reproductive health [267].

Functional foods like coffee, tea, and cocoa contain bioactive compounds that can inhibit white adipogenesis and promote brown adipogenesis and lipolysis, preventing obesity. Some compounds, like caffeine and chlorogenic acid, are specific to each type [268].

Tea is steeped in an ancient and rich history, having been drunk for millennia, notably in China. Of the numerous types of tea, non-Camellia types—often called herbal tea—date back to the Tang Dynasty. Uniquely different from the conventional tea prepared from Camellia sinensis, herbal teas are produced by infusing or boiling parts of plants like roots, stems, leaves, flowers, fruits, seeds, bark, or even entire plants. Some teas can also be prepared by soaking the ingredients in cold water, particularly those made with green tea and additional leaves, flowers, or fruits [269]. Bioactive substances such as polyphenols, flavonoids, terpenoids, volatile oils, alkaloids, organic acids, and polysaccharides make up herbal teas. They are in charge of the numerous biological properties of herbal teas, including their anti-inflammatory, anti-bacterial, antidiabetic, antioxidant, and anticancer properties. Herbal tea's functional and therapeutic potential is demonstrated by the fact that it is mostly made from the leaves, buds, flowers, and fruits of medicinal plants [270-273].

SUMMARY

Carotenoids are made up of isoprene units. Different carotenoids like α and β-carotene, lycopene, xanthophylls, and lutein have multiple applications as nutraceuticals. α and β-carotene have antioxidant potential; however, β-carotene is a more versatile nutraceutical due to its multiple applications in decreasing the risk of some cancers, cardiovascular disease, age-related macular degeneration, and cataracts, and increasing immune response. Lycopene has a cancer-protective effect; xanthophylls like zeaxanthin and lutein have protective effects in retinal function and the prevention of different eye diseases. Phenolic compounds like tocopherols, tocotrienols, and resveratrol have free radical scavenging activity, anticancer, cardioprotective, and neuroprotective effects. Anticancer effects and antihyperlipidemic role of diallyl sulfides and allyl trisulfide are reported in many studies (Fig. **24**). Flavonoids are the most studied and reported compounds for various health benefits. Flavonoids like rutin, naringin, quercetin, anthocyanidins, catechins, and flavones have been clinically tested in many clinical studies. Phytoestrogens like isoflavones and daidzein are extensively studied in postmenopausal women for the management of the risk of breast cancer and coronary artery disease. Functional foods, including oats, wheat bran, rice bran, seafoods, coffee, and tea, are also captured in this chapter for their benefits on microbiota, brain health due to PUFA, and obesity management.

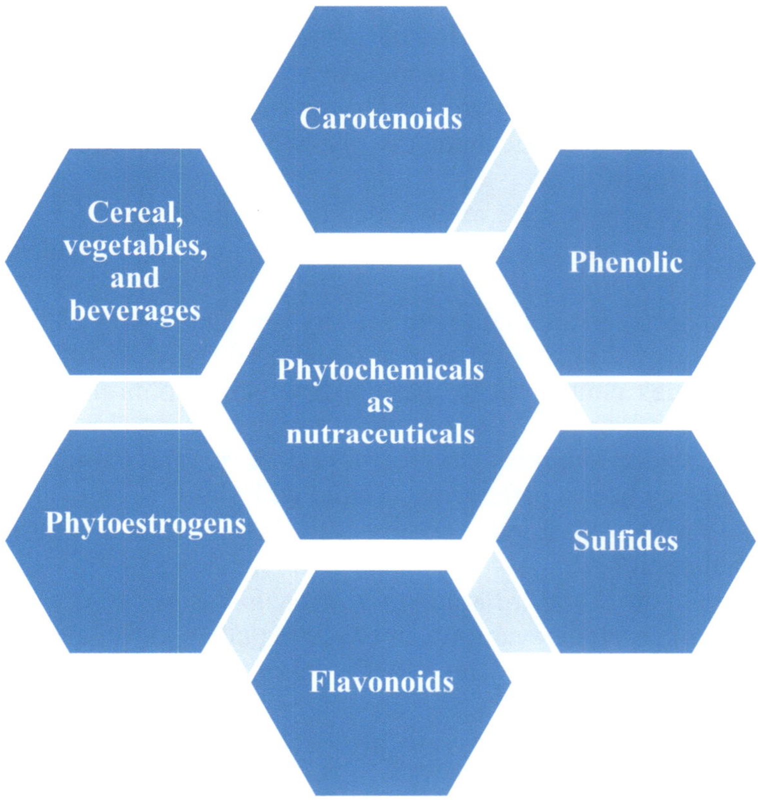

Fig. (24). Phytochemicals as nutraceuticals.

EXERCISE

1. Define the term "nutraceutical" and explain how phytochemicals fit into this category.
2. What is the primary distinction between a nutraceutical and a functional food?
3. Discuss the general mechanisms by which phytochemicals exert their beneficial health effects.
4. Why is it often recommended to obtain phytochemicals from whole foods rather than isolated supplements?
5. Name two major carotenoids found in common fruits and vegetables.
6. Explain the primary biological function of β-carotene in the human body.
7. Beyond its antioxidant properties, what specific health benefits are attributed to lycopene?

8. Differentiate between the chemical structures of α-carotene and β-carotene.
9. Which specific eye health benefits are associated with lutein, and what is its primary dietary source?
10. Describe the general pathway by which carotenoids are absorbed and metabolized in the human body.
11. What is the chemical classification of tocopherols and tocotrienols?
12. Compare and contrast the antioxidant efficacy of tocopherols and tocotrienols.
13. Name a significant natural source of resveratrol.
14. Discuss the proposed mechanisms by which resveratrol contributes to cardiovascular health.
15. Explain why tocopherols are often added to food products.
16. From which plant family are diallyl sulfides and allyl trisulfide primarily derived?
17. What is the characteristic biological activity associated with diallyl sulfides?
18. Describe a potential pharmaceutical application for allyl trisulfide.
19. How do sulfides contribute to the characteristic aroma and flavor of their source plants?
20. Identify the general chemical structure that defines a flavonoid.
21. What are the key health benefits associated with rutin?
22. From which fruit is naringin predominantly extracted, and what is its notable taste characteristic?
23. Discuss the potential anti-inflammatory mechanisms of quercetin.
24. Explain the role of anthocyanidins in imparting color to fruits and vegetables.
25. Differentiate between catechins and flavones based on their chemical structure.
26. Name a food source rich in catechins and describe their significance as nutraceuticals.
27. What is the significance of the "hydroxyl group" arrangement in flavonoids for their biological activity?
28. Define "phytoestrogen" and explain its general mechanism of action in the human body.
29. Name two common dietary sources of isoflavones.
30. How does genistein differ from daidzein in terms of its chemical structure and primary biological activity?
31. What potential health benefits are associated with lignans?
32. Discuss the concept of "selective estrogen receptor modulation" in the context of phytoestrogens.
33. Identify the primary beneficial phytochemicals found in oats.
34. Explain how wheat bran contributes to gut health.
35. What unique lipids are found in rice bran, and what are their purported health benefits?

36. Discuss the role of omega-3 fatty acids in seafood as nutraceuticals.
37. Name two major phytochemicals present in coffee and tea, respectively.
38. Beyond caffeine, what other health-promoting compounds are found in coffee?
39. How do the processing methods of tea influence its phytochemical profile?
40. What are the key differences in the fiber content and types of phytochemicals between oats and rice bran?

Case 1: *Mrs. Sharma, a 65-year-old, has been advised by her doctor to increase her intake of antioxidants due to a family history of cardiovascular disease. She enjoys cooking and often incorporates tomatoes into her meals. She reads online that lycopene, a powerful antioxidant, is abundant in tomatoes. However, she is confused about whether fresh tomatoes or processed tomato products (like tomato paste or sauce) are better sources of bioavailable lycopene.*

Discussion Questions

1. Explain to Mrs. Sharma why lycopene's bioavailability might differ between fresh and processed tomatoes.
2. What specific health benefits, beyond general antioxidant activity, are attributed to lycopene that would be relevant to Mrs. Sharma's concerns?
3. Suggest practical ways Mrs. Sharma can maximize the absorption of lycopene from her diet.
4. Are there any potential interactions between lycopene and common medications that Mrs. Sharma should be aware of (assume she is on statins for cholesterol management)?

Case 2: *Mr. Gupta, a 40-year-old, drinks several cups of green tea daily, believing it offers significant health benefits. He has heard about catechins and their antioxidant properties. Recently, he started experiencing some mild digestive discomfort and is wondering if his tea consumption could be a factor, or if there's an optimal way to consume green tea for maximum benefit.*

Discussion Questions

1. Identify the primary class of phytochemicals in green tea responsible for its antioxidant properties and name a specific example.
2. Explain the proposed mechanisms by which these phytochemicals contribute to health.
3. What are some potential interactions between green tea catechins and other compounds, including iron absorption?

4. Advise Mr. Gupta on how to optimize his green tea consumption for maximal health benefits while minimizing any potential digestive issues.

Case 3: *Ms. Devi, a 52-year-old executive, is experiencing menopausal symptoms, including hot flashes and mood swings. She is reluctant to use hormone replacement therapy and is exploring natural alternatives. She has read about the potential benefits of soy products and flaxseeds due to their phytoestrogen content.*

Discussion Questions

1. Explain what phytoestrogens are and how they might alleviate menopausal symptoms. Name two specific types of phytoestrogens found in soy and flaxseeds.
2. Discuss the concept of "selective estrogen receptor modulation" in the context of phytoestrogens and its relevance to Ms. Devi's situation.
3. What are the key differences between isoflavones (found in soy) and lignans (found in flaxseeds) in terms of their chemical structure and primary dietary sources?
4. What are some considerations or potential risks Ms. Devi should be aware of when increasing her intake of phytoestrogen-rich foods?

Case 4: *Mr. Ali, a 58-year-old, has a long-standing tradition of consuming raw garlic daily, attributing it to his good health and strong immune system. He often mentions "sulfur compounds" as the reason for garlic's benefits. His doctor is impressed by his dedication but wants to understand the scientific basis of his practice.*

Discussion Questions

1. Identify the main class of phytochemicals responsible for the characteristic odor and health benefits of garlic. Name two specific compounds within this class.
2. Describe the process by which these sulfur compounds are formed in garlic after crushing or cutting.
3. Discuss the purported mechanisms of action for diallyl sulfides and allyl trisulfide in promoting human health.
4. Are there any potential drug interactions or contraindications Mr. Ali should be aware of, given his regular consumption of raw garlic (assume he is on an anticoagulant medication)?

Case 5: *Ms. Priya, a 30-year-old, is keen on a holistic approach to health and has been incorporating various "superfoods" into her diet, including oats, wheat bran, and a variety of colourful fruits and vegetables. She is particularly interested in understanding how these diverse food sources contribute to overall well-being through their phytochemical content.*

Discussion Questions

1. Describe the primary types of phytochemicals found in oats and wheat bran, and explain their distinct contributions to gut health.
2. How do the phytochemicals present in colourful fruits (*e.g.*, anthocyanidins) and vegetables (*e.g.*, lutein) complement each other in providing a broad spectrum of health benefits?
3. If Ms. Priya were to choose between rice bran and oats for their specific lipid-related benefits, what key differences in their phytochemical profiles would she consider?
4. Discuss the importance of dietary diversity in obtaining a wide range of phytochemicals, illustrating with examples from Ms. Priya's diet.

REFERENCES

[1] Pandey MM, Rastogi S, Rawat AKS. Indian traditional ayurvedic system of medicine and nutritional supplementation. Evid Based Complement Alternat Med 2013; 2013: 1-12. [http://dx.doi.org/10.1155/2013/376327] [PMID: 23864888]

[2] Kumar A, Sakhare K, Bhattacharya D, *et al.* Communication in non-communicable diseases (NCDs) and the role of immunomodulatory nutraceuticals in their management. Front Nutr 2022; 9: 966152. [http://dx.doi.org/10.3389/fnut.2022.966152]

[3] Britton G, Liaaen-Jensen S, Pfander H. Carotenoids volume 5: nutrition and health. 2009. [http://dx.doi.org/10.1007/978-3-7643-7501-0]

[4] Sesso HD, Gaziano JM. Carotenoids in health and disease. New York, NY: Marcel Dekker 2005; p. 473.

[5] Rüttimann A. Dienolether condensations–a powerful tool in carotenoid synthesis. Pure Appl Chem 1999; 71(12): 2285-93. [http://dx.doi.org/10.1351/pac199971122285]

[6] G. Britton, S. Liaaen-Jensen, H. Pfander, Carotenoids. Vol. 2: Synthesis, Birkhäuser, Basel, 1996.

[7] Meléndez-Martínez AJ, Mandić AI, Bantis F, *et al.* A comprehensive review on carotenoids in foods and feeds: status quo, applications, patents, and research needs. Crit Rev Food Sci Nutr 2022; 62: 1999-2049. [http://dx.doi.org/10.1080/10408398.2020.1867959] [PMID: 28455059]

[8] Tanumihardjo SA. Carotenoids: Health effects, editor(s): benjamin caballero, encyclopedia of human nutrition (third Edition), Academic Press; 2013: 292-297.

[9] Azevedo-Meleiro CH, Rodriguez-Amaya DB. Qualitative and quantitative differences in carotenoid composition among Cucurbita moschata, Cucurbita maxima, and Cucurbita pepo. J Agric Food Chem 2007; 55(10): 4027-33. [http://dx.doi.org/10.1021/jf063413d] [PMID: 17444652]

[10] Gallicchio L, Boyd K, Matanoski G, *et al.* Carotenoids and the risk of developing lung cancer: a systematic review. Am J Clin Nutr 2008; 88(2): 372-83.
[http://dx.doi.org/10.1093/ajcn/88.2.372] [PMID: 18689373]

[11] Huang Y, Chen H, Su Y, Liu H, Hu J, Hong K. Increased blood alpha-carotene, all-trans-Be-a-carotene and lycopene levels are associated with beneficial changes in heart rate variability: a CVD-stratified analysis in an adult population-based study. Nutr J 2021; 20(1): 43.
[http://dx.doi.org/10.1186/s12937-021-00700-w] [PMID: 33971890]

[12] Johnson EJ. The role of carotenoids in human health. Nutr Clin Care 2002; 5(2): 56-65.
[http://dx.doi.org/10.1046/j.1523-5408.2002.00004.x] [PMID: 12134711]

[13] Mayne ST. Beta-carotene, carotenoids, and disease prevention in humans. FASEB J 1996; 10(7): 690-701.
[http://dx.doi.org/10.1096/fasebj.10.7.8635686] [PMID: 8635686]

[14] Silalahi J. Anticancer and health protective properties of citrus fruit components. Asia Pac J Clin Nutr 2002; 11(1): 79-84.
[http://dx.doi.org/10.1046/j.1440-6047.2002.00271.x] [PMID: 11890643]

[15] Bhaskarachary K. Functional foods and Nutraceutical Available from: https://epgp.inflibnet.ac.in/epgpdata/uploads/epgp_content/S000444FN/P000556/M012441/ET/1459416151et35.pdf

[16] McMILLAN DC, Talwar D, Sattar N, Underwood M, St J O'Reilly D, McARDLE COLIN. The relationship between reduced vitamin antioxidant concentrations and the systemic inflammatory response in patients with common solid tumours. Clin Nutr 2002; 21(2): 161-4.
[http://dx.doi.org/10.1054/clnu.2001.0527] [PMID: 12056790]

[17] DellaPenna D, Pogson BJ. Vitamin synthesis in plants: tocopherols and carotenoids. Annu Rev Plant Biol 2006; 57(1): 711-38.
[http://dx.doi.org/10.1146/annurev.arplant.56.032604.144301] [PMID: 16669779]

[18] Krinsky NI. Effects of carotenoids in cellular and animal systems. Am J Clin Nutr 1991; 53(1) (Suppl.): 238S-46S.
[http://dx.doi.org/10.1093/ajcn/53.1.238S] [PMID: 1985393]

[19] Fayaz M, Namitha KK, Murthy KNC, *et al.* Chemical composition, iron bioavailability, and antioxidant activity of *Kappaphycus alvarezzi* (Doty). J Agric Food Chem 2005; 53(3): 792-7.
[http://dx.doi.org/10.1021/jf0493627] [PMID: 15686435]

[20] Kolb N, Vallorani L, Milanovic N, Stocchi V. Evaluation of marine algae wakame (*Undaria pinnatifida*) and kombu (*Laminaria digitata* japonica) as food supplements. Food Technol Biotechnol 2004; 42: 57-61.

[21] Norziah MH, Ching CY. Nutritional composition of edible seaweed *Gracilaria changgi.* Food Chem 2000; 68(1): 69-76.
[http://dx.doi.org/10.1016/S0308-8146(99)00161-2]

[22] Ratana-Arporn P, Chirapart A. Nutritional evaluation of tropical green seaweeds *Caulerpa lentillifera* and *Ulva reticulata.* Witthayasan Kasetsat Witthayasat 2006; 40 (Suppl.): 75-8.

[23] Saini RK, Nile SH, Park SW. Carotenoids from fruits and vegetables: Chemistry, analysis, occurrence, bioavailability and biological activities. Food Res Int 2015; 76(Pt 3): 735-50.
[http://dx.doi.org/10.1016/j.foodres.2015.07.047] [PMID: 28455059]

[24] Raghuvanshi S, Reed V, Blaner WS, Harrison EH. Cellular localization of β-carotene 15,15′ oxygenase-1 (BCO1) and β-carotene 9′,10′ oxygenase-2 (BCO2) in rat liver and intestine. Arch Biochem Biophys 2015; 572: 19-27.
[http://dx.doi.org/10.1016/j.abb.2014.12.024] [PMID: 25575786]

[25] Sánchez C, Baranda AB, Martínez de Marañón I. The effect of high pressure and high temperature

processing on carotenoids and chlorophylls content in some vegetables. Food Chem 2014; 163: 37-45. [http://dx.doi.org/10.1016/j.foodchem.2014.04.041] [PMID: 24912693]

[26] Hemila¨ H, Virtamo J, Albanes D, Kaprio J. Vitamin E and beta-carotene supplementation and hospital-treated pneumonia incidence in male smokers. Chest 2004; 125(2): 557-65. [http://dx.doi.org/10.1378/chest.125.2.557] [PMID: 14769738]

[27] Hemilä H, Virtamo J, Albanes D, Kaprio J. Physical activity and the common cold in men administered vitamin E and β-carotene. Med Sci Sports Exerc 2003; 35(11): 1815-20. [http://dx.doi.org/10.1249/01.MSS.0000093616.60899.92] [PMID: 14600543]

[28] Kazi N, Radvany R, Oldham T, *et al.* Immunomodulatory effect of β-carotene on T lymphocyte subsets in patients with resected colonic polyps and cancer. Nutr Cancer 1997; 28(2): 140-5. [http://dx.doi.org/10.1080/01635589709514566] [PMID: 9290119]

[29] Fryburg DA, Mark RJ, Griffith BP, Askenase PW, Patterson TF. The effect of supplemental beta-carotene on immunologic indices in patients with AIDS: a pilot study. Yale J Biol Med 1995; 68(1-2): 19-23.
[PMID: 8748463]

[30] Garewal HS, Ampel NM, Watson RR, Prabhala RH, Dols CL. A preliminary trial of beta-carotene in subjects infected with the human immunodeficiency virus. J Nutr 1992; 122(3) (Suppl.): 728-32. [http://dx.doi.org/10.1093/jn/122.suppl_3.728] [PMID: 1347316]

[31] Nishida K, Sugimoto M, Ikeda S, Kume S. Effects of supplemental β-carotene on mucosal IgA induction in the jejunum and ileum of mice after weaning. Br J Nutr 2014; 111(2): 247-53. [http://dx.doi.org/10.1017/S0007114513002195] [PMID: 23830034]

[32] Gollnick HPM, Hopfenmu¨ller W, Hemmes C, *et al.* Systemic beta carotene plus topical UV-sunscreen are an optimal protection against harmful effects of natural UV-sunlight: results of the Berlin-Eilath study. Eur J Dermatol 1996; 6(3): 219-38.

[33] Hughes DA, Wright AJA, Finglas PM, *et al.* The effect of β-carotene supplementation on the immune function of blood monocytes from healthy male nonsmokers. J Lab Clin Med 1997; 129(3): 309-17. [http://dx.doi.org/10.1016/S0022-2143(97)90179-7] [PMID: 9042816]

[34] Heywood R, Palmer AK, Gregson RL, Hummler H. The toxicity of beta-carotene. Toxicology 1985; 36(2-3): 91-100.
[http://dx.doi.org/10.1016/0300-483X(85)90043-5] [PMID: 4049434]

[35] Boon CS, McClements DJ, Weiss J, Decker EA. Factors influencing the chemical stability of carotenoids in foods. Crit Rev Food Sci Nutr 2010; 50(6): 515-32. [http://dx.doi.org/10.1080/10408390802565889] [PMID: 20544442]

[36] Gerester H. Anticarcinogenic effect of common carotenoids. Int J Vitam Nutr Res 1993; 15: 1507-16.

[37] Walter P. The scientific basis for vitamin intake in human nutrition, Bibliotheca Nutritio at Dieta n°52. Basel: Karger 1995.

[38] Talsma EF, Brouwer ID, Verhoef H, *et al.* Biofortified yellow cassava and vitamin A status of Kenyan children: a randomized controlled trial. Am J Clin Nutr 2016; 103(1): 258-67. [http://dx.doi.org/10.3945/ajcn.114.100164] [PMID: 26675768]

[39] Meydani M, Martin A, Ribaya-Mercado JD, Gong J, Blumberg JB, Russell RM. β-carotene supplementation increases antioxidant capacity of plasma in older women. J Nutr 1994; 124(12): 2397-403.
[http://dx.doi.org/10.1093/jn/124.12.397] [PMID: 16856320]

[40] Micozzi MS, Brown ED, Edwards BK, *et al.* Plasma carotenoid response to chronic intake of selected foods and β-carotene supplements in men. Am J Clin Nutr 1992; 55(6): 1120-5. [http://dx.doi.org/10.1093/ajcn/55.6.1120] [PMID: 1595584]

[41] Dutta D, Raychaudhuri U, Chakarborty R. Structure, health benefits, antioxidant property and

processing and storage of carotenoids. Afr J Biotechnol 2005; 4: 1510-20. a

[42] Schunck CA. The xanthophyll group of yellow colouring matters. Proc R Soc Lond 1904; 72(477-486): 165-76.
[http://dx.doi.org/10.1098/rspl.1903.0035]

[43] Clinton SK, Emenhiser C, Schwartz SJ, *et al.* cis-trans lycopene isomers, carotenoids, and retinol in the human prostate. Cancer Epidemiol Biomarkers Prev 1996; 5(10): 823-33.
[PMID: 8896894]

[44] Shi J, Le Maguer M. Lycopene in tomatoes: chemical and physical properties affected by food processing. Crit Rev Biotechnol 2000; 20(4): 293-334.
[http://dx.doi.org/10.1080/07388550091144212] [PMID: 11192026]

[45] Nguyen ML, Schwartz SJ. Lycopene stability during food processing. Exp Biol Med (Maywood) 1998; 218(2): 101-5.
[http://dx.doi.org/10.3181/00379727-218-44274] [PMID: 9605205]

[46] Nguyen M, Francis D, Schwartz S. Thermal isomerisation susceptibility of carotenoids in different tomato varieties. J Sci Food Agric 2001; 81(9): 910-7.
[http://dx.doi.org/10.1002/jsfa.911]

[47] Unlu NZ, Bohn T, Francis DM, Nagaraja HN, Clinton SK, Schwartz SJ. Lycopene from heat-induced *cis* -isomer-rich tomato sauce is more bioavailable than from all- *trans* -rich tomato sauce in human subjects. Br J Nutr 2007; 98(1): 140-6.
[http://dx.doi.org/10.1017/S0007114507685201] [PMID: 17391568]

[48] Kopec RE, Cooperstone JL, Schweiggert RM, *et al.* Avocado consumption enhances human postprandial provitamin A absorption and conversion from a novel high-β-carotene tomato sauce and from carrots. J Nutr 2014; 144(8): 1158-66.
[http://dx.doi.org/10.3945/jn.113.187674] [PMID: 24899156]

[49] Hof KH, de Boer BCJ, Tijburg LBM, *et al.* Carotenoid bioavailability in humans from tomatoes processed in different ways determined from the carotenoid response in the triglyceride-rich lipoprotein fraction of plasma after a single consumption and in plasma after four days of consumption. J Nutr 2000; 130(5): 1189-96.
[http://dx.doi.org/10.1093/jn/130.5.1189] [PMID: 10801917]

[50] R. Watson, B. Dokken, Glucose intake and utilization in pre-diabetes and diabetes, Academic Press. 2014.

[51] Story EN, Kopec RE, Schwartz SJ, Harris GK. An update on the health effects of tomato lycopene. Annu Rev Food Sci Technol 2010; 1(1): 189-210.
[http://dx.doi.org/10.1146/annurev.food.102308.124120] [PMID: 22129335]

[52] Stahl W, Sies H. Bioactivity and protective effects of natural carotenoids. Biochim Biophys Acta Mol Basis Dis 2005; 1740(2): 101-7.
[http://dx.doi.org/10.1016/j.bbadis.2004.12.006]

[53] Rao A, Rao L. Carotenoids and human health. Pharmacol Res 2007; 55(3): 207-16.
[http://dx.doi.org/10.1016/j.phrs.2007.01.012] [PMID: 17349800]

[54] Kucuk O, Sarkar FH, Sakr W, *et al.* Lycopene in the treatment of prostate cancer. Pure Appl Chem 2002; 74(8): 1443-50.
[http://dx.doi.org/10.1351/pac200274081443]

[55] Kucuk O, Sarkar FH, Djuric Z, *et al.* Effects of lycopene supplementation in patients with localized prostate cancer. Exp Biol Med (Maywood) 2002; 227(10): 881-5.
[http://dx.doi.org/10.1177/153537020222701007] [PMID: 12424329]

[56] Burton-Freeman B, Talbot J, Park E, Krishnankutty S, Edirisinghe I. Protective activity of processed tomato products on postprandial oxidation and inflammation: A clinical trial in healthy weight men and women. Mol Nutr Food Res 2012; 56(4): 622-31.

[http://dx.doi.org/10.1002/mnfr.201100649] [PMID: 22331646]

[57] Li YF, Chang YY, Huang HC, Wu YC, Yang MD, Chao PM. Tomato juice supplementation in young women reduces inflammatory adipokine levels independently of body fat reduction. Nutrition 2015; 31(5): 691-6.
[http://dx.doi.org/10.1016/j.nut.2014.11.008] [PMID: 25837214]

[58] Biddle MJ, Lennie TA, Bricker GV, Kopec RE, Schwartz SJ, Moser DK. Lycopene dietary intervention: a pilot study in patients with heart failure. J Cardiovasc Nurs 2015; 30(3): 205-12.
[http://dx.doi.org/10.1097/JCN.0000000000000108] [PMID: 24651682]

[59] Markovits N, Ben Amotz A, Levy Y. The effect of tomato-derived lycopene on low carotenoids and enhanced systemic inflammation and oxidation in severe obesity. Isr Med Assoc J 2009; 11(10): 598-601.
[PMID: 20077945]

[60] Grether-Beck S, Marini A, Jaenicke T, Stahl W, Krutmann J. Molecular evidence that oral supplementation with lycopene or lutein protects human skin against ultraviolet radiation: results from a double-blinded, placebo-controlled, crossover study. Br J Dermatol 2017; 176(5): 1231-40.
[http://dx.doi.org/10.1111/bjd.15080] [PMID: 27662341]

[61] Li XN, Lin J, Xia J, Qin L, Zhu SY, Li JL. Lycopene mitigates atrazine-induced cardiac inflammation *via* blocking the NF-κB pathway and NO production. J Funct Foods 2017; 29: 208-16.
[http://dx.doi.org/10.1016/j.jff.2016.12.029]

[62] Róvero Costa M, Leite Garcia J, Cristina Vágula de Almeida Silva C, *et al.* Lycopene modulates pathophysiological processes of non-alcoholic fatty liver disease in obese rats 2019.
[http://dx.doi.org/10.3390/antiox8080276]

[63] Leh HE, Mohd Sopian M, Abu Bakar MH, Lee LK. The role of lycopene for the amelioration of glycaemic status and peripheral antioxidant capacity among the Type II diabetes mellitus patients: a case–control study. Ann Med 2021; 53(1): 1060-6.
[http://dx.doi.org/10.1080/07853890.2021.1943515] [PMID: 34180336]

[64] Gong M, Bassi A. Carotenoids from microalgae: A review of recent developments. Biotechnol Adv 2016; 34(8): 1396-412.
[http://dx.doi.org/10.1016/j.biotechadv.2016.10.005] [PMID: 27816618]

[65] Peng J, Yuan JP, Wu CF, Wang JH. Fucoxanthin, a marine carotenoid present in brown seaweeds and diatoms: metabolism and bioactivities relevant to human health. Mar Drugs 2011; 9(10): 1806-28.
[http://dx.doi.org/10.3390/md9101806] [PMID: 22072997]

[66] Guerin M, Huntley ME, Olaizola M. Haematococcus astaxanthin: applications for human health and nutrition. Trends Biotechnol 2003; 21(5): 210-6.
[http://dx.doi.org/10.1016/S0167-7799(03)00078-7] [PMID: 12727382]

[67] Desmarchelier C, Borel P. Overview of carotenoid bioavailability determinants: From dietary factors to host genetic variations. Trends Food Sci Technol 2017; 69: 270-80.
[http://dx.doi.org/10.1016/j.tifs.2017.03.002]

[68] Bernstein PS, Li B, Vachali PP, *et al.* Lutein, zeaxanthin, and meso-zeaxanthin: The basic and clinical science underlying carotenoid-based nutritional interventions against ocular disease. Prog Retin Eye Res 2016; 50: 34-66.
[http://dx.doi.org/10.1016/j.preteyeres.2015.10.003] [PMID: 26541886]

[69] Johnson EJ. A possible role for lutein and zeaxanthin in cognitive function in the elderly. Am J Clin Nutr 2012; 96(5): 1161S-5S.
[http://dx.doi.org/10.3945/ajcn.112.034611] [PMID: 23053547]

[70] Chasan-Taber L, Willett WC, Seddon JM, *et al.* A prospective study of carotenoid and vitamin A intakes and risk of cataract extraction in US women. Am J Clin Nutr 1999; 70(4): 509-16.
[http://dx.doi.org/10.1093/ajcn/70.4.509] [PMID: 10500020]

[71] Demmig-Adams B, Adams WW III. The role of xanthophyll cycle carotenoids in the protection of photosynthesis. Trends Plant Sci 1996; 1(1): 21-6.
[http://dx.doi.org/10.1016/S1360-1385(96)80019-7]

[72] Mares-Perlman JA, Millen AE, Ficek TL, Hankinson SE. The body of evidence to support a protective role for lutein and zeaxanthin in delaying chronic disease. Overview. J Nutr 2002; 132(3): 518S-24S.
[http://dx.doi.org/10.1093/jn/132.3.518S] [PMID: 11880585]

[73] Barros MP, Marin DP, Bolin AP, *et al.* Combined astaxanthin and fish oil supplementation improves glutathione-based redox balance in rat plasma and neutrophils. Chem Biol Interact 2012; 197(1): 58-67.
[http://dx.doi.org/10.1016/j.cbi.2012.03.005] [PMID: 22465178]

[74] Fisher AEO, Naughton DP. Why nutraceuticals do not prevent or treat Alzheimer's disease. Nutr J 2005; 4(1): 14.
[http://dx.doi.org/10.1186/1475-2891-4-14] [PMID: 15826313]

[75] Dall'Osto L, Cazzaniga S, Bressan M, *et al.* Two mechanisms for dissipation of excess light in monomeric and trimeric light-harvesting complexes. Nat Plants 2017; 3(5): 17033.
[http://dx.doi.org/10.1038/nplants.2017.33] [PMID: 28394312]

[76] Bone RA, Landrum JT, Tarsis SL. Preliminary identification of the human macular pigment. Vision Res 1985; 25(11): 1531-5.
[http://dx.doi.org/10.1016/0042-6989(85)90123-3] [PMID: 3832576]

[77] Harold H. Schmitz, Christopher L. Poor, Eric T. Gugger, John W. Erdman, Analysis of carotenoids in human and animal tissues. Methods in Enzymology, Academic Press 1993; 214: 102-16.

[78] Gruszecki WI, Strzałka K. Carotenoids as modulators of lipid membrane physical properties. Biochim Biophys Acta Mol Basis Dis 2005; 1740(2): 108-15.
[http://dx.doi.org/10.1016/j.bbadis.2004.11.015] [PMID: 15949676]

[79] Krinsky NI, Johnson EJ. Carotenoid actions and their relation to health and disease. Mol Aspects Med 2005; 26(6): 459-516.
[http://dx.doi.org/10.1016/j.mam.2005.10.001] [PMID: 16309738]

[80] González S, Astner S, An W, Pathak MA, Goukassian D. Dietary lutein/zeaxanthin decreases ultraviolet B-induced epidermal hyperproliferation and acute inflammation in hairless mice. J Invest Dermatol 2003; 121(2): 399-405.
[http://dx.doi.org/10.1046/j.1523-1747.2003.12355.x] [PMID: 12880433]

[81] Chung RWS, Leanderson P, Lundberg AK, Jonasson L. Lutein exerts anti-inflammatory effects in patients with coronary artery disease. Atherosclerosis 2017; 262: 87-93.
[http://dx.doi.org/10.1016/j.atherosclerosis.2017.05.008] [PMID: 28527371]

[82] Corvi F, Souied EH, Falfoul Y, *et al.* Pilot evaluation of short-term changes in macular pigment and retinal sensitivity in different phenotypes of early age-related macular degeneration after carotenoid supplementation. Br J Ophthalmol 2017; 101(6): 770-3.
[http://dx.doi.org/10.1136/bjophthalmol-2016-309115] [PMID: 27587715]

[83] Xu XR, Zou ZY, Xiao X, Huang YM, Wang X, Lin XM. Effects of lutein supplement on serum inflammatory cytokines, ApoE and lipid profiles in early atherosclerosis population. J Atheroscler Thromb 2013; 20(2): 170-7.
[http://dx.doi.org/10.5551/jat.14365] [PMID: 23154578]

[84] Saha SK, Ermis H, Murray P. Marine microalgae for potential lutein production. Appl Sci (Basel) 2020; 10(18): 6457.
[http://dx.doi.org/10.3390/app10186457]

[85] Richer S, Stiles W, Statkute L, *et al.* Double-masked, placebo-controlled, randomized trial of lutein and antioxidant supplementation in the intervention of atrophic age-related macular degeneration: the Veterans LAST study (Lutein Antioxidant Supplementation Trial). Optometry 2004; 75(4): 216-29.

[http://dx.doi.org/10.1016/S1529-1839(04)70049-4] [PMID: 15117055]

[86] Richer S, Devenport J, Lang JC. LAST II: Differential temporal responses of macular pigment optical density in patients with atrophic age-related macular degeneration to dietary supplementation with xanthophylls. Optometry 2007; 78(5): 213-9.
[http://dx.doi.org/10.1016/j.optm.2006.10.019] [PMID: 17478338]

[87] Weigert G, Kaya S, Pemp B, *et al.* Effects of lutein supplementation on macular pigment optical density and visual acuity in patients with age-related macular degeneration 2011.
[http://dx.doi.org/10.1167/iovs.11-7522]

[88] Murray IJ, Makridaki M, van der Veen RLP, Carden D, Parry NRA, Berendschot TTJM. Lutein supplementation over a one-year period in early AMD might have a mild beneficial effect on visual acuity: the CLEAR study. Invest Ophthalmol Vis Sci 2013; 54(3): 1781-8.
[http://dx.doi.org/10.1167/iovs.12-10715] [PMID: 23385792]

[89] Moeller SM, Parekh N, Tinker L, *et al.* Associations between intermediate age-related macular degeneration and lutein and zeaxanthin in the Carotenoids in Age-related Eye Disease Study (CAREDS): ancillary study of the Women's Health Initiative. Arch Ophthalmol 2006; 124(8): 1151-62.
[http://dx.doi.org/10.1001/archopht.124.8.1151] [PMID: 16908818]

[90] Zhang PC, Wu CR, Wang ZL, *et al.* Effect of lutein supplementation on visual function in nonproliferative diabetic retinopathy. Asia Pac J Clin Nutr 2017; 26(3): 406-11.
[http://dx.doi.org/10.6133/apjcn.032016.13] [PMID: 28429904]

[91] Brazionis L, Rowley K, Itsiopoulos C, O'Dea K. Plasma carotenoids and diabetic retinopathy. Br J Nutr 2009; 101(2): 270-7.
[http://dx.doi.org/10.1017/S0007114508006545] [PMID: 18554424]

[92] Rubin LP, Chan GM, Barrett-Reis BM, *et al.* Effect of carotenoid supplementation on plasma carotenoids, inflammation and visual development in preterm infants. J Perinatol 2012; 32(6): 418-24.
[http://dx.doi.org/10.1038/jp.2011.87] [PMID: 21760585]

[93] Williams KM, Bentham GCG, Young IS, *et al.* Association between myopia, ultraviolet b radiation exposure, serum vitamin d concentrations, and genetic polymorphisms in vitamin d metabolic pathways in a multicountry european study. JAMA Ophthalmol 2017; 135(1): 47-53.
[http://dx.doi.org/10.1001/jamaophthalmol.2016.4752] [PMID: 27918775]

[94] Tanito M, Obana A, Gohto Y, Okazaki S, Gellermann W, Ohira A. Macular pigment density changes in Japanese individuals supplemented with lutein or zeaxanthin: quantification *via* resonance Raman spectrophotometry and autofluorescence imaging. Jpn J Ophthalmol 2012; 56(5): 488-96.
[http://dx.doi.org/10.1007/s10384-012-0157-0] [PMID: 22699751]

[95] Karppi J, Laukkanen JA, Kurl S. Plasma lutein and zeaxanthin and the risk of age-related nuclear cataract among the elderly Finnish population. Br J Nutr 2012; 108(1): 148-54.
[http://dx.doi.org/10.1017/S0007114511005332] [PMID: 22005336]

[96] Pratyusha S. Phenolic compounds in the plant development and defense: an overview. IntechOpen 2022.
[http://dx.doi.org/10.5772/intechopen.102873]

[97] Shahidi F, De Camargo A. Tocopherols and tocotrienols in common and emerging dietary sources: occurrence, applications, and health benefits. Int J Mol Sci 2016; 17(10): 1745.
[http://dx.doi.org/10.3390/ijms17101745] [PMID: 27775605]

[98] Szewczyk K, Chojnacka A, Górnicka M. Tocopherols and tocotrienols—bioactive dietary compounds; what is certain, what is doubt? Int J Mol Sci 2021; 22(12): 6222.
[http://dx.doi.org/10.3390/ijms22126222] [PMID: 34207571]

[99] Ali SS, Ahsan H, Zia MK, Siddiqui T, Khan FH. Understanding oxidants and antioxidants: classical team with new players. J Food Biochem 2020; 44(3): e13145.

[http://dx.doi.org/10.1111/jfbc.13145] [PMID: 31960481]

[100] Mathur P, Ding Z, Saldeen T, Mehta JL. Tocopherols in the prevention and treatment of atherosclerosis and related cardiovascular disease. Clin Cardiol 2015; 38(9): 570-6. [http://dx.doi.org/10.1002/clc.22422] [PMID: 26272221]

[101] Lewis ED, Meydani SN, Wu D. Regulatory role of vitamin E in the immune system and inflammation. IUBMB Life 2019; 71(4): 487-94. [http://dx.doi.org/10.1002/iub.1976] [PMID: 30501009]

[102] Age-Related Eye Disease Study Research Group. A randomized, placebo-controlled, clinical trial of high-dose supplementation with vitamins C and E, beta carotene, and zinc for age-related macular degeneration and vision loss: AREDS report no. 8. Archives of ophthalmology (Chicago, Ill.: 1960), 2001; 119(10), 1417–1436. [http://dx.doi.org/10.1001/archopht.119.10.1417]

[103] Browne D, McGuinness B, Woodside JV, McKay GJ. Vitamin E and Alzheimer's disease: what do we know so far? Clin Interv Aging 2019; 14: 1303-17. [http://dx.doi.org/10.2147/CIA.S186760] [PMID: 31409980]

[104] Pervez MA, Khan DA, Ijaz A, Khan S. Effects of delta-tocotrienol supplementation on liver enzymes, inflammation, oxidative stress and hepatic steatosis in patients with nonalcoholic fatty liver disease. Turk J Gastroenterol 2018; 29(2): 170-6. [http://dx.doi.org/10.5152/tjg.2018.17297] [PMID: 29749323]

[105] Tan S, Chiew Y, Ahmad B, Kadir K. Tocotrienol-rich vitamin e from palm oil (tocovid) and its effects in diabetes and diabetic nephropathy: a pilot phase ii clinical trial. Nutrients 2018; 10(9): 1315. [http://dx.doi.org/10.3390/nu10091315] [PMID: 30227659]

[106] Gopalan Y, Shuaib IL, Magosso E, *et al.* Clinical investigation of the protective effects of palm vitamin E tocotrienols on brain white matter. Stroke 2014; 45(5): 1422-8. [http://dx.doi.org/10.1161/STROKEAHA.113.004449] [PMID: 24699052]

[107] Nesaretnam K, Selvaduray KR, Abdul Razak G, Veerasenan SD, Gomez PA. Effectiveness of tocotrienol-rich fraction combined with tamoxifen in the management of women with early breast cancer: a pilot clinical trial. Breast Cancer Res 2010; 12(5): R81. [http://dx.doi.org/10.1186/bcr2726] [PMID: 20929592]

[108] Soon HK, Abdul R. Potential of mixed tocotrienol supplementation to reduce cholesterol and cytokines level in adults with metabolic syndrome. Malays J Nutr 2015; 21(2): 231-43.

[109] Shen CL, Wang S, Yang S, *et al.* A 12-week evaluation of annatto tocotrienol supplementation for postmenopausal women: safety, quality of life, body composition, physical activity, and nutrient intake. BMC Complement Altern Med 2018; 18(1): 198-0. [http://dx.doi.org/10.1186/s12906-018-2263-0] [PMID: 29954374]

[110] Salehi B, Mishra AP, Nigam M, *et al.* Resveratrol: A double-edged sword in health benefits. Biomedicines 2018; 6(3): 91. [http://dx.doi.org/10.3390/biomedicines6030091] [PMID: 30205595]

[111] Lee PS, Chiou YS, Ho CT, Pan MH. Chemoprevention by resveratrol and pterostilbene: Targeting on epigenetic regulation. Biofactors 2018; 44(1): 26-35. [http://dx.doi.org/10.1002/biof.1401] [PMID: 29220106]

[112] Iuga C, Alvarez-Idaboy JR, Russo N. Antioxidant activity of trans-resveratrol toward hydroxyl and hydroperoxyl radicals: a quantum chemical and computational kinetics study. J Org Chem 2012; 77(8): 3868-77. [http://dx.doi.org/10.1021/jo3002134] [PMID: 22475027]

[113] Varoni EM, Lo Faro AF, Sharifi-Rad J, Iriti M. Anticancer molecular mechanisms of resveratrol. Front Nutr 2016; 3: 8. [http://dx.doi.org/10.3389/fnut.2016.00008] [PMID: 27148534]

[114] Kundu JK, Surh YJ. Cancer chemopreventive and therapeutic potential of resveratrol: Mechanistic perspectives. Cancer Lett 2008; 269(2): 243-61.
[http://dx.doi.org/10.1016/j.canlet.2008.03.057] [PMID: 18550275]

[115] Riba A, Deres L, Sumegi B, Toth K, Szabados E, Halmosi R. Cardioprotective effect of resveratrol in a postinfarction heart failure model. Oxid Med Cell Longev 2017; 2017(1): 6819281.
[http://dx.doi.org/10.1155/2017/6819281] [PMID: 29109832]

[116] Bastianetto S, Ménard C, Quirion R. Neuroprotective action of resveratrol. Biochim Biophys Acta Mol Basis Dis 2015; 1852(6): 1195-201.
[http://dx.doi.org/10.1016/j.bbadis.2014.09.011] [PMID: 25281824]

[117] Zhou ZX, Mou SF, Chen XQ, Gong LL, Ge WS. Anti-inflammatory activity of resveratrol prevents inflammation by inhibiting NF-κB in animal models of acute pharyngitis. Mol Med Rep 2017; 17(1): 1269-74.
[http://dx.doi.org/10.3892/mmr.2017.7933] [PMID: 29115472]

[118] Abba Y, Hassim H, Hamzah H, Noordin MM. Antiviral Activity of Resveratrol against Human and Animal Viruses. Adv Virol 2015; 2015: 1-7.
[http://dx.doi.org/10.1155/2015/184241] [PMID: 26693226]

[119] Timmers S, Konings E, Bilet L, *et al.* Calorie restriction-like effects of 30 days of resveratrol supplementation on energy metabolism and metabolic profile in obese humans. Cell Metab 2011; 14(5): 612-22.
[http://dx.doi.org/10.1016/j.cmet.2011.10.002] [PMID: 22055504]

[120] Chen S, Zhao X, Ran L, *et al.* Resveratrol improves insulin resistance, glucose and lipid metabolism in patients with non-alcoholic fatty liver disease: A randomized controlled trial. Dig Liver Dis 2015; 47(3): 226-32.
[http://dx.doi.org/10.1016/j.dld.2014.11.015] [PMID: 25577300]

[121] Pasinetti GM, Wang J, Ho L, Zhao W, Dubner L. Roles of resveratrol and other grape-derived polyphenols in Alzheimer's disease prevention and treatment. Biochim Biophys Acta Mol Basis Dis 2015; 1852(6): 1202-8.
[http://dx.doi.org/10.1016/j.bbadis.2014.10.006] [PMID: 25315300]

[122] Zhu W, Qin W, Zhang K, *et al.* Trans-resveratrol alters mammary promoter hypermethylation in women at increased risk for breast cancer. Nutr Cancer 2012; 64(3): 393-400.
[http://dx.doi.org/10.1080/01635581.2012.654926] [PMID: 22332908]

[123] Ramirez DA, Locatelli DA, González RE, Cavagnaro PF, Camargo AB. Analytical methods for bioactive sulfur compounds in Allium: An integrated review and future directions. J Food Compos Anal 2017; 61: 4-19.
[http://dx.doi.org/10.1016/j.jfca.2016.09.012]

[124] Rao PSS, Midde N, Miller D, Chauhan S, Kumar A, Kumar S. Diallyl sulfide: potential use in novel therapeutic interventions in alcohol, drugs, and disease mediated cellular toxicity by targeting cytochrome P450 2E1. Curr Drug Metab 2015; 16(6): 486-503.
[http://dx.doi.org/10.2174/1389200216666150812123554] [PMID: 26264202]

[125] Wang G, Yang Y, Wang C, *et al.* Exploring the role and mechanisms of diallyl trisulfide and diallyl disulfide in chronic constriction-induced neuropathic pain in rats. Korean J Pain 2020; 33(3): 216-25.
[http://dx.doi.org/10.3344/kjp.2020.33.3.216] [PMID: 32606266]

[126] Quintero-Fabián S, Ortuño-Sahagún D, Vázquez-Carrera M, López-Roa RI. Alliin, a garlic (Allium sativum) compound, prevents LPS-induced inflammation in 3T3-L1 adipocytes. Mediators Inflamm 2013; 2013: 1-11.
[http://dx.doi.org/10.1155/2013/381815] [PMID: 24453416]

[127] Wu CC, Chung JG, Tsai SJ, Yang JH, Sheen LY. Differential effects of allyl sulfides from garlic essential oil on cell cycle regulation in human liver tumor cells. Food Chem Toxicol 2004; 42(12):

1937-47.
[http://dx.doi.org/10.1016/j.fct.2004.07.008] [PMID: 15500931]

[128] Seki T, Hosono T, Hosono-Fukao T, *et al.* Anticancer effects of diallyl trisulfide derived from garlic. Asia Pac J Clin Nutr 2008; 17 (Suppl. 1): 249-52.
[PMID: 18296348]

[129] National Center for Biotechnology Information. PubChem Compound Summary for CID 16315, Diallyl trisulfide. Retrieved May 6, 2024, Available from: https://pubchem.ncbi.nlm.nih.gov/compound/Diallyl-trisulfide

[130] Mandal SK, Das A, Dey S, *et al.* Bioactivities of Allicin and related organosulfur compounds from garlic: Overview of the literature since 2010. Egypt J Chem 2019; 62: 2-3.
[http://dx.doi.org/10.21608/ejchem.2019.15787.1954]

[131] Xiao D, Lew KL, Kim YA, *et al.* Diallyl trisulfide suppresses growth of PC-3 human prostate cancer xenograft *in vivo* in association with Bax and Bak induction. Clin Cancer Res 2006; 12(22): 6836-43.
[http://dx.doi.org/10.1158/1078-0432.CCR-06-1273] [PMID: 17121905]

[132] Marni R, Kundrapu DB, Chakraborti A, Malla R. Insight into drug sensitizing effect of diallyl disulfide and diallyl trisulfide from Allium sativum L. on paclitaxel-resistant triple-negative breast cancer cells. J Ethnopharmacol 2022; 296: 115452.
[http://dx.doi.org/10.1016/j.jep.2022.115452] [PMID: 35690339]

[133] Chung JG, Hsu SC, Huang AC, Lee JH. Diallyl sulfide, diallyl disulfide and diallyl trisulfide inhibit Ras, ERK, JNK, Cox-2 and NF-κB led to decrease MDR and Mrps expressions in human colon cancer colo 205 cells. FASEB J 2007; 21(6): A793-4.
[http://dx.doi.org/10.1096/fasebj.21.6.A793-d]

[134] Puccinelli M. Effect of diallyl trisulfide on hedgehog signaling in pancreatic cancer cells 2016. Available from: https://docs.lib.purdue.edu/open_access_theses/1132

[135] Mathan SV, Singh R, Kim SH, Singh SV, Singh RP. Diallyl trisulfide induces ros-mediated mitotic arrest and apoptosis and inhibits hnscc tumor growth and cancer stemness. Cancers (Basel) 2024; 16(2): 378.
[http://dx.doi.org/10.3390/cancers16020378] [PMID: 38254868]

[136] Hosono T, Fukao T, Ogihara J, *et al.* Diallyl trisulfide suppresses the proliferation and induces apoptosis of human colon cancer cells through oxidative modification of beta-tubulin. J Biol Chem 2005; 280(50): 41487-93.
[http://dx.doi.org/10.1074/jbc.M507127200] [PMID: 16219763]

[137] Liu Y, Zhu P, Wang Y, *et al.* Antimetastatic therapies of the polysulfide diallyl trisulfide against triple-negative breast cancer (tnbc) *via* suppressing mmp2/9 by blocking nf-κb and erk/mapk signaling pathways. PLoS One 2015; 10(4): e0123781.
[http://dx.doi.org/10.1371/journal.pone.0123781] [PMID: 25927362]

[138] Wang HC, Yang JH, Hsieh SC, Sheen LY. Allyl sulfides inhibit cell growth of skin cancer cells through induction of DNA damage mediated G2/M arrest and apoptosis. J Agric Food Chem 2010; 58(11): 7096-103.
[http://dx.doi.org/10.1021/jf100613x] [PMID: 20459099]

[139] Yu CS, Huang C, Lai KC, *et al.* Diallyl trisulfide induces apoptosis in human primary colorectal cancer cells. Oncol Rep 2012; 28(3): 949-54.
[http://dx.doi.org/10.3892/or.2012.1882] [PMID: 22736270]

[140] Rodríguez De Luna SL, Ramírez-Garza RE, Serna Saldívar SO. Environmentally friendly methods for flavonoid extraction from plant material: Impact of their operating conditions on yield and antioxidant properties. ScientificWorldJournal 2020; 2020: 1-38.
[http://dx.doi.org/10.1155/2020/6792069] [PMID: 32908461]

[141] Saini N, Gahlawat SK, Lather V. Flavonoids: A nutraceutical and its role as anti-inflammatory and

anticancer agent. In: Gahlawat S, Salar R, Siwach P, Duhan J, Kumar S, Kaur P, Eds. Plant Biotechnology: Recent Advancements and Developments. Singapore: Springer 2017. [http://dx.doi.org/10.1007/978-981-10-4732-9_13]

[142] Manach C, Scalbert A, Morand C, Rémésy C, Jiménez L. Polyphenols: food sources and bioavailability. Am J Clin Nutr 2004; 79(5): 727-47. [http://dx.doi.org/10.1093/ajcn/79.5.727] [PMID: 15113710]

[143] Tsao R. Chemistry and biochemistry of dietary polyphenols. Nutrients 2010; 2(12): 1231-46. [http://dx.doi.org/10.3390/nu2121231] [PMID: 22254006]

[144] Santos EL, Maia BHLNS, Ferriani AP, Teixeira SD. Flavonoids: classification, biosynthesis and chemical ecology. InTech 2017. [http://dx.doi.org/10.5772/67861]

[145] Gonzales GB, Smagghe G, Grootaert C, Zotti M, Raes K, Camp JV. Flavonoid interactions during digestion, absorption, distribution and metabolism: a sequential structure–activity/property relationship-based approach in the study of bioavailability and bioactivity. Drug Metab Rev 2015; 47(2): 175-90. [http://dx.doi.org/10.3109/03602532.2014.1003649] [PMID: 25633078]

[146] Nabavi SM, Šamec D, Tomczyk M, *et al.* Flavonoid biosynthetic pathways in plants: Versatile targets for metabolic engineering. Biotechnol Adv 2020; 38: 107316. [http://dx.doi.org/10.1016/j.biotechadv.2018.11.005] [PMID: 30458225]

[147] Ganeshpurkar A, Saluja AK. The pharmacological potential of rutin. Saudi Pharm J 2017; 25(2): 149-64. [http://dx.doi.org/10.1016/j.jsps.2016.04.025] [PMID: 28344465]

[148] Pandey P, Khan F, Qari HA, Oves M. Rutin (bioflavonoid) as cell signaling pathway modulator: prospects in treatment and chemoprevention. pharmaceuticals (basel). 2021; 14(11): 1069. Published 2021 Oct 22. [http://dx.doi.org/10.3390/ph14111069]

[149] Gęgotek A, Rybałtowska-Kawałko P, Skrzydlewska E. Rutin as a mediator of lipid metabolism and cellular signaling pathways interactions in fibroblasts altered by uva and uvb radiation. Oxid Med Cell Longev 2017; 2017(1): 4721352. [http://dx.doi.org/10.1155/2017/4721352] [PMID: 28168010]

[150] Babazadeh A, Ghanbarzadeh B, Hamishehkar H. Phosphatidylcholine-rutin complex as a potential nanocarrier for food applications. J Funct Foods 2017; 33: 134-41. [http://dx.doi.org/10.1016/j.jff.2017.03.038]

[151] Dehelean CA, Coricovac D, Pinzaru I, *et al.* Rutin bioconjugates as potential nutraceutical prodrugs: An *in vitro* and *in ovo* toxicological screening. Front Pharmacol 2022; 13: 1000608. [http://dx.doi.org/10.3389/fphar.2022.1000608] [PMID: 36210849]

[152] Prasad R, Prasad SB. A review on the chemistry and biological properties of Rutin, a promising nutraceutical agent. Asian J Pharm Pharmacol 2019; 5(S1): 1-20. [http://dx.doi.org/10.31024/ajpp.2019.5.s1.1]

[153] Boyle SP, Dobson VL, Duthie SJ, Hinselwood DC, Kyle JAM, Collins AR. Bioavailability and efficiency of rutin as an antioxidant: a human supplementation study. Eur J Clin Nutr 2000; 54(10): 774-82. [http://dx.doi.org/10.1038/sj.ejcn.1601090] [PMID: 11083486]

[154] Chen P, Yuan C, Hong Z, *et al.* Revealing the mechanism of "Huai Hua San" in the treatment of ulcerative colitis based on network pharmacology and experimental study. J Ethnopharmacol 2021; 281: 114321. [http://dx.doi.org/10.1016/j.jep.2021.114321] [PMID: 34118340]

[155] Roy D, Mukherjee D, Ghosh M, Adhikari D, Rangra NK, Singh A. Rutin's efficacy as a potent

flavonoid in the management of colitis. Nature Cell and Science 2024; (3): 121-132. [http://dx.doi.org/10.61474/ncs.2024.00027]

[156] Bazyar H, Zare Javid A, Ahangarpour A, *et al.* The effects of rutin supplement on blood pressure markers, some serum antioxidant enzymes, and quality of life in patients with type 2 diabetes mellitus compared with placebo 2023. [http://dx.doi.org/10.3389/fnut.2023.1214420]

[157] Stabrauskiene J, Kopustinskiene DM, Lazauskas R, Bernatoniene J. Naringin and naringenin: their mechanisms of action and the potential anticancer activities. Biomedicines 2022; 10(7): 1686. [http://dx.doi.org/10.3390/biomedicines10071686] [PMID: 35884991]

[158] Sharma A, Bhardwaj P, Arya SK. Naringin: A potential natural product in the field of biomedical applications. Carbohydrate Polymer Technologies and Applications 2021; 2: 100068. [http://dx.doi.org/10.1016/j.carpta.2021.100068]

[159] Singh S, Sharma A, Monga V, Bhatia R. Compendium of naringenin: potential sources, analytical aspects, chemistry, nutraceutical potentials and pharmacological profile. Crit Rev Food Sci Nutr 2023; 63(27): 8868-99. [http://dx.doi.org/10.1080/10408398.2022.2056726] [PMID: 35357240]

[160] Massaro L, Raguzzini A, Aiello P, Valencia DV. The potential role of naringin and naringenin as nutraceuticals against metabolic syndrome. Endocr Metab Immune Disord Drug Targets 2023; 23(4): 428-45. [http://dx.doi.org/10.2174/1871530322666220827141203] [PMID: 36043734]

[161] Saxena D, Sharma U, Rawat A. A review of naringenin's nutraceutical properties: a boon in the sustainable food system, 2024.

[162] Rajadurai M, Prince PSM. Naringin ameliorates mitochondrial lipid peroxides, antioxidants and lipids in isoproterenol-induced myocardial infarction in Wistar rats. Phytother Res 2009; 23(3): 358-62. [http://dx.doi.org/10.1002/ptr.2632] [PMID: 18844325]

[163] Reshef N, Hayari Y, Goren C, Boaz M, Madar Z, Knobler H. Antihypertensive effect of sweetie fruit in patients with stage I hypertension. Am J Hypertens 2005; 18(10): 1360-3. [http://dx.doi.org/10.1016/j.amjhyper.2005.05.021] [PMID: 16202862]

[164] Toth PP, Patti AM, Nikolic D, *et al.* Bergamot reduces plasma lipids, atherogenic small dense LDL, and subclinical atherosclerosis in subjects with moderate hypercholesterolemia: A 6 months prospective study. Front Pharmacol 2016; 6: 299. [http://dx.doi.org/10.3389/fphar.2015.00299] [PMID: 26779019]

[165] Mollace V, Sacco I, Janda E, *et al.* Hypolipemic and hypoglycaemic activity of bergamot polyphenols: From animal models to human studies. Fitoterapia 2011; 82(3): 309-16. [http://dx.doi.org/10.1016/j.fitote.2010.10.014] [PMID: 21056640]

[166] Habauzit V, Verny MA, Milenkovic D, *et al.* Flavanones protect from arterial stiffness in postmenopausal women consuming grapefruit juice for 6 mo: a randomized, controlled, crossover trial. Am J Clin Nutr 2015; 102(1): 66-74. [http://dx.doi.org/10.3945/ajcn.114.104646] [PMID: 26016866]

[167] Naeini F, Namkhah Z, Tutunchi H, *et al.* Effects of naringenin supplementation in overweight/obese patients with non-alcoholic fatty liver disease: study protocol for a randomized double-blind clinical trial. Trials 2021; 22(1): 801. [http://dx.doi.org/10.1186/s13063-021-05784-7] [PMID: 34774104]

[168] Rebello CJ, Beyl RA, Lertora JJL, *et al.* Safety and pharmacokinetics of naringenin: A randomized, controlled, single-ascending-dose clinical trial. Diabetes Obes Metab 2020; 22(1): 91-8. [http://dx.doi.org/10.1111/dom.13868] [PMID: 31468636]

[169] Soliman NA, Abdel Ghafar MT, AbuoHashish NA, *et al.* The possible role of naringenin in the prevention of alcohol-induced neurochemical and neurobehavioral deficits. Neurochem Res 2023;

48(2): 537-50.
[http://dx.doi.org/10.1007/s11064-022-03775-x] [PMID: 36242717]

[170] Boots AW, Haenen GRMM, Bast A. Health effects of quercetin: From antioxidant to nutraceutical. Eur J Pharmacol 2008; 585(2-3): 325-37.
[http://dx.doi.org/10.1016/j.ejphar.2008.03.008] [PMID: 18417116]

[171] Aghababaei F, Hadidi M. Recent advances in potential health benefits of quercetin. Pharmaceuticals (Basel) 2023; 16(7): 1020.
[http://dx.doi.org/10.3390/ph16071020] [PMID: 37513932]

[172] Shabir I, Kumar Pandey V, Shams R, *et al.* Promising bioactive properties of quercetin for potential food applications and health benefits: A review. Front Nutr 2022; 9: 999752.
[http://dx.doi.org/10.3389/fnut.2022.999752] [PMID: 36532555]

[173] Zahedi M, Ghiasvand R, Feizi A, Asgari G, Darvish L. Does quercetin improve cardiovascular risk factors and inflammatory biomarkers in women with type 2 diabetes: A double-blind randomized controlled clinical trial. Int J Prev Med 2013; 4(7): 777-85.
[PMID: 24049596]

[174] Pfeuffer M, Auinger A, Bley U, *et al.* Effect of quercetin on traits of the metabolic syndrome, endothelial function and inflammation in men with different APOE isoforms. Nutr Metab Cardiovasc Dis 2013; 23(5): 403-9.
[http://dx.doi.org/10.1016/j.numecd.2011.08.010] [PMID: 22118955]

[175] Hickson LJ, Langhi Prata LGP, Bobart SA, *et al.* Senolytics decrease senescent cells in humans: Preliminary report from a clinical trial of Dasatinib plus Quercetin in individuals with diabetic kidney disease. EBioMedicine 2019; 47: 446-56.
[http://dx.doi.org/10.1016/j.ebiom.2019.08.069] [PMID: 31542391]

[176] Sajadi Hezaveh Z, Azarkeivan A, Janani L, Hosseini S, Shidfar F. The effect of quercetin on iron overload and inflammation in β-thalassemia major patients: A double-blind randomized clinical trial. Complement Ther Med 2019; 46: 24-8.
[http://dx.doi.org/10.1016/j.ctim.2019.02.017] [PMID: 31519283]

[177] Javadi F, Ahmadzadeh A, Eghtesadi S, *et al.* The effect of quercetin on inflammatory factors and clinical symptoms in women with rheumatoid arthritis: a double-blind, randomized controlled trial. J Am Coll Nutr 2017; 36(1): 9-15.
[http://dx.doi.org/10.1080/07315724.2016.1140093] [PMID: 27710596]

[178] Rezvan N, Moini A, Gorgani-Firuzjaee S, Hosseinzadeh-Attar MJ. Oral quercetin supplementation enhances adiponectin receptor transcript expression in polycystic ovary syndrome patients: A randomized placebo-controlled double-blind clinical trial. Cell J 2018; 19(4): 627-33.
[http://dx.doi.org/10.22074/cellj.2018.4577] [PMID: 29105398]

[179] Hussain SA, Ahmed ZA, Mahwi TO, Aziz TA. Quercetin dampens postprandial hyperglycemia in type 2 diabetic patients challenged with carbohydrates load. Int J Diabetes Res 2012; 1: 32-5.
[http://dx.doi.org/10.5923/j.diabetes.20120103.01]

[180] Dehghani F, Sezavar Seyedi Jandaghi SH, Janani L, Sarebanhassanabadi M, Emamat H, Vafa M. Effects of quercetin supplementation on inflammatory factors and quality of life in post-myocardial infarction patients: A double blind, placebo-controlled, randomized clinical trial. Phytother Res 2021; 35(4): 2085-98.
[http://dx.doi.org/10.1002/ptr.6955] [PMID: 33216421]

[181] Jan R, Khan M, Asaf S, Lubna , Asif S, Kim KM. Bioactivity and therapeutic potential of kaempferol and quercetin: new insights for plant and human health. Plants 2022; 11(19): 2623.
[http://dx.doi.org/10.3390/plants11192623] [PMID: 36235488]

[182] Bharathy P, Thanikachalam PV. Pharmacological relevance of Anthocyanin derivative: A review. Pharmacological Research -. Zhongguo Xiandai Zhongyao 2024; 100565.

[183] Posadino AM, Giordo R, Ramli I, *et al.* An updated overview of cyanidins for chemoprevention and cancer therapy. Biomed Pharmacother 2023; 163: 114783.
[http://dx.doi.org/10.1016/j.biopha.2023.114783] [PMID: 37121149]

[184] Posadino AM, Giordo R, Ramli I, *et al.* An updated overview of cyanidins for chemoprevention and cancer therapy. Biomedicine & Pharmacotherapy 2023; 163: 114783.
[http://dx.doi.org/10.1016/J.BIOPHA.2023.114783]

[185] Bub A, Watzl B, Heeb D, Rechkemmer G, Briviba K. Malvidin-3-glucoside bioavailability in humans after ingestion of red wine, dealcoholized red wine and red grape juice. Eur J Nutr 2001; 40(3): 113-20.
[http://dx.doi.org/10.1007/s003940170011] [PMID: 11697443]

[186] Lapidot T, Harel S, Granit R, Kanner J. Bioavailability of red wine anthocyanins as detected in human urine. J Agric Food Chem 1998; 46(10): 4297-302.
[http://dx.doi.org/10.1021/jf980007o]

[187] Alvarez-Suarez JM, Giampieri F, Tulipani S, *et al.* One-month strawberry-rich anthocyanin supplementation ameliorates cardiovascular risk, oxidative stress markers and platelet activation in humans. J Nutr Biochem 2014; 25(3): 289-94.
[http://dx.doi.org/10.1016/j.jnutbio.2013.11.002] [PMID: 24406274]

[188] Shim SH, Kim JM, Choi CY, Kim CY, Park KH. Ginkgo biloba extract and bilberry anthocyanins improve visual function in patients with normal tension glaucoma. J Med Food 2012; 15(9): 818-23.
[http://dx.doi.org/10.1089/jmf.2012.2241] [PMID: 22870951]

[189] Miyake S, Takahashi N, Sasaki M, Kobayashi S, Tsubota K, Ozawa Y. Vision preservation during retinal inflammation by anthocyanin-rich bilberry extract: cellular and molecular mechanism. Lab Invest 2012; 92(1): 102-9.
[http://dx.doi.org/10.1038/labinvest.2011.132] [PMID: 21894150]

[190] Ohguro H, Ohguro I, Katai M, Tanaka S. Two-year randomized, placebo-controlled study of black currant anthocyanins on visual field in glaucoma. Ophthalmologica 2012; 228(1): 26-35.
[http://dx.doi.org/10.1159/000335961] [PMID: 22377796]

[191] Aboonabi A, Aboonabi A. Anthocyanins reduce inflammation and improve glucose and lipid metabolism associated with inhibiting nuclear factor-kappaB activation and increasing PPAR-γ gene expression in metabolic syndrome subjects. Free Radic Biol Med 2020; 150: 30-9.
[http://dx.doi.org/10.1016/j.freeradbiomed.2020.02.004] [PMID: 32061902]

[192] Aboonabi A, Meyer RR, Gaiz A, Singh I. Anthocyanins in berries exhibited anti-atherogenicity and antiplatelet activities in a metabolic syndrome population. Nutr Res 2020; 76: 82-93.
[http://dx.doi.org/10.1016/j.nutres.2020.02.011] [PMID: 32217379]

[193] Anuyahong T, Chusak C, Thilavech T, Adisakwattana S. Postprandial effect of yogurt enriched with anthocyanins from riceberry rice on glycemic response and antioxidant capacity in healthy adults. Nutrients 2020; 12(10): 2930.
[http://dx.doi.org/10.3390/nu12102930] [PMID: 32987943]

[194] Feng RC, Dong YH, Hong XL, Su Y, Wu XV. Effects of anthocyanin-rich supplementation on cognition of the cognitively healthy middle-aged and older adults: a systematic review and meta-analysis of randomized controlled trials. Nutr Rev 2023; 81(3): 287-303.
[http://dx.doi.org/10.1093/nutrit/nuac055] [PMID: 35960187]

[195] Sergio Davinelli PhD, Juan Carlos Bertoglio MD, PhD, Armando ZarrelliPhD, Riccardo Pina PhD and Giovanni Scapagnini MD, PhD. A Randomized Clinical TrialEvaluating the Efficacy of an Anthocyanin–Maqui Berry Extract (Delphinol®) on OxidativeStress Biomarkers, Journal of the American College of Nutrition, 2015; 34:sup1, 28-33.

[196] Kizawa Y, Sekikawa T, Kageyama M, Tomobe H, Kobashi R, Yamada T. Effects of anthocyanin, astaxanthin, and lutein on eye functions: a randomized, double-blind, placebo-controlled study. J Clin

Biochem Nutr 2021; 69(1): 77-90.
[http://dx.doi.org/10.3164/jcbn.20-149] [PMID: 34376917]

[197] Niemeyer ED, Brodbelt JS. Isomeric differentiation of green tea catechins using gas-phase hydrogen/deuterium exchange reactions. J Am Soc Mass Spectrom 2007; 18(10): 1749-59.
[http://dx.doi.org/10.1016/j.jasms.2007.07.009] [PMID: 17702600]

[198] Bae J, Kim N, Shin Y, Kim SY, Kim YJ. Activity of catechins and their applications. Biomed Dermatol 2020; 4(1): 8.
[http://dx.doi.org/10.1186/s41702-020-0057-8]

[199] Gadkari PV, Balaraman M. Catechins: Sources, extraction and encapsulation: A review. Food Bioprod Process 2015; 93: 122-38.
[http://dx.doi.org/10.1016/j.fbp.2013.12.004]

[200] Ding Y, Li H, Cao S, Yu Y. Effects of catechin on the malignant biological behavior of gastric cancer cells through the PI3K/Akt signaling pathway. Toxicol Appl Pharmacol 2024; 490: 117036.
[http://dx.doi.org/10.1016/j.taap.2024.117036] [PMID: 39009138]

[201] Sistanipour E, Meshkini A, Oveisi H. Catechin-conjugated mesoporous hydroxyapatite nanoparticle: A novel nano-antioxidant with enhanced osteogenic property. Colloids Surf B Biointerfaces 2018; 169: 329-39.
[http://dx.doi.org/10.1016/j.colsurfb.2018.05.046] [PMID: 29800908]

[202] Kaur R, Rajput R, Nag P, Kumar S, Rachana MS, Singh M. Synthesis, characterization and evaluation of antioxidant properties of catechin hydrate nanoparticles. J Drug Deliv Sci Technol 2017; 39: 398-407.
[http://dx.doi.org/10.1016/j.jddst.2017.04.030]

[203] Abdulsalam M. Kassem, May Almukainzi, Tarek M. *et al.* A pH-sensitive silica nanoparticles for colon-specific delivery and controlled release of catechin: Optimization of loading efficiency and *in vitro* release kinetics. Eur J Pharm Sci 2024; 192: 106652.

[204] Mahmoodi M, Hosseini R, Kazemi A, Ofori-Asenso R, Mazidi M, Mazloomi SM. Effects of green tea or green tea catechin on liver enzymes in healthy individuals and people with nonalcoholic fatty liver disease: A systematic review and meta-analysis of randomized clinical trials. Phytother Res 2020; 34(7): 1587-98.
[http://dx.doi.org/10.1002/ptr.6637] [PMID: 32067271]

[205] Xu R, Yang K, Li S, Dai M, Chen G. Effect of green tea consumption on blood lipids: a systematic review and meta-analysis of randomized controlled trials 2020.
[http://dx.doi.org/10.1186/s12937-020-00557-5]

[206] Samavat H, Newman AR, Wang R, Yuan JM, Wu AH, Kurzer MS. Effects of green tea catechin extract on serum lipids in postmenopausal women: a randomized, placebo-controlled clinical trial. Am J Clin Nutr 2016; 104(6): 1671-82.
[http://dx.doi.org/10.3945/ajcn.116.137075] [PMID: 27806972]

[207] Yoshitomi R, Yamamoto M, Kumazoe M, *et al.* The combined effect of green tea and α-glucosyl hesperidin in preventing obesity: a randomized placebo-controlled clinical trial. Sci Rep 2021; 11(1): 19067.
[http://dx.doi.org/10.1038/s41598-021-98612-6] [PMID: 34561541]

[208] Amit Baran Das VV. Goud, Chandan Das, 9 - Phenolic compounds as functional ingredients in beverages, editor(s): alexandru mihai grumezescu, alina maria holban, value-added ingredients and enrichments of beverages, Academic Press. 2019: 285-323.

[209] Jiang N, Doseff A, Grotewold E. Flavones: from biosynthesis to health benefits. Plants 2016; 5(2): 27.
[http://dx.doi.org/10.3390/plants5020027] [PMID: 27338492]

[210] Punia Bangar S, Kajla P, Chaudhary V, Sharma N, Ozogul F. Luteolin: A flavone with myriads of bioactivities and food applications. Food Biosci 2023; 52: 102366.

[http://dx.doi.org/10.1016/j.fbio.2023.102366]

[211] Xue JC, Yuan S, Meng H, *et al.* The role and mechanism of flavonoid herbal natural products in ulcerative colitis. Biomed Pharmacother 2023; 158: 114086. [http://dx.doi.org/10.1016/j.biopha.2022.114086] [PMID: 36502751]

[212] D'Ascanio L, Vitelli F, Cingolani C, Maranzano M, Brenner MJ, Di Stadio A. Randomized clinical trial "olfactory dysfunction after COVID-19: olfactory rehabilitation therapy *vs.* intervention treatment with Palmitoylethanolamide and Luteolin": preliminary results. Eur Rev Med Pharmacol Sci 2021; 25(11): 4156-62. [http://dx.doi.org/10.26355/eurrev_202106_26059] [PMID: 34156697]

[213] Hsu YL, Hou MF, Tsai EM, Kuo PL. Tricetin, a dietary flavonoid, induces apoptosis through the reactive oxygen species/c-Jun NH2-terminal kinase pathway in human liver cancer cells. J Agric Food Chem 2010; 58(23): 12547-56. [http://dx.doi.org/10.1021/jf103159r] [PMID: 21067180]

[214] Nagy-Pénzes M, Hajnády Z, Regdon Z, *et al.* Tricetin reduces inflammation and acinar cell injury in cerulein-induced acute pancreatitis: the role of oxidative stress-induced dna damage signaling. Biomedicines. 2022; 10(6): 1371. Published 2022 Jun 10. [http://dx.doi.org/10.3390/biomedicines10061371]

[215] Ko KP. Isoflavones: chemistry, analysis, functions and effects on health and cancer. Asian Pac J Cancer Prev 2014; 15(17): 7001-10. [http://dx.doi.org/10.7314/APJCP.2014.15.17.7001] [PMID: 25227781]

[216] Dakora FD, Phillips DA. Diverse functions of isoflavonoids in legumes transcend anti-microbial definitions of phytoalexins. Physiol Mol Plant Pathol 1996; 49(1): 1-20. [http://dx.doi.org/10.1006/pmpp.1996.0035]

[217] Křížová L, Dadáková K, Kašparovská J, Kašparovský T. Isoflavones. Molecules. 2019; 24(6): 1076. Published 2019 Mar 19. [http://dx.doi.org/10.3390/molecules24061076]

[218] Shu XO, Zheng Y, Cai H, *et al.* Soy food intake and breast cancer survival. JAMA 2009; 302(22): 2437-43. [http://dx.doi.org/10.1001/jama.2009.1783] [PMID: 19996398]

[219] Yan L, Spitznagel EL. Soy consumption and prostate cancer risk in men: a revisit of a meta-analysis. Am J Clin Nutr 2009; 89(4): 1155-63. [http://dx.doi.org/10.3945/ajcn.2008.27029] [PMID: 19211820]

[220] Wiseman H, O'Reilly JD, Adlercreutz H, *et al.* Isoflavone phytoestrogens consumed in soy decrease F2-isoprostane concentrations and increase resistance of low-density lipoprotein to oxidation in humans. Am J Clin Nutr 2000; 72(2): 395-400. [http://dx.doi.org/10.1093/ajcn/72.2.395] [PMID: 10919933]

[221] Sakai E, Farhana F, Yamaguchi Y, Tsukuba T. Chapter 1 - Potentials of natural antioxidants from plants as antiosteoporotic agents, Editor(s): Atta-ur-Rahman. Studies in Natural Products Chemistry, Elsevier. 2022; 72: 1-28.

[222] Nabavi S, Nabavi S, Daglia M, *et al.* Daidzein and its effects on brain. Curr Med Chem 2017; 24(4): 365-75. [http://dx.doi.org/10.2174/0929867323666161101140214] [PMID: 27804870]

[223] Komrakova M, Klara Stuermer E, Michael Stuermer K, Sehmisch S. Isoflavones: chemistry, analysis, function and effects. The Royal Society of Chemistry 2012; pp. 597-610. [http://dx.doi.org/10.1039/9781849735094-00597]

[224] Sirotkin AV, Alwasel SH, Harrath AH. The influence of plant isoflavones daidzein and equol on female reproductive processes 2021. [http://dx.doi.org/10.3390/ph14040373]

[225] Ubaid M. Salauddin, Shadani MA, *et al.* Daidzein from dietary supplement to a drug candidate: An evaluation of potential. *ACS Omega.* 2023; 8(36): 32271-32293. Published 2023; 27. [http://dx.doi.org/10.1021/acsomega.3c03741]

[226] Dijkstra SC, Lampe SC, Ray RM, *et al.* Biomarkers of dietary exposure are associated with lower risk of breast fibroadenomas in Chinese women. J Nutr 2010; 140(7): 1302-10. [http://dx.doi.org/10.3945/jn.109.119727] [PMID: 20484550]

[227] Bitto A, Polito F, Squadrito F, *et al.* Genistein aglycone: a dual mode of action anti-osteoporotic soy isoflavone rebalancing bone turnover towards bone formation. Curr Med Chem 2010; 17(27): 3007-18. [http://dx.doi.org/10.2174/092986710791959738] [PMID: 20629630]

[228] Lazarevic B, Hammarström C, Yang J, *et al.* The effects of short-term genistein intervention on prostate biomarker expression in patients with localised prostate cancer before radical prostatectomy. Br J Nutr 2012; 108(12): 2138-47. [http://dx.doi.org/10.1017/S0007114512000384] [PMID: 22397815]

[229] Yasuda M, Sugahara K, Zhang J, Shuin T, Kodama H. Effect of cisplatin treatment on the urinary excretion of guanidinoacetic acid, creatinine and creatine in patients with urinary tract neoplasm, and on superoxide generation in human neutrophils. Physiol Chem Phys Med NMR 2000; 32(2): 119-25. [PMID: 11383133]

[230] Löhr JM, Karimi M, Omazic B, *et al.* A phase I dose escalation trial of AXP107-11, a novel multi-component crystalline form of genistein, in combination with gemcitabine in chemotherapy-naive patients with unresectable pancreatic cancer. Pancreatology 2016; 16(4): 640-5. [http://dx.doi.org/10.1016/j.pan.2016.05.002] [PMID: 27234064]

[231] Marini H, Bitto A, Altavilla D, *et al.* Efficacy of genistein aglycone on some cardiovascular risk factors and homocysteine levels: A follow-up study. Nutr Metab Cardiovasc Dis 2010; 20(5): 332-40. [http://dx.doi.org/10.1016/j.numecd.2009.04.012] [PMID: 19631515]

[232] Squadrito F, Marini H, Bitto A, *et al.* Genistein in the metabolic syndrome: results of a randomized clinical trial. J Clin Endocrinol Metab 2013; 98(8): 3366-74. [http://dx.doi.org/10.1210/jc.2013-1180] [PMID: 23824420]

[233] Okamura S, Sawada Y, Satoh T, *et al.* Pueraria mirifica phytoestrogens improve dyslipidemia in postmenopausal women probably by activating estrogen receptor subtypes. Tohoku J Exp Med 2008; 216(4): 341-51. [http://dx.doi.org/10.1620/tjem.216.341] [PMID: 19060449]

[234] R. W, e Silva MLA, Sola Veneziani RC, Ricardo S, Kenupp J. Lignans: Chemical and biological properties [Internet]. Phytochemicals - A Global Perspective of Their Role in Nutrition and Health. InTech; 2012. [http://dx.doi.org/10.5772/28471]

[235] Mukhija M, Joshi BC, Bairy PS, Bhargava A, Sah AN. Lignans: a versatile source of anticancer drugs. Beni Suef Univ J Basic Appl Sci 2022; 11(1): 76. [http://dx.doi.org/10.1186/s43088-022-00256-6] [PMID: 35694188]

[236] Demark-Wahnefried W, Robertson CN, Walther PJ, Polascik TJ, Paulson DF, Vollmer RT. Pilot study to explore effects of low-fat, flaxseed-supplemented diet on proliferation of benign prostatic epithelium and prostate-specific antigen. Urology 2004; 63(5): 900-4. [http://dx.doi.org/10.1016/j.urology.2003.12.010] [PMID: 15134976]

[237] Peterson J, Dwyer J, Adlercreutz H, Scalbert A, Jacques P, McCullough ML. Dietary lignans: physiology and potential for cardiovascular disease risk reduction. Nutr Rev 2010; 68(10): 571-603. [http://dx.doi.org/10.1111/j.1753-4887.2010.00319.x] [PMID: 20883417]

[238] Hu Y, Li Y, Sampson L, *et al.* Lignan intake and risk of coronary heart disease. J Am Coll Cardiol 2021; 78(7): 666-78.

[http://dx.doi.org/10.1016/j.jacc.2021.05.049] [PMID: 34384548]

[239] Nowak DA, Snyder DC, Brown AJ, Demark-Wahnefried W. The effect of flaxseed supplementation on hormonal levels associated with polycystic ovarian syndrome: a case study. Curr Top Nutraceutical Res 2007; 5(4): 177-81.
[PMID: 19789727]

[240] Wang S, Hu Y, Liu B, Li Y, Wang M, Sun Q. Lignan intake and type 2 diabetes incidence among us men and women. JAMA Netw Open 2024; 7(8): e2426367.
[http://dx.doi.org/10.1001/jamanetworkopen.2024.26367] [PMID: 39110458]

[241] Abuajah CI, Ogbonna AC, Osuji CM. Functional components and medicinal properties of food: a review. J Food Sci Technol 2015; 52(5): 2522-9.
[http://dx.doi.org/10.1007/s13197-014-1396-5] [PMID: 25892752]

[242] Safety assessment and potential health benefits of food components based on selected scientific criteria. Crit Rev Food Sci Nutr 1999; 39(3): 203-6.
[http://dx.doi.org/10.1080/10408699991279169] [PMID: 10367185]

[243] Paudel D, Dhungana B, Caffe M, Krishnan P. A review of health-beneficial properties of oats 2021.
[http://dx.doi.org/10.3390/foods10112591]

[244] Djorgbenoo R, Hu J, Hu C, Sang S. Fermented oats as a novel functional food 2023.
[http://dx.doi.org/10.3390/nu15163521]

[245] Xu D, Feng M, Chu Y, *et al.* The prebiotic effects of oats on blood lipids, gut microbiota, and short-chain fatty acids in mildly hypercholesterolemic subjects compared with rice: a randomized, controlled trial. Front Immunol 2021; 12: 787797.
[http://dx.doi.org/10.3389/fimmu.2021.787797] [PMID: 34956218]

[246] Onipe OO, Jideani AIO, Beswa D. Composition and functionality of wheat bran and its application in some cereal food products. Int J Food Sci Technol 2015; 50(12): 2509-18.
[http://dx.doi.org/10.1111/ijfs.12935]

[247] Yao W, Gong Y, Li L, Hu X, You L. The effects of dietary fibers from rice bran and wheat bran on gut microbiota: An overview. Food Chem X 2022; 13: 100252.
[http://dx.doi.org/10.1016/j.fochx.2022.100252]

[248] Li C, Stump M, Wu W, Li Y. Exploring the chemical composition, antioxidant potential, and bread quality effects of the nutritional powerhouse: Wheat bran – A mini-review. Journal of Agriculture and Food Research 2023; 14: 100898.
[http://dx.doi.org/10.1016/j.jafr.2023.100898]

[249] Shen X, Zhao T, Zhou Y, Shi X, Zou Y, Zhao G. Effect of oat β-glucan intake on glycaemic control and insulin sensitivity of diabetic patients: a meta-analysis of randomized controlled trials. Nutrients 2016; 8(1): 39.
[http://dx.doi.org/10.3390/nu8010039] [PMID: 26771637]

[250] Keenan JM, Goulson M, Shamliyan T, Knutson N, Kolberg L, Curry L. The effects of concentrated barley β-glucan on blood lipids in a population of hypercholesterolaemic men and women. Br J Nutr 2007; 97(6): 1162-8.
[http://dx.doi.org/10.1017/S0007114507682968] [PMID: 17445284]

[251] Gul K, Yousuf B, Singh AK, Singh P, Wani AA. Rice bran: Nutritional values and its emerging potential for development of functional food—A review. Bioactive Carbohydrates and Dietary Fibre 2015; 6(1): 24-30.
[http://dx.doi.org/10.1016/j.bcdf.2015.06.002]

[252] Alauddin Md, Islam J, Shirakawa H, Koseki T. Ardiansyah, komai m rice bran as a functional food: an overview of the conversion of rice bran into a superfood/functional food. Superfood and Functional Food - An Overview of Their Processing and Utilization. InTech 2017. Internet
[http://dx.doi.org/10.5772/66298]

[253] Ardiansyah SH, Shirakawa H, Shimeno T, *et al.* Adenosine, an identified active component from the Driselase-treated fraction of rice bran, is effective at improving metabolic syndrome in stroke-prone spontaneously hypertensive rats. J Agric Food Chem 2009; 57(6): 2558-64. [http://dx.doi.org/10.1021/jf803347c] [PMID: 19292472]

[254] Ardiansyah OY, Ohsaki Y, Shirakawa H, Koseki T, Komai M. Novel effects of a single administration of ferulic acid on the regulation of blood pressure and the hepatic lipid metabolic profile in stroke-prone spontaneously hypertensive rats. J Agric Food Chem 2008; 56(8): 2825-30. [http://dx.doi.org/10.1021/jf072896y] [PMID: 18345632]

[255] Manzoor A, Pandey VK, Dar AH, *et al.* Rice bran: Nutritional, phytochemical, and pharmacological profile and its contribution to human health promotion. Food Chemistry Advances 2023; 2: 100296. [http://dx.doi.org/10.1016/j.focha.2023.100296]

[256] Alauddin Md. Sadia Rahman, Jahidul Islam, Hitoshi Shirakawa, Michio Komai, Md Zakir Hossen Howlader. Chapter 8 - Development of Rice Bran Functional Food and Evaluation of Its Healthful Properties. Editor(s): Ling-Zhi Cheong, Xuebing Xu. Rice Bran and Rice Bran Oil. AOCS Press. 2019: 183-206.

[257] Hongu N, Kitts DD, Zawistowski J, *et al.* Pigmented rice bran and plant sterol combination reduces serum lipids in overweight and obese adults. J Am Coll Nutr 2014; 33(3): 231-8. [http://dx.doi.org/10.1080/07315724.2013.869772] [PMID: 24955613]

[258] Ito Y, Nakashima Y, Matsuoka S. Rice bran extract containing acylated steryl glucoside fraction decreases elevated blood LDL cholesterol level in obese Japanese men. J Med Invest 2015; 62(1.2): 80-4. [http://dx.doi.org/10.2152/jmi.62.80] [PMID: 25817289]

[259] Nhung BT, Tuyen LD, Linh VA, *et al.* Rice bran extract reduces the risk of atherosclerosis in post-menopausal Vietnamese women. J Nutr Sci Vitaminol (Tokyo) 2016; 62(5): 295-302. [http://dx.doi.org/10.3177/jnsv.62.295] [PMID: 27928115]

[260] Edrisi F, Salehi M, Ahmadi A, Fararoei M, Rusta F, Mahmoodianfard S. Effects of supplementation with rice husk powder and rice bran on inflammatory factors in overweight and obese adults following an energy-restricted diet: a randomized controlled trial. Eur J Nutr 2018; 57(2): 833-43. [http://dx.doi.org/10.1007/s00394-017-1555-3] [PMID: 29063186]

[261] Qureshi AA, Sami SA, Khan FA. Effects of stabilized rice bran, its soluble and fiber fractions on blood glucose levels and serum lipid parameters in humans with diabetes mellitus Types I and II. J Nutr Biochem 2002; 13(3): 175-87. [http://dx.doi.org/10.1016/S0955-2863(01)00211-X] [PMID: 11893482]

[262] Chauhan K, Yadav N, Singh R, Kumar A, Mandakini H, Kumar N. Seafood as functional food ingredients and nutraceuticals. In: Bashir K, Jan K, Ahmad FJ, Eds. Functional Foods and Nutraceuticals: Chemistry, Health Benefits and the Way Forward. Cham: Springer 2024. [http://dx.doi.org/10.1007/978-3-031-59365-9_10]

[263] Shahidi F, Ambigaipalan P. Novel functional food ingredients from marine sources. Curr Opin Food Sci 2015; 2: 123-9. [http://dx.doi.org/10.1016/j.cofs.2014.12.009]

[264] Gormley T. Ronan. Fish as a functional food. Food Sci Technol (Campinas) 2006; 20(3): 25-8.

[265] He K, Song Y, Daviglus M L, *et al.* Accumulated evidence on fish consumption and coronary heart disease mortality: a meta-analysis of cohort studies 2004. [http://dx.doi.org/10.1161/01.CIR.0000132503.19410.6B]

[266] Dórea JG, da Costa THM. Is coffee a functional food? Br J Nutr 2005; 93(6): 773-82. [http://dx.doi.org/10.1079/BJN20051370] [PMID: 16022745]

[267] Wang Q, Hu GL, Qiu MH, Cao J, Xiong WY. Coffee, tea, and cocoa in obesity prevention: Mechanisms of action and future prospects. Current Research in Food Science 2024; 8: 100741.

[http://dx.doi.org/10.1016/j.crfs.2024.100741] [PMID: 38694556]

[268] Ye L, Wang H, Duncan SE, Eigel WN, O'Keefe SF. Antioxidant activities of Vine Tea (Ampelopsis grossedentata) extract and its major component dihydromyricetin in soybean oil and cooked ground beef. Food Chem 2015; 172: 416-22.
[http://dx.doi.org/10.1016/j.foodchem.2014.09.090] [PMID: 25442572]

[269] Liu Y, Guo C, Zang E, *et al.* Review on herbal tea as a functional food: classification, active compounds, biological activity, and industrial status. Journal of Future Foods 2023; 3(3): 206-19.
[http://dx.doi.org/10.1016/j.jfutfo.2023.02.002]

[270] Wink M. Modes of action of herbal medicines and plant secondary metabolites. Medicines 2015; 2(3): 251-86.
[http://dx.doi.org/10.3390/medicines2030251]

[271] McKay DL, Blumberg JB. A review of the bioactivity and potential health benefits of herbal teas. Phytother Res 2007; 21(6): 519-30.
[http://dx.doi.org/10.1002/ptr.2072]

[272] Crozier A, Jaganath IB, Clifford MN. Dietary phenolics: chemistry, bioavailability and effects on health. Nat Prod Rep 2009; 26(8): 1001-43.
[http://dx.doi.org/10.1039/b802662a]

[273] Poswal FS, Russell G, Mackonochie M, MacLennan E, Adukwu EC, Rolfe V. Herbal teas and their health benefits: A scoping review. Plant Foods Hum Nutr 2019; 74(3): 266-76.
[http://dx.doi.org/10.1007/s11130-019-00750-w]

CHAPTER 9

Herbs as Nutraceuticals

Mukesh Singh Sikarwar[1,*], **Vaibhav Kumar Rathi**[2] and **Maulshree Bhandari**[3]

[1] *Amity Institute of Pharmacy, Amity University, Gwalior, Madhya Pradesh, India*

[2] *Department of Pharmacy, Quantum University, Roorkee (Haridwar), Uttarakhand, India*

[3] *Invertis Institute of Pharmacy, Invertis University, Bareilly, Uttar Pradesh, India*

Abstract: Herbal drugs are best utilized as nutraceuticals due to the presence of a variety of phytochemicals. Nutraceuticals are gaining popularity due to their pivotal role in the management of chronic diseases, especially noncommunicable diseases. Inflammation and oxidative stress are the underlying causes for multiple diseases, including diabetes, cardiovascular disease, cancer, and liver diseases. Most of the herbs contain pigments like chlorophyll in leaves, flavonoids in fruits and flowers, tannins in bark (stem and roots), carbohydrates in exudates like gum and mucilage, and alkaloids in different parts of the plants. These phytochemicals are extensively studied for their reactive oxygen species quenching potential and prevention of low-grade inflammation, hence used as nutraceuticals in the prevention and management of diseases as an adjuvant to the primary treatment. This chapter compiles the pharmacognostical and chemical background, including pharmacological and clinical studies on these herbs. Popular herbal drugs like Andrographis, Ashwagandha, Bramhi, Boswellia, fenugreek, garlic, ginger, gingko, ginseng, kelp, milk thistle, psyllium husk, St. John's Wort, turmeric, valerian, spirulina, wheatgrass, chlorella, and Lingzhi mushroom, along with other herbs, are covered in this chapter. Most of these herbs are used as Ayurveda and clinical nutraceuticals; however, the dosage form and dose are key factors for the successful outcome of these nutraceuticals. The marker compounds of the herbs and their percentages in standardized dosage form contribute to their possible role in prevention and treatment.

Keywords: Clinical studies, Drug interaction, Nutraceuticals, Pharmacological use.

INTRODUCTION

Herbal nutraceuticals are plant-derived supplements that enhance well-being and treat illnesses caused by bad dietary choices. Nutraceuticals are extracted from

* **Corresponding author Mukesh Singh Sikarwar:** Amity Institute of Pharmacy, Amity University, Gwalior, Madhya Pradesh, India; E-mail: mukeshsikarwar@gmail.com

Mukesh Singh Sikarwar, Arunachalam Muthuraman & Sohrab A. Shaikh (Eds.)

oils, roots, seeds, berries, or flowers. Herbal nutraceuticals come in many forms, such as capsules, tablets, powders, liquids, and gels. Prebiotics, probiotics, herbal formulations, dietary fiber, proteins, and other natural resources are readily accessible and have a large commercial value. Nutraceuticals are of increasing interest due to their potential nutritional, safety, and therapeutic advantages, potentially altering gene expression, antioxidant defenses, cell proliferation, and mitochondrial integrity [1]. Herbal bioactive components, including flavonoids, terpenoids, saponins, and polyphenols, are vital nutraceuticals with health-promoting therapeutic qualities, typically utilised as dietary supplements in traditional healthcare. The following plants are examined in as much detail as possible as nutraceuticals.

HAWTHORN

Hawthorn, a fragile plant from the Rosaceae family and Crataegus genus, originated from the Mediterranean, North Africa, Europe, and Central Asia. With approximately 200 species worldwide, few, such as C. *oxycantha, C. laevigata, C. monogyna, C. orientalis, and C. pinnatifida*, are well studied or used medicinally (Fig. **1**). Since ancient times, its leaves, flowers, and fruits have been employed in extracts or tinctures. Today, hawthorn is legally acknowledged as an herbal medication in pharmacopoeias of nations including China, England, Germany, and France [2]. Hawthorn preparations are standardized according to the number of flavonoids and oligomeric proanthocyanidins they contain. These compounds have important diuretic, inotropic, and vasodilator properties. Numerous Crataegus species have demonstrated encouraging benefits in treating peripheral vascular disease, hypertension, angina, congestive heart failure, hyperlipidemia, and diabetes mellitus, according to extensive research on both humans and animals [3].

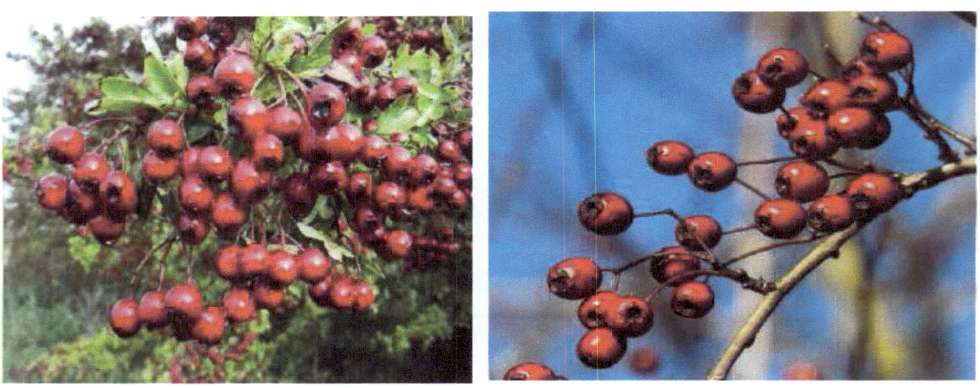

Fig. (1). Hawthorn berries.

Ethnopharmacology of Hawthorn

The hawthorn has been used as a medicine for many years. The berries and leaves were thought to have medicinal properties in the thirteenth century, when they were used to cure digestive disorders like vomiting and diarrhoea. Hawthorn was utilized by the Chinese to treat dyspnoea, regulate hyperlipidaemia, reduce "fullness of the stomach," and enhance digestion by reducing food stasis. Utilization for kidney stones and as a diuretic dates back to the eighteenth century. In Europe, use for a range of cardiovascular conditions was first documented in the late 1800s. Hawthorn was not widely used in American medicine until 1896. These days, hawthorn is mostly utilized as an alternative treatment for several cardiovascular conditions, including hypertension, arrhythmias, angina, the New York Heart Association's (NYHA) functional class II Congestive Heart Failure (CHF), and hyperlipidaemia. The berries, blossoms, and leaves of hawthorn have been considered the plant's most active parts since the 1800s [4].

Chemical Constituents

Hawthorn includes catechins, amines, triterpene saponins, oligomeric procyanidins, and flavonoids (*e.g.*, hyperoside, quercetin, quercitrin, hyperine) as well as flavon-C-glycosides (*e.g.*, vitexin, isovitexin, orientin, isoorientin). Crataegus acid, a triterpene carboxylic acid prevalent in hawthorn berries, is considered to contribute to its coronary vasodilator properties. Amines are presumably inactive after consumption owing to fast breakdown in the stomach. The flavonoids and oligomeric procyanidins are regarded as the key drivers of hawthorn's pharmacological actions. In animal studies, hawthorn increases oxygen consumption, demonstrates positive inotropic action, strengthens blood vessel walls, and promotes coronary blood flow, with flavonoids predominantly responsible for these cardiovascular effects. Human studies imply that increased flavonoid consumption decreases coronary heart disease risk. Additionally, oligomeric procyanidins in hawthorn's leaves and blossoms may inhibit Human Neutrophil Elastase (HNE) and scavenge free radicals, thus minimizing myocardial damage during ischemia and lowering the risk of cardiac failure [5].

Clinical Trials of Hawthorn

Congestive heart failure: Hawthorn has shown potential in treating congestive heart failure in both controlled and uncontrolled clinical investigations. The largest trial to date was an uncontrolled, multicenter, observational investigation of the therapeutic benefits of hawthorn extract WS 1442 (Crataegutt novo 450, Willmar Schwabe) in 1011 patients with NYHA functional class II CHF [6 - 8]. Each individual got one tablet with 84.3 mg of procyanidin twice a day for 24 weeks. Clinical complaints, including exercise dyspnoea, palpitations, and exhaustion, as well as performance on an exercise tolerance test and ejection fraction (which increased in 196 participants from 47% at baseline to 51% at week 24), all showed improvements. The authors came to the conclusion that hawthorn is a safe, efficient treatment for NYHA functional class II CHF and that patients experience an improvement in well-being after starting medication. Similar outcomes were observed by Eichstadt *et al.* in their uncontrolled experiment [9]. Several placebo-controlled experiments have assessed the effectiveness of hawthorn in treating heart failure, and in nearly all of them, a positive effect has been noted. A randomized, double-blind, placebo-controlled trial involving 85 patients with NYHA functional class II CHF was the only one that showed no effect. When used for a minimum of six weeks, hawthorn seems to help patients with NYHA functional class II CHF and has good tolerance. Its effectiveness and long-term safety remain unknown. The leaves and blossoms of the hawthorn plant have been used in preparations that have been evaluated thus far; the effectiveness of using other plant components in goods is unknown. Further studies examining higher dosages used for longer durations will aid in clarifying the function of hawthorn in CHF treatment [10].

Hypercholesterolemia: In addition to decreasing the participants' total cholesterol, low-density lipoprotein cholesterol, and the ratio of total cholesterol to high-density lipoprotein cholesterol, the study by Eiff *et al.* investigated the effects of hawthorn-passionflower extract on their capacity for exercise [11]. Iron, zinc, B1, and C vitamins were added to the beverage, which had very little sugar or salt. For a month, thirty hyperlipidemic individuals, aged 43 to 59, were administered 250 mL of the beverage twice daily. Venous blood samples were taken when the patient was fasting at the beginning and end of the therapy session. The findings showed a substantial decrease in lipid peroxide malonic dialdehyde, total cholesterol, serum triglycerides, LDL cholesterol, and apolipoprotein B. No appreciable changes were observed in HDL [11].

Dosage and administration: The recommended daily dose is 160–900 mg of a natural water-ethanol extract of hawthorn leaves. 3.5–20 mg of epicatechin or flavonoids from flowers (30–169 equivalents) administered in two or more servings [7]. Based on the flavonoid hyperoside, a daily dosage of 12–15 mg (300–900 mg of dry extract per day) has been suggested for the treatment of cardiac insufficiency. The suggested daily dosage for treating cardiac insufficiency is 45–90 mg (240–560 mg of dry extract), which is based on oligomeric procyanidins. Due to variances in strength, drinking brewed hawthorn tea is not recommended. Because Hawthorn's benefits take time to show, the suggested daily dosage should be taken for at least six weeks in three separate doses [12].

Adverse Effects: Hawthorn's tolerance has fared well in clinical trials. No notable adverse effects have been linked to lower doses. When taken therapeutically, hawthorn may cause mild rash, headache, sweating, palpitations, dizziness, sleepiness, agitation, and gastrointestinal problems. Large dosages caused arrhythmias, hypotension, and sleepiness in the animals [13].

Drug Interactions

- When hawthorn is taken along with medications that dilate blood vessels, like theophylline, papaverine, caffeine, sodium nitrate, and adenosine, there may be an increase in vasodilation [14].
- Hawthorn may enhance or decrease the effects of medications used to treat arrhythmias, hypertension, angina, and heart failure. Digoxin may have increased effects, which could call for lowering the dosage [15].
- Digoxin's effects can be amplified, requiring a potential digoxin dosage reduction. Avoid combining hawthorn with other cardiac-active herbs, as this may intensify its effects. Such herbs include black hellebore, mate, ginger, cola, squill, pheasant's eye herb, motherwort, lily-of-the-valley roots, strophanthus, and shepherd's purse [16].

Precautions and contraindications: Hawthorn usage should be avoided in children under the age of twelve and in pregnant and lactating women. Patients who are hypersensitive to any product ingredients or who have experienced an adverse reaction should not use hawthorn. Hyperlipidemia, arrhythmias, and congestive heart failure are serious medical disorders that require a physician's evaluation. Hawthorn self-medication should never be done by patients without first seeing a doctor [17].

GRAPE SEEDS

The grapevine, or *Vitis vinifera* L., is a significant fruit crop grown worldwide; in 2013, its yield was said to have exceeded 75.1 million tonnes. Grapes are commonly cultivated for winemaking but occasionally utilized as table grapes or dried to produce raisins (Fig. **2**). The species is rich in phytochemicals, particularly phenolic compounds, with antioxidant activities, and provides health effects through scavenging free radicals. Interestingly, these bioactive phenolics can be obtained at an affordable cost from grape peels and seeds, which are otherwise considered low-value residues of the production of wine and juice [18]. Grape seeds have a significantly higher polyphenol content (60–70%) compared to fruit pulp (10%) and peels (28%–35%). *Vitis vinifera* has been valued for its medicinal and nutritional properties for almost 6,000 years. Greek philosophers and ancient Egyptian consumers alike praised the virtues of the plant, often in the form of wine [19 - 21]. Ripe grapes were used to treat a variety of ailments, including cholera, smallpox, cancer, nausea, infections, and diseases of the skin, kidneys, liver, and circulatory system, as well as bleeding, dyspepsia, dysuria, bronchitis, and gout. Unripe grapes soothed sore throats, dried grapes (raisins) alleviated thirst and constipation, and grapevine sap was utilized in traditional European medicines for eye and skin illnesses. The food and pharmaceutical industries are especially concerned with the medical and health effects of epicatechin, gallic acid, and catechin, and also polymeric and oligomeric procyanidins, which are the main polyphenolic chemicals in grape seeds [22].

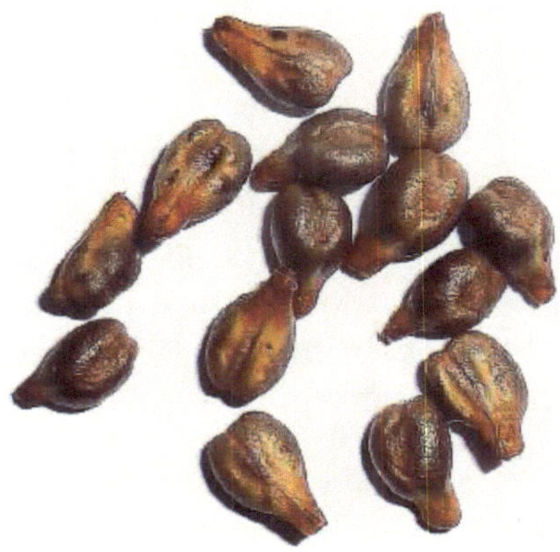

Fig. (2). Grape seeds.

Macroscopic Characters

In the transverse section of the seeds from both types, which were determined to be nearly identical, cuticle and epidermis; massive parenchymatous cells make up the outer integument, or soft seed coat; the medium integument, or hard seed coat, is made up of inner integument; (v) endosperm and embryo; two layers of cells. In the initial observation, the epidermis was thin, and the cuticle was composed of cells that were rectangular in shape. There was an outer integument of cells called parenchymatous. The outer integument and the epidermis were composed of a thin layer of cells that enveloped the seed. This tissue's dorsal aspect contained the raphe. The medium tissue, also known as the medium integument, was made up of two layers of thin-walled, rectangular cells. The endosperm and the medium integument are separated by the inner integument. Enchymatous tissue, covered in integuments, populated the core of the seed, housing the embryo sac [23].

Chemical Constituents: Grape seeds include a complex nutritional composition, including water (7%), minerals (3%), fiber (35%), and protein (11%), alongside a fat content varying from 7 to 20%. Additionally, grape seed extracts are characterized by a complex composition of proanthocyanidin-containing chemicals, comprising polymers (11–39%), oligomers (17–63%), and monomers

(5–30%). Proanthocyanidins, the principal ingredients of these extracts, lend the distinctive red hue and astringent flavor to grape seed extracts. However, higher proanthocyanidin levels may impact the color and sensory qualities of derived goods [24 - 26].

Therapeutic Activities of Grape Seeds: Hydrogen peroxide, superoxide, and hydroxyl radicals are examples of common Reactive Oxygen Species (ROS). These ROS are often produced by the body as a signal molecule that supports the immune system and homeostasis. These antioxidant enzymes, including glutathione peroxidase, catalase, and superoxide dismutase, can overcome this process [27]. An imbalance between ROS and antioxidants, which are connected to oxidative stress-related lung and cardiovascular disorders, as well as degenerative diseases, and Type 2 Diabetes Mellitus (T2DM), is brought on by an excess of ROS. Quercetin, resveratrol, procyanidins, and other phenolic compounds with anti-inflammatory and antioxidant qualities are therefore found in grapes and their metabolites [28].

Grape seed antioxidant activity: The most prominent bioactive feature of phenolic compounds is their capacity to lessen oxidative stress. Many studies have examined grape seed extracts' capacity to scavenge Reactive Oxygen Species (ROS) and prevent lipid oxidation [29]. The high antioxidant activity of grape seed and seed oil is linked to the high content of procyanidins, epicatechin, gallic acid, and other phenolic compounds; this might be the result of their synergistic interaction [30]. The biological mechanisms underlie the antioxidant's capacity to chelate metals and neutralise free radicals, particularly hydroxyl radicals, both of which affect cell signalling and the immune system. This is particularly important given grape seed extract's capacity to reduce oxidative stress, Lower Low-density Lipoprotein (LDL) levels, and minimise the inflammatory process associated with certain disorders [31]. It has been shown that defatted milled grape seed, a byproduct of wine production, protects the cell membrane from oxidative damage, preventing the oxidation of proteins and lipids from the extraction of grape seed oil [32]. Globally, greater rates of morbidity and mortality are usually associated with chronic conditions. Inflammatory processes, which are often difficult to control with current measures and treatments [33]. Arachidonic Acid (AA) is required for the synthesis of prostaglandins and leukotrienes, and its release initiates the inflammatory response. Grape seed oil contains polyphenols that can stop this process [34].

Grape seed oil's function in cell cycle regulation: Grape seed oil contains certain phenolic compounds that have anticancer effects, alter the cell cycle, and make tumour cells lethal without posing a threat to healthy cells [35]. Proanthocyanidins, which are polymers of flavan-3-ol, inhibit the growth of cancer cells [36]. The biological mechanisms that have been suggested include the deactivation of the phosphoinositide 3-kinase (PI3K)/Protein Kinase B (PKB) signalling pathway, which triggers apoptosis in colon cancer cells, and the decrease in the expression of pro-angiogenic factors, such as vascular endothelial growth factor and angiopoietins. Furthermore, the chemotherapeutic medication 5-fluorouracil was more lethal to these cells when the low molecular weight procyanidins in ripe grape seeds were present, suggesting that these components may be used as supplements to treat colon cancer [37, 38]. This study evaluated the effectiveness of lipid nanocarriers based on grape seed oil and laurel leaf oil in scavenging free radicals and eliminating certain tumour cells. The nanocarriers' capacity to scavenge over 98% of oxygen-free radicals inhibited the development of tumour cells even in the absence of an anticancer drug [39]. The MDA-MB-231 and HeLa tumour cells had a 40% mortality rate, whereas the normal B16 cells had a 20% death rate, according to the survival profile of tumour and normal cells. The study suggests that lipid nanocarriers derived from laurel leaf oil and grape seed oil may improve the anticancer drug's therapeutic performance in clinical settings while reducing the toxicity of delivery methods [40]. A number of authors have suggested that the anticancer activity of lipid nanocarriers may be due to the many bioactive compounds present in grape seed and laurel oils; this action is the result of multiple cellular mechanisms and processes [41].

Microbiological properties of grape seed oil: Grape seed oil may have antibacterial properties since it is poisonous to some microorganisms. It was discovered that the oil extracted from grape seeds inhibited the development of Staphylococcus aureus and *Escherichia coli* [42]. Resveratrol is one example of a phenolic molecule that exhibits antimicrobial action by causing oxidative damage to the membranes of bacteria, especially *E. coli*, without causing harm to host cells. According to these results, resveratrol may be used in addition to conventional therapies when antibiotics are not working [41, 42].

Trials on Humans

According to research with 35,239 male participants, using grape seed extract on a daily basis was linked to a 41% lower chance of developing prostate cancer overall. In the same cohort, however, there was no discernible link between the use of grape seed supplements and either lung or colorectal cancer. The VITAL trial did not assess grape seed oil as a cancer-preventive agent. In humans, the effects of grape seed oil intake on insulin resistance and inflammation were assessed in women who were overweight or obese. Insulin resistance scores, TNF-α, and ultrasensitive C-Reactive Protein (us-CRP) all decreased in the grape seed oil group, although only us-CRP significantly decreased as compared to the sunflower oil group. In comparison to peanut oil, grape seed oil has also shown a reduction in platelet aggregation. In adults, consuming up to 45 g of grape seed oil per day appeared to lower LDL cholesterol levels by 7% and raise HDL-c by 13%. However, there are contradictory findings about how using grape seed oil alters the lipid profiles of the muscles, liver, and serum. To assess how grape seed oil affects a person's lipid profile, well-planned, randomised clinical studies are required [42].

KELP

Biological Source: Kelp is a brown alga obtained from the dried ribbon-like thallus of *Laminaria japonica* belonging to the family *Laminariaceae.* Brown algae of the Laminaria J.V. Lamour species are well-known. The food, cosmetic, and pharmaceutical industries all make extensive use of them. The genus name of Laminaria plants originates from the Latin term "lamina," which translates to "plate." Additionally, it shows the algal thallus's lamellar shape. The seaweed Laminaria is a member of the brown class. The algae belong to the Laminariaceae family (lat. Phaeophyceae). Thirty kelp species exist, three of which are found in the southern hemisphere's waters, and the remainder in the northern hemisphere's waters. The majority of kelp (Fig. **3**) species can be found in the Pacific [43].

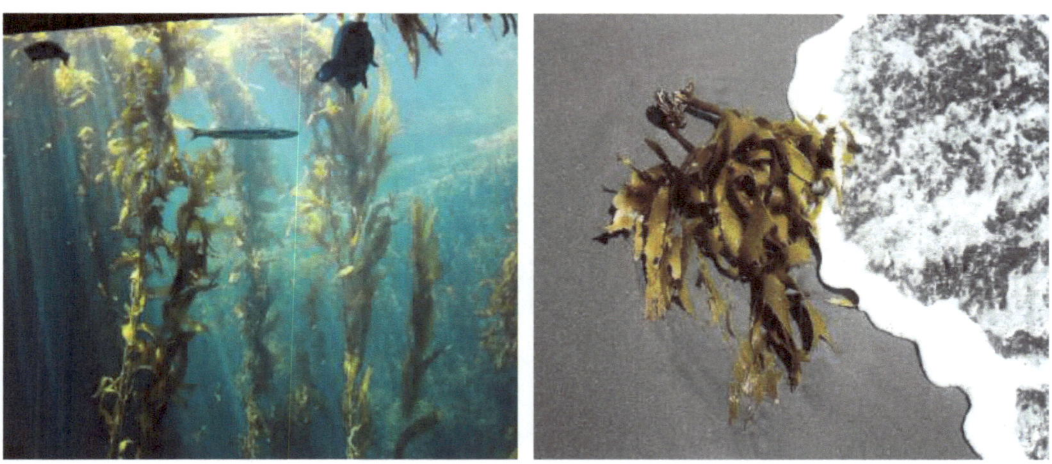

Fig. (3). Kelp.

Cultivation and collection: The dried kelp thallus of brown seaweed, specifically saccharine and Japanese kelp, the pharmacognostic features are given in Table **1**. The kelp is harvested between June and October and utilized as raw herbal medicine (also known as medicinal plant raw materials, or MPRM). As a valuable food and medicinal plant, kelp is widely cultivated in Japan, Korea, China, and the Far East of Russia. For patients suffering from persistent atonic constipation, especially those with hyperlipidemia, kelp thallus is utilized as a mild laxative.

The Laminaria species is recommended as a supplementary treatment for atherosclerosis, as well as for the management and prophylaxis of endemic goiter, hyperthyroidism, and mild variants of Graves' disease [44].

Table 1. Pharmacognostical characteristics.

Macroscopic Characters	
Stature	Ribbon like
Length	1-12 m long
Wide	10-35 cm
Texture	Kelp plate is linear, Mucous, soft, with wavy edges.
colour	Greenish brown
Cultivation	late autumn and grows again in winter
Life expectancy of kelp	2-4 years, depending upon climatic conditions

Clinical Trials of Kelp

Thyroid cancer patients: The survey was created as an observational study by the researchers with advice from specialists in health information technology, CAM research, and thyroid cancer. They methodically examined earlier surveys that concentrate on cancer patients' use of CAM. The survey is based on National Health Interview data from 2007. Supplemental Questionnaire for Survey on Alternative Medicine. This covers all 27 regularly used CAM therapies. Here, ten different provider-based CAM types are utilized in the US, as well as 17 CAM therapies that are self-administered. The online survey was tested on a limited number of thyroid patients with cancer (n = 5). There were four primary groups: general state of health, demographic data, and inquiries about CAM use and general inquiries on CAM use. Inquiries concerning the respondents' use of kelp were made, in addition to an empty space to keep a record of whether they use other forms of supplement.

The majority of kelp users have had thyroid hormone replacement therapy, radioactive iodine treatment, and surgery; they frequently combine complementary and alternative medicine (CAM) with traditional therapies for differentiated thyroid cancer. In addition to using kelp for therapy, people with differentiated thyroid cancer frequently use it to address associated symptoms, including pain and exhaustion. Physicians are aware of CAM usage since excessive iodine consumption can interfere with whole-body scans and radioactive iodine therapy. Seaweeds have a wide range of iodine contents, with varying levels that can be absorbed. Although the safety of kelp supplementation in individuals with thyroid cancer is unknown, Japan has a lower incidence of thyroid cancer than the US and a high daily intake of seaweed. Although the study shows a slight prevalence of kelp usage among patients with thyroid cancer, it also emphasises the necessity of better CAM communication. The study emphasises how important it is for patients and doctors to have regular conversations on kelp, CAM usage, and traditional therapy [45]. *Pregnancy:* As the general safety has not been reported, kelp is not recommended during pregnancy and breastfeeding [46]. *Contraindications:* Studies have shown that using kelp supplements along with thyroid drugs, lithium, and amiodarone should be avoided [46].

MILK THISTLE

Biological Source: Milk thistle is obtained from the seeds of *Silybum marianum,* belonging to the family Composite or *Asteraceae.* In ancient Greece, milk thistle (*Silybum marianum*) was used to cure gallbladder and liver illnesses and to safeguard the liver against poisons. It has lately been looked for use as an anticarcinogen, cytoprotectant, and a liver damage supportive treatment from poisoning with Amanita phalloides. It's in the motion component, known as silymarin. It is mostly present in the seeds. Silymarin experiences a hepatic recirculation, which causes liver cells to contain more of the substance than serum does. It is composed of substances known as flavonolignans, the most typical being silybin [47]. Asteraceae, often known as Compositae, is the family of asters that includes artichokes and daisies. *Silybum marianum* is a member of this family. Originally brought to North America by European colonists early in their migration, milk thistle (Fig. **4**) is today widely distributed throughout Europe and is also found in South America, California, and the eastern United States [48]. The term "milk thistle" comes from the leaves' distinctive spikes and white veins, which were supposedly meant to convey the milk of the Virgin Mary [47, 48]. The same tradition gives rise to the Latin name. The plant features a profusion of sturdy spines in addition to huge, brilliant purple flowers. Because of the latter quality, it can be used in some places in place of barbed wire. Commercial milk thistle is planted all throughout the United States; it likes sunny spots with well-drained soil [49].

Geographical Source: It is farmed commercially in a number of nations, such as Pakistan and Iran. It has also been explored as a potential biomass crop for the generation of bioenergy, at least in Sardinia. In Russia, it was commonly grown as an oil-seed plant up until the 1930s [50]. Its demand fluctuates between 18 and 20 tons annually, and its average sale is approximately USD 8 billion [51]. These days, the extract is sold as silymarin and silybinin pills and capsules with increased bioavailability under brand names including Legalon, Indena, Livergol, and Silipder [50].

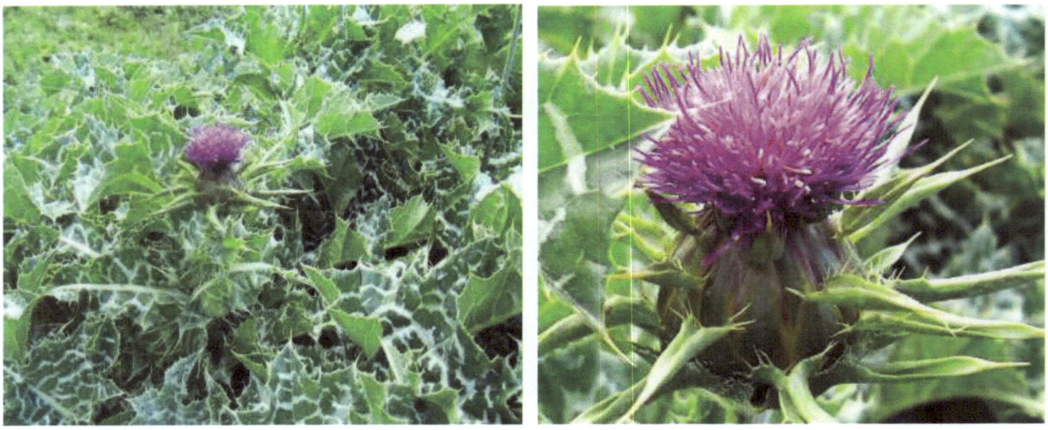

Fig. (4). Milk thistle.

Ethnopharmacology: Since the time of Greek herbalist Dioscorides, who claimed that drinking a tea made from milk thistle seeds could heal a poisonous snake bite, milk thistle extracts have been utilized as medicinal treatments. Plant juice and honey combined worked wonders for "carrying off bile". The "best remedy against melancholy" or "black bile" is milk thistle. Milk thistle was promoted as a liver disease remedy. Infusions made from fresh root and seeds were effective in treating jaundice, shattering and expelling stones, and treating blockages of the liver and spleen in the late sixteenth century. Rademacher made "Rademacher's Tincture," an ethanol extract from the seeds intended to treat hepatosplenic diseases, popular between 1772 and 1850. In accordance with this custom, a medical school began employing milk thistle extracts at the turn of the 20th century to treat conditions such as "liver congestion," varicose veins, irregular menstruation, and spleen and kidney abnormalities [52].

Chemical Constituents: Silybin, also referred to as silybinin or silibinin, was the first flavonolignan isolated from milk thistle and is a component of a complex mixture encompassing silydianin, silychristin (also known as silicristin or silychristin A), isosilybin A–D, isosilychristin, 3-deoxyflavonolignans (such as silandrin and silymonin), silyhermin (including neosilyhermine A and B), 2,3-dehydrosilybin, 2,3-cis-silybin A and B, neusilychristin, isosilandrin A and B, silychristin B (a diastereomer of silychristin A), and silyamadin [53 - 57]. Additionally, mariamides A and B, characterized by hydroxy-methoxyphenyl and acrylamido groups, are bioactive compounds within this matrix. Other notable constituents include coniferin, kaempferol, taxifolin, dihydrokaempferol, dihydroquercetin-4′-methylether, naringenin (and its glucoside), N, N′-1,4-butanediylbis(4-hydroxybenzamide), 4,4′-diphenylmethanebis(methyl)carbamates, and 3-methylcarboxymethylindole-1-N-β-D-glucopyranoside. Further significant compounds comprise (1R,7R,10R,11R)-12-hydroxy anhuienosol, 2-hydroxymethyl-5-(2-hydroxypropan-2-yl) phenol, donepezil, rutin, quercetin, and morin [58 - 63].

Clinical Trials of Milk Thistle

In one scientific experiment, both male and female healthy volunteers who took 140 mg of standardised silymarin orally three times a day for 28 days saw no negative side effects. Another investigation was conducted when 50 healthy mothers were breastfeeding [64]. For 63 days, 420 mg of micronized silymarin was administered orally every day as part of this experiment. It has outstanding tolerance and no negative side effects. For 10 days, 22 healthy, normal volunteers took 400 mg of silymarin and 295 mg of L-arginine; they had no adverse effects [65]. Tests on blood and urine samples collected on Days 0, 10, and 27 showed that silymarin was safe [66]. In a different trial, taking capsules with 175 mg of milk thistle extract orally three times a day for 14 days did not cause any significant side effects or toxicity in healthy participants [67].

Patients with Liver Disease: 24 men and women with Hepatitis C Virus (HCV) infections whose hepatitis was not cured by interferon therapy were included in the research. Patients received dosages of 140, 280, 560, and 700 mg of oral silymarin three times a day for seven days. At 280 mg of the drug, headaches and nausea were seen [68]. However, no adverse drug-related side effects were reported. The patients in this other clinical study received interferon alfa 2b, PEGylated ribavirin, and a daily supplement consisting of 94 mg of silybin, vitamin E, and phospholipids for a year. This study found no serious adverse effects, despite a number of symptoms, such as weight loss, joint discomfort, muscular soreness, irritability, hyperglycemia, and hypercholesterolaemia [69]. Furthermore, 27 male and female patients who were treated with ribavirin and interferon but had detectable hepatitis C virus ribonucleic acids received intravenous silymarin (20 mg/kg) for 14 or 21 days as part of a different experiment including these patients. Their blood was taken on Days 1, 8, 15, and 22, and every four weeks. Although 12 patients reported a burning feeling and 15 patients reported gastrointestinal problems during medication, this study demonstrated that silymarin did not indicate substantial harm. The bilirubin levels in all study participants increased slightly, from 0.98 ± 0.35 to 2.12 ± 0.99 mg/dl. Additionally, in Kalantari, Shahshahan, and Hejazi, taking 630 mg of silymarin orally daily for 24 weeks was safe for both male and female patients. When given intravenously to hepatitis C patients for two days during PEGylated-interferon alpha-2a therapy, silymarin (1,400 mg/day silymarin over 120–360 min) was well tolerated; nevertheless, a few moderate adverse effects, such as diarrhoea, vomiting, stomach discomfort, and hot feeling, were recorded [70]. Before the patients encountered these issues, more than two days had gone by, and giving patients oral dosages of 700 and 420 mg silymarin three times a day for 24 weeks was shown to be safe in another investigation. Therefore, it may be concluded that a high dosage was well tolerated by hepatitis C patients [71].

NAFLD, or non-alcoholic fatty liver disease: According to a meta-analysis study on people with non-alcoholic fatty liver disease, taking 140 mg of silymarin twice daily for 12 weeks was safe and did not cause any negative side effects or toxicities. In patients with acute hepatitis, treatment with 140 mg silymarin three times a day for four weeks was well tolerated, and no adverse effects were noted. Following silymarin medication, the participants in this experimental research were monitored for a further four weeks. For a whole year, individuals with non-alcoholic fatty liver disease who received 94 mg of silybin, 194 mg of phosphatidylcholine made with 89.28 mg of vitamin E twice daily, saw no significant adverse effects. However, several short-term adverse effects were seen, such as diarrhoea, pruritus, and dysgeusia [72].

Rhinitis due to allergies: In 94 individuals with allergic rhinitis and a positive skin prick test, symptoms decreased after taking 140 mg of silymarin orally three times a day for a month. There was no significant danger. Unfavourable reactions were seen. Due to its antioxidant properties, the purpose of this experiment was to assess how silymarin affected the symptoms of allergic rhinitis [73].

Ulcerative Colitis: To assess the possible advantages of silymarin, a randomised, double-blind clinical study was carried out on patients with ulcerative colitis. They received silymarin as part of their usual treatment regimen; six months later, the medication was given orally at a rate of 140 mg per day. Headache, nausea, diarrhoea, and stomach discomfort were the most frequent adverse effects of silymarin. However, silymarin showed no discernible toxicity, and any adverse effects were transient [74].

Tuberculosis: Patients with TB who had been treated with antituberculosis medicine were given one silymarin (140 mg) tablet every eight hours. There were no significant adverse effects associated with silymarin during the second or fourth weeks of the study. In another research, this dosage of silymarin had no adverse effects for eight weeks. Additionally, there were no adverse effects from taking 140 mg of silymarin orally twice a day for eight weeks. In a double-blind clinical trial, individuals with TB who took 140 mg of silymarin orally three times a day for two weeks saw no serious adverse effects. Anorexia and nausea were among the gastrointestinal issues [75].

Arthritis: To assess silymarin's anti-inflammatory properties, individuals with osteoarthritis in their knees were given 300 mg of the drug orally every day for eight weeks. Comparison tests between silymarin and nonsteroidal anti-inflammatory drugs were conducted on 220 subjects (79 males and 141 women). Consequently, there was no toxicity observed, good silymarin tolerance, and a reduction in the patients' elevated interleukin levels [76]. In a double-blind clinical study, 30 males and 30 females with recurring arthritic diseases were treated for three months with 120 mg of silibinin twice a day and 12 mg of methotrexate each week. The toxicity and side effects of silibinin were not recorded in this trial [77 - 79].

Topical Silymarin Safety and Side Effects in Humans: Patients with melasma were treated with topical silymarin cream (0.1% and 0.2%) used twice a day for four weeks [80]. There were no adverse consequences observed. In a randomised, double-blind, placebo-controlled study, patients with gastric cancer who developed hand-foot syndrome due to capecitabine did not report any adverse effects by using 1% silymarin gel twice a day for nine weeks [81]. Patients with breast cancer who used topical silymarin for 5.5 weeks, two hours before radiation therapy, experienced no adverse effects, and the medication proved effective in avoiding dermatitis brought on by radiation therapy [82].

Pregnancy: In one clinical study, a woman with chronic hepatitis B took oral 150 mg silymarin twice a day after taking lamivudine both before and during her pregnancy. During the thirteenth week of pregnancy, no foetal abnormalities or adverse consequences were seen. It was safe to utilise specific doses of lamivudine and silymarin while pregnant. There is presently inadequate information on silymarin's safety during human pregnancy; thus, more study is required [83].

PSYLLIUM HUSK

Biological Source: It is obtained from the whole seed husk of *Plantago ovata,* belonging to the family *Plantaginaceae,* commonly called Isapgol. Psyllium husk (Fig. **5**), which is derived from Plantago ovata seeds, is composed of highly branched, gel-forming arabinoxylan, a polymer that is rich in xylose and arabinose but difficult for humans to digest. However, because certain components of the intestinal microbiota may use these oligosaccharides and the sugars they contain as an energy source, psyllium might be considered to have prebiotic potential [84]. Prebiotics often promote the development of good bacteria in the host and boost the synthesis of Short-Chain Fatty Acids (SCFA), such as propionate and butyrate, which have been shown to improve colon health. By retaining water in the small intestine, psyllium can also enhance the passage of water into the ascending colon. The resulting increase in intestinal fluidity may be the reason for psyllium husk's effectiveness in relieving constipation. In addition to softening and increasing frequency, the presence of free water in the faeces alters the environmental conditions in the colon [85].

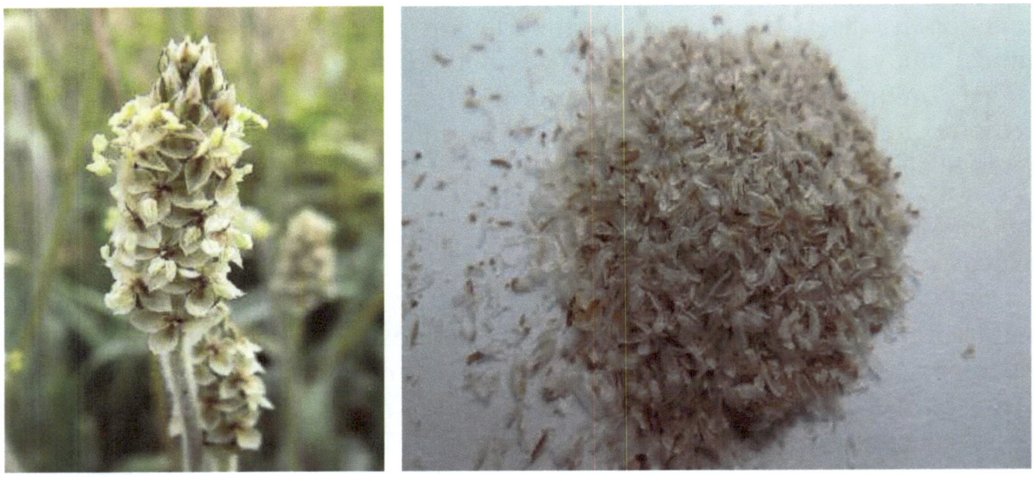

Fig. (5). *Psyllium.*

Nutritional Quality

Psyllium husk is obtained from the Plantago species and is a vegetable source of food with higher-quality nutritional content than cereals and legumes. It contains 6.83% protein, 0.94% fat, 4.07% ash, and 84.98% total carbohydrates. The seed oil of Plantago is high in linoleic acid (40.6%) and oleic acid (39.1%), with a lesser component of linolenic acid (6.9%). Rat bioassays for high nutritional efficiency were 89.6% dry matter digestibility, 86.0% apparent digestibility, 88.1% true digestibility, and a corrected net protein ratio (NPRc) of 4.40. Psyllium husk hydrogel is rigid, resistant to breakage, and rapidly dissolving, and its hydrophobicity and viscosity vary with temperature, pH, concentration, and shear rate [86]. Psyllium mucilage, the colorless gelling agent, creates a high-viscosity, gel-like network in water, the cause of much of its health value, *i.e.*, prevention and control of chronic diseases. Its functionality makes it a most useful dietary fiber for uses as a thickener in ice cream and frozen desserts [87]. Technical-grade psyllium functions as a hydrocolloidal agent to facilitate water retention in recently seeded turf and transplant survival of woody plants. Moreover, psyllium mucilage acts as a natural dietary fiber in animal feed, with dehusked seeds being used in India as poultry and cattle feed [88].

Clinical Trials of Psyllium Husk

A study was done to ascertain the pharmacological underpinnings of psyllium husk (Ispaghula) use as medicine for diseases of gastrointestinal motility. Mice were employed in *in vitro* tests, while extracted rabbit jejunum and guinea-pig ileum were used in *in vivo* investigations. The research shows that ispaghula has two distinct effects on the gut: one is gut-stimulatory, partially mediated by activation of muscarinic and 5-HT4 receptors, which may enhance the laxative effect of its fiber content; the other is gut-inhibitory, potentially mediated by blockade of Ca^{2+} channels and activation of NO-cyclic guanosine monophosphate pathways. Results point to the presence of unidentified and gut-stimulatory components in psyllium husk, as well as gut-inhibitory components that may involve the CCB and NO-cGMP pathways and be mediated through muscarinic or 5-HT4 receptor activation. This could account for psyllium husk's dual benefits in treating constipation and diarrhoea [89].

Effect of *Psyllium* Husk on Intestinal Microbiota in Constipated Patients and Healthy Controls

Eight healthy volunteers and sixteen constipated patients participated in a double-blind, randomised, placebo-controlled clinical study that examined the effects of seven days of psyllium *vs* a placebo (maltodextrin). We evaluated the patients' Short-Chain Fatty Acid (SCFA), faecal water content, gastrointestinal (GI) transit, and stool microbial composition. Psyllium supplementation increased Veillonella and decreased Subdoligranulum in healthy adults, but the effects were more noticeable in constipated subjects, who also showed changes in acetate and propionate levels and an increase in Lachnospira, Faecalibacterium, Phascolarctobacterium, Veillonella, and Sutterella, and a decrease in uncultured Coriobacteria and Christensenella. We found that many taxa were associated with altered faecal water content, SCFAs, and GI transit in these individuals. Higher faecal water is associated with notable increases in three taxa that are known to generate butyrate: Lachnospira, Roseburia, and Faecalibacterium. In conclusion, supplementing with psyllium resulted in substantial changes in microbiota and increased stool water, with the most noticeable changes happening in individuals who were constipated [90].

Interactions: It is advisable to avoid taking ispaghula 30 to 60 minutes before taking any other prescription since it may decrease the absorption of other drugs. Ispaghula should not be used with mesalazine since it lowers colonic pH and may reduce the medication's efficacy, even if no interactions have been reported. The bioavailability of lithium and carbamazepine may be reduced when ispaghula is taken with them [91].

Contraindications: It is not recommended for children under the age of six for constipation or under the age of twelve for other uses due to a lack of conclusive evidence of efficacy. Ispaghula husk should not be taken just before bed. It is not recommended for those who have sudden changes in bowel habits that last for more than two weeks, have inexplicable rectal bleeding, or have trouble voiding after using a laxative. Not recommended for people who have trouble swallowing [91].

ST. JOHN'S WORT

Biological Source: It is obtained from the flowering part of *Hypericum perforatum,* which belongs to the family *Hypericaceae* (Fig. **6**). Known widely as St. John's wort, the flowering plant Hypericum perforatum is a widespread weed in the United States. Historically, plant extracts have been used to treat "insomnia and other mental conditions". Its golden blossom was customarily gathered for St. John the Baptist's supper, and its popular name is derived from the fact that "wort" is the ancient English word for plant [92].

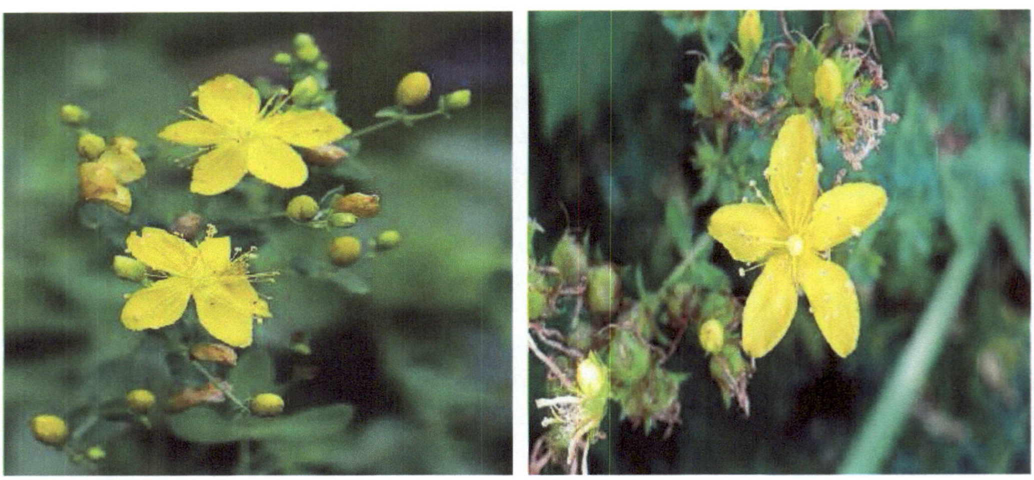

Fig. (6). St. John's wort.

Clinical Trials on St. John's Wort

It has been demonstrated that hypericum extract contains at least 10 chemicals with biological action, including β-sitosterol, quercetin, xanthones, monoterpenes, hypericin, pseudohypericin, and catechin. Numerous medications have been demonstrated to attach to neuroreceptors in the brain and prevent the absorption of certain neurotransmitters that are believed to play a role in depression. Recent data from the National Institutes of Health cast doubt on the importance of hypericin, which was once thought to be the main active component of the hypericum plant. However, the amount of hypericin in various hypericum formulations is constant. It would be wise to subject hypericum extract to the same dietary and medication combination limitations as this class of medications because it has been identified as a Monoamine Oxidase (MAO) inhibitor. However, a number of recent investigations have demonstrated that hypericum extract's relative inhibitory potential on the MAO system is extremely low, far lower than that of the widely used MAO inhibitors [93, 94].

Methodological Quality

Eight high-quality efficacy studies were included in the evaluation: each one included baseline depression assessments and comparison demographic data for the control and treatment groups. Six of the studies used the Hamilton Rating Scale for Depression (HAMD) to define "responder" arbitrarily, provided a full list of subject dropouts, and described methods for successful blinding. With a mean age of 47, the trials included both men and women aged 19 to 75. Clinics in internal medicine, neurology, psychiatry, and general practice were among the several venues from which participants were recruited. However, failing to do an intention-to-treat analysis and failing to determine if the differences in responder rates between the active and placebo groups were statistically significant were the two most common methodological errors [95].

Efficacy Compared with Placebo

Patients using hypericum extract showed a substantial improvement in their HAMD scores, according to four trials comparing the extract to a placebo. Additionally, compared to placebo, three found a greater response rate among hypericum patients. At the conclusion of six weeks, a higher percentage of patients on hypericum extract were responders in the largest experiment. Compared to the placebo group, the active treatment group's mean HAMD scores are decreased more. With an 81% response rate in hypericum extract patients and a 26% response rate in placebo patients, the mean HAMD scores decreased in both groups in a subsequent experiment [96].

Efficacy Compared with Other Antidepressants

Tricyclic antidepressants (TCAs) were used as a control therapy in four trials where Hypericum extract was compared to the drug. However, relatively low dosages of TCAs were delivered in the studies, which is not the norm in practical settings. Even at a low dosage of amitriptyline hydrochloride, the response rate in the amitriptyline group was higher than that in the hypericum group in one of the experiments. The amitriptyline group saw a greater mean decrease in the overall HAMD score. In a second research, 209 individuals suffering from severe depression were given either 50 mg of imipramine hydrochloride three times a day or 600 mg of a hypericum extract containing 0.3% hypericin three times a day. After six weeks, both groups had modest response rates, with the imipramine group experiencing a larger decline in their overall HAMD score [97].

Safety: Tricyclic antidepressants (TCAs) served as a control in four experiments that contrasted hypericum extract with them. However, the studies' most significant fault was that they used incredibly low dosages of TCA. Due to the severe degree of baseline depression, three of these studies used fixed dosages of TCAs that were at or below the manufacturer's recommended starting doses. This is not typical in practice. Even with a modest dosage of amitriptyline hydrochloride, the hypericum group's responder rate was lower than that of the amitriptyline group in a Wheatley study. Additionally, the amitriptyline group had a greater decline in their overall HAMD score. At the sixth week of a trial involving 209 patients suffering from severe depression, neither group responded well. The imipramine group saw a larger mean decrease in their total HAMD score (-12.7 *vs.* -10.9) [98].

Pregnancy: A 38-year-old woman allegedly started. She took 900 mg of St. John's wort every day throughout the 24th week of her pregnancy, and she took the last dosage 24 hours before giving birth in 1998. The pregnancy went smoothly except for the delayed onset of thrombocytopenia. Another example was a 43-year-old woman who stopped taking fluoxetine and methylphenidate after becoming pregnant and started taking 900 mg of St. John's wort per day. Although any negative conditions would have been highlighted, the report makes no indication of the pregnancy's outcome. A crude aqueous extract of St. John's wort has been shown to have a modest uterotonic impact on rabbits and guinea pigs. Due to the absence of toxicity evidence, St. John's wort usage during pregnancy is not advised [99].

TRIBULUS

Biological Source: It is obtained from the seeds of *Tribulus terrestris* L., which belongs to the family *Zygophyllaceae*. Known as devil's thorn commonly. It is discovered that *Tribulus terrestris* L. (Fig. **7**) grows in subtropical regions worldwide. It is a widely widespread member of the *Zygophyllaceae* family, generally referred to as Gokhru all around India. *T. terrestris* L. fruits have been utilized in conventional Chinese medicine to treat ocular problems, edema, distention of the abdomen, emission, severe leucorrhea, impotence, and veiling. Origins and Fruits help with piles, rheumatism, kidney, and vein problems. Menorrhagia, calculi, impotence, and premature ejaculation, as well as overall weakness, *etc*. Luteinizing Hormone (LH), which tells the body to produce additional testosterone autonomously, is stimulated naturally by *T. terrestris*. A clinical study found that T. terrestris augmented libido, ovulation, and reproductive function by raising the level of hormones such as estradiol and only slightly impacted testosterone [100].

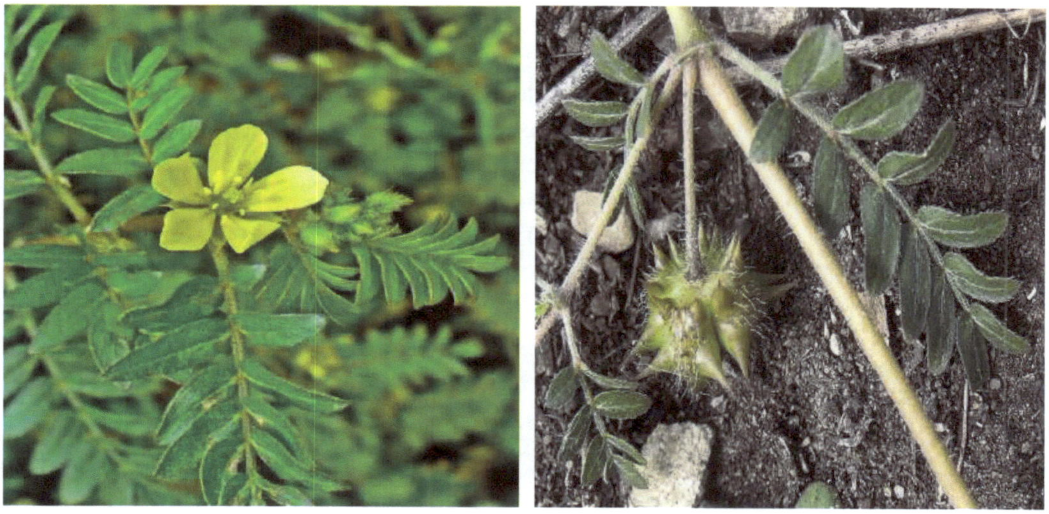

Fig. (7). *Tribulus terrestris* L.

Pharmacognostical Characteristics

In cooler areas, this herbaceous perennial plant with tap roots thrives as an annual summer plant. The stems, which frequently branch, extend outward from the crown to a diameter of between 10 cm and more than 1 m. Typically, they are prostrate and form flat patches, although in shade or among taller plants, they may climb more upwardly. With leaflets shorter than a quarter of an inch in length, the leaves are paraxially compound. The flowers have five lemon-yellow petals and are 4 to 10 mm in width [101]. Every flower blooms for one week, and then a fruit that readily splits into four or five single-seeded nutlets appears. This herb spreads and trails and is heavily covered with tiny hair. Compound leaves have three to six pairs of oppositely oriented, up to eight-centimetre-long leaflets. Usually, single, smooth, white or yellow flowers grow from the leaf axils. Bloom rapidly, with short and dense hair. Fruits are globose, tuberculate, spinous, or nearly glabrous, with two pairs of long, stiff spines on each pair, one longer than the other [102]. They are also frequently muriculate and woodi cocci. Fruit frequently sticks to animals' bodies and clothing. Woodi cocci contain a lot of seeds. The plant is extensively found throughout India, reaching elevations of up to 3,000 meters [103].

Chemical Constituents: This plant yields diosgenin and steroidal saponin. It has a high calcium and protein content. Semi-drying oil, peroxides, diastase, protein, resins, traces of glycosides, and a significant amount of inorganic debris are all present in dried fruit. Additionally, β-sitosterol and stigmasterol were extracted from the roots, stem, and leaves [104].

Pharmacological Activities: Tribulus terrestris displays a broad spectrum of pharmacological activity, including astringent, analgesic, alterative, emmenagogue, nervine tonic, demulcent, anti-inflammatory, antibacterial, diuretic, and aphrodisiac properties. Infusions or decoctions of its spiny fruits and plant parts are used to treat numerous genitourinary ailments, such as postpartum uterine disorders, gravel, renal illnesses, impotence, gout, urinary issues, calculus disorders, chronic cystitis, gleet, gonorrhea, phosphaturia, and spermatorrhea. Additionally, in northern India, it is employed in controlling cough and heart illnesses [105].

Clinical Trial of Tribulus

For erectile dysfunction in Men: Clinical investigations investigating the effectiveness of *Tribulus Terrestris* (TT) extracts in males have focused on two key outcome categories. Some studies primarily analyse the therapy of erectile dysfunction, measuring erection quality and desire intensity, while others measure changes in baseline testosterone secretion by comparing post-trial levels to beginning values. However, current data have not completely settled concerns surrounding TT's genuine efficacy, due to subjective endpoint judgements and uneven findings, even for objectively measurable measures like testosterone, dihydrotestosterone, and pituitary gonadotropin levels [106]. In a recent phase IV, prospective, randomized, double-blind, placebo-controlled clinical trial, Kamenov *et al.* investigated the safety and efficacy of a standardized TT extract (Tribestan®, Sopharma AD; 250 mg coated tablets, equivalent to ≥112.5 mg furostanol saponins) in men with mild to moderate erectile dysfunction, with or without hypoactive sexual desire disorder [105]. The study featured 90 patients per group (treatment *vs.* placebo), a 12-week treatment length with a daily dosage of three coated tablets, with the primary endpoint being the change in International Index of Erectile Function (IIEF) score at the trial's completion. The treatment group revealed substantial increases in erection, libido, and orgasmic function, with no variations in side effect profiles compared to the placebo [107]. *Dose:* Active doses used in clinical situations range from 750-1500 mg/day [108].

TURMERIC

Biological Source: It is obtained from the dried roots of *Curcuma longa,* belonging to the family *Zingiberaceae*. Turmeric (Fig. **8**), which originates from plants, has been found to offer medicinal advantages. Owing to these benefits, a variety of turmeric dietary supplements with diverse formulations and health claims (increasing joint comfort, enhancing cognitive function, encouraging flexibility and mobility, and delivering cardiovascular health advantages [109]. Originally from India, turmeric (Curcuma longa) is a plant that belongs to the ginger family (*Zingiberaceae*) and is currently farmed all over the world, particularly in Southeast Asia, China, and Latin America. In India and other Asian nations, curries are typically cooked with turmeric due to its flavor and color. India is the leading exporter and the greatest producer of turmeric. According to research, the global turmeric market was valued at over 1.7 million metric tons, and by 2027, it was predicted to rise drastically. The global curcumin market was valued at over half a billion US dollars in 2016 and is predicted to grow at a Compound Annual Growth Rate (CAGR) of 13% between 2018 and 2025 [110].

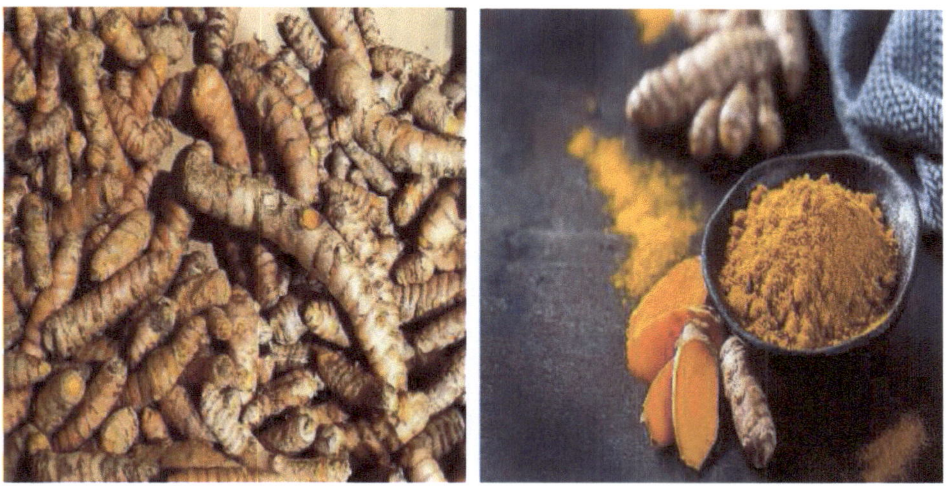

Fig. (8). Turmeric.

Chemical Constituents: Turmeric (*Curcuma longa*) possesses a complex chemical composition, consisting of approximately 70% carbohydrates, 13% moisture, 6% protein, 6% essential oils (including borneol, phellandrene, sabinene, cineol, zingiberene, and sesquiterpenes), 5% fat, 3% minerals (potassium, calcium, phosphorus, iron, and sodium), 3–5% curcuminoids, and trace amounts of vitamins B1, B2, C, and niacin [111]. The curcuminoid fraction includes around 77% curcumin (CUR), 17% demethoxycurcumin (DMC), and 3–6% bisdemethoxycurcumin (BMC). Curcumin was initially obtained from C. longa rhizomes by Vogel and Pelletier in 1815. Curcumin comes in two tautomeric forms-enol and keto- with the keto form prevailing in neutral and acidic pH settings, while the enol form, stabilized by intramolecular hydrogen bonding, is prominent in alkaline situations [112, 113]. Due to its lipophilic nature (log P = 3.0), curcumin is largely insoluble in aqueous solutions at neutral or acidic pH but dissolves rapidly in organic solvents such as methanol, ethanol, acetone, and dimethyl sulfoxide. In alkaline aqueous solutions, curcumin's solubility rises;

however, it degrades fast in both neutral and alkaline settings. Maximum absorption of curcumin occurs at 430 nm in methanol and at 415–420 nm in acetone [114].

Clinical Trials of Turmeric

Inflammation and Pain: Biliary illnesses, abnormalities of the liver. Oppenheimer performed the first clinical trial of curcumin in 1937 to evaluate the effects of "curcumen" or "curcunat" (contains 0.1 to 0.25 g), 0.1 g of calcium cholate, and sodium curcumin on biliary diseases in humans. An intravenous injection of 5% sodium curcumin solution was provided to healthy persons, causing the gallbladder to empty fast. During a lengthy period of monitoring, one patient notably exhibited a complete recovery. In a separate experiment, the administration of Chologam F Nattermann (dry extracts from Curcuma and Schöllkraut) substantially alleviated the symptoms of biliary dyskinesia [115].

Bronchial Asthma: It has also been discovered that curcumin works incredibly well for bronchial asthma. Abidi *et al.* looked into how well patients with bronchial asthma responded to curcumin as an adjuvant treatment. The mean forced expiratory volume 1s (FEV1) values improved after taking curcumin pills, indicating a reduction in airway blockage. Additionally, better haematological parameters were attained [116]. *Gingivitis:* An infection with Helicobacter pylori in the stomach induces the release of a number of inflammatory cytokines, which in turn produce gastritis. In research, Koosirirat and colleagues studied the influence of curcumin on the production of IL-8, IL-1β, TNF-α, and COX-2 in the stomach mucosa of patients with gastritis infected with Helicobacter pylori. Curcumin has a limited influence on inflammatory cytokine production induced by H. pylori, as indicated by its failure to suppress the production of these cytokines. However, according to other studies, the curcumin drug relieved these patients [117].

Curcumin for Skin Diseases: Additionally, curcumin has demonstrated remarkable efficacy against a range of skin conditions, including vitiligo and psoriasis [118]. *Psoriasis:* An autoimmune disorder called psoriasis is marked by irregularly formed skin patches. Curcumin was demonstrated to have an antipsoriatic impact in a clinical investigation *via* modulating PhK activity. In a recent clinical intervention that was double-blind, randomized, and placebo-controlled, those who took the curcumin formulation Meriva revealed improved health results. When these people took topical steroids in combination, it further exacerbated their antipsoriatic effects. As a consequence, it was observed that it was highly beneficial when taken as an adjuvant treatment for psoriasis vulgaris and that it greatly lowered blood levels of IL-22. Furthermore, in a phase II, open-label, two-stage Simon trial, the safety and efficacy of curcumin were reported. Patients with plaque psoriasis got 4.5 g of oral curcuminoid C3 complex once a day [119].

Dermatitis: Curcumin has been tested in a randomized, double-blind, placebo-controlled clinical study to see if it might diminish the severity of radiation-associated dermatitis in 30 women with breast cancer who developed dermatitis. A decrease in the Radiation dermatitis severity was noticed in those Patients who are taking 6 g/day of curcumin p.o. after sessions of radiation [120]. *Curcumin for Infectious Diseases:* Curcumin has demonstrated considerable effects in the treatment of infectious disorders. Hepatitis B, Hepatitis C, alcoholic liver disease, non-alcoholic fatty liver disease, drug-induced hepatotoxicity, liver cancer, biliary cirrhosis, and primary sclerosing cholangitis are among the several liver disease that curcumin has been found to protect against. Curcumin's capacity to decrease NF-κB and function as an antioxidant is vital for its ability to prevent a number of liver illnesses. In a number of animal models of liver injury, curcumin was found to decrease liver damage. It was shown that the herbal combination of C. longa and Tinospora cordifolia greatly decreased hepatotoxicity brought on by anti-tuberculosis medicine without having any severe side effects [121]. *Other Diseases:* Curcumin has promise for treating several disorders, including arsenic carcinogenicity and dyspepsia. Its antioxidant qualities can decrease arsenic's harmful effects, suppress exercise-induced oxidative stress, and lower premenstrual syndrome severity in women. Curcuminoids can help prevent oxidative damage in β-thalassemia/Hb E patients. It has been proven to enhance post-operative results in patients receiving laparoscopic cholecystectomy. Curcumin's anti-inflammatory properties help reduce pruritus and enhance the quality of life in individuals with lupus nephritis and MGUS. Oral use of curcumin can help regulate renal inflammation and lower paraprotein levels in individuals with MGUS and multiple myeloma. Overall, curcumin's multitargeting potential is substantial (Table **2**) [122].

Table 2. Clinical Trials of *Curcuma longa* [123 - 127].

Disease/Condition	Formulation Used	Study Type	Key Outcome
General Curcumin Absorption	Curcumin + hydrophilic carrier, cellulose derivatives, antioxidants	Human study (12 healthy volunteers)	Curcuminoid levels in blood increased compared to regular curcumin.
Solid Tumor	Meriva® (curcumin + phosphatidylcholine)	Clinical trial (80 chemotherapy patients)	Reduced inflammation markers (TNF-α and IL-6).
Diabetes	Meriva®	Clinical trial (38 patients)	Improved blood flow and reduced swelling in limbs

(Table 2) cont.....

Disease/Condition	Formulation Used	Study Type	Key Outcome
Osteoarthritis	Meriva®	Clinical trial (100 patients)	Better clinical results and improvement in biochemical markers
Neuronal Damage	Solid lipid nanoparticles	Animal study (male mice)	Decreased brain toxicity caused by aluminum chloride (AlCl3)

Dosage: It is well acknowledged that curcumin does not result in substantial short-term toxicity at doses up to 8 g, based on human research. Day 1. This curcumin dosage is thought to be appropriate for clinical investigations. It involves the brief administration of curcumin. Curcumin at this dosage is not entirely safe, though. Since research on humans has indicated that curcumin at dosages varying from 0.9 to 3.6 g day~1 for 1-4 months is the source of certain negative consequences, such as nausea and diarrhea, and results in an elevation of lactate dehydrogenase and alkaline phosphatase in the serum [128].

VITEX

Biological Source: It is obtained from the dried fruits of *Vitex agnus-castus,* belonging to the family *Lamiaceae*. According to traditional applications, the Vitex (Fig. **9**) species have been employed as a folk remedy to treat a variety of diseases. Under the subheading "Alternative and complementary medicinal uses," Vitex species are highlighted as a medication that doctors prescribe to treat a variety of illnesses. Additionally, it lists the applications for which Vitex species, or their commercially available preparations, are used. The Vitex species are listed alphabetically under each area [129].

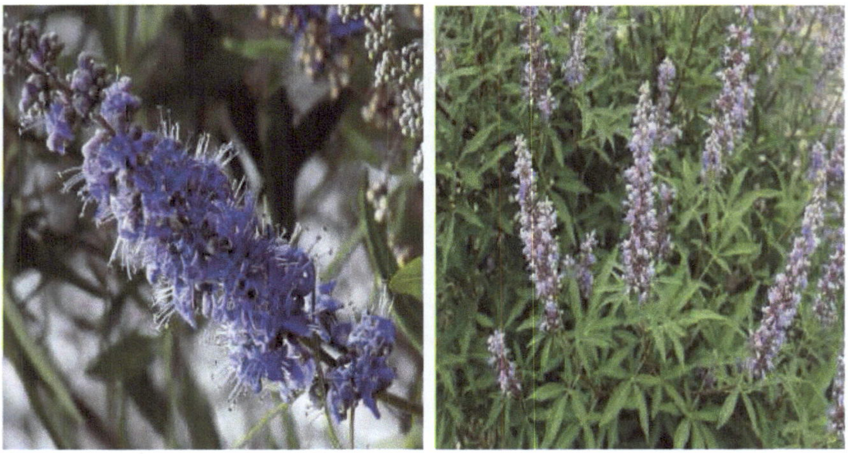

Fig. (9). Vitex.

Geographical Source: The biggest genus in the Verbenaceae family, Vitex, has 250 species of deciduous shrubs dispersed globally. Notable medicinal species include *V. agnus-castus* Linn. and *V. negundo* Linn. The Chaste Tree (*V. agnus-castus*) typically grows along riverbanks and shorelines in Central Asia, Southern Europe, and the Mediterranean. *V. negundo* is mostly found in Pakistan, India, and Sri Lanka. V. rotundifolia Linn. occurs throughout China's coastline from north to south, as well as in the Mediterranean and Central Asia. *V. trifolia* is prevalent in Vietnam and other Asian nations [130].

Morphology: Known by the common names monk's pepper and chaste tree, *Vitex agnus castus* is a member of the Verbenaceae family, which is found in Central Asia, the Mediterranean area, and Southern Europe. It is also harvested in various locations around the continent. It is a massive shrub or small deciduous tree that may grow to a height of 1.5 to 2 meters on average [131]. The leaves have five to seven finger-like leaflets and range in diameter from 7.6 to 10 cm. They have a gray-green tinge on top, a lighter bottom, and a fragrant top. From July through early October, purple-blackberries that yield fruit produce clusters of fragrant, violet, blue, and deep purple blossoms. Because the dried leaves and fruit berries have been used medicinally, it is considered an herbal plant product. The medicinal component of *Vagnus-castus* is in its fruit [132].

Traditional Use

Another name for the *Vitex agnus-castus* tree is "chaste lamb" in Latin, which describes the decrease in sexual drive that follows ingestion of a beverage prepared from the plant's seeds. The fruits have been used for more than 2500 years in ancient Egypt, Greece, Iran, and Rome to cure a variety of gynaecologic conditions. It has also been used because it is said to reduce libido. In traditional Persian medicine, the berries of *V. agnus-castus* can be used in lieu of pepper, and the leaves and fruits are good options for adding flavour and spice to cuisine. In addition to its antiepileptic, carminative, energiser, sedative, anticonvulsant, and tranquillizing properties, the fruit has been proposed as a hormone-like remedy for menstruation difficulties and digestive disorders. In addition to treating acne, snakebites, scorpion stings, inadequate breastfeeding, menstrual discomfort, eye diseases, spasmodic dysmenorrhea, and stomach pains, this plant is used as an emmenagogue, an anaphrodisiac, and an antispasmodic in the ethnomedicine of various nations [133].

Chemical Constituents

Vitex agnus-castus fruits contain a range of chemical components, including essential oils, flavonoids, iridoid glycosides, diterpenoids (such as agnuside), isoflavonoids, and phenolic compounds. The major active chemicals include flavonoids such as apigenin, vitexin, isovitexin, luteolin, orientin, and isoorientin, along with numerous others, such as 6″-caffeoylisoorientin, viteagnusins, vitexlactams, and viteagnuside [134]. *In-vitro* studies on the fruits also discovered that they contain isoflavonoid vitexcarpan and phenolic substances such as agnucastoside C, p-hydroxybenzoic acid, and its glucose ester. Linoleic acid, another component, may have estrogen-like actions by binding to estrogen receptors and activating particular genes. The essential oil of Vitex agnus-castus comprises chemicals such as (Z)-β-farnesene, 1,8-cineole, sabinene, α-pinene, and α-terpinyl acetate. Standard preparations of the plant employ essential reference chemicals such as vitexilactone, casticin, aucubin, and agnuside for quality control [135].

Pharmacological Activities

Vitex agnus-castus is mostly used to treat menstrual abnormalities, menopausal problems, and PMS because of its hormonal properties. Additional benefits include anti-inflammatory, anti-tumoricidal, antimutagenic, antimicrobial, antifungal, insect repellent, larvicidal, osteopenic, antinociceptive, opioidergic, antiepileptic, oxidative stress, antioxidant qualities, and prevention of non-alcoholic fat liver disease (Tables **3** and **4**) [136].

Table 3. Pharmacological activities of vitex.

Effect	Plant Part Used	Key Chemical Compounds	Experimental Model	Refs.
Neuroprotective	Ethanolic extract of fruits (seeds)	Linoleic acid	*In vitro*	[137]
Antimicrobial	Methanolic leaf extract, seed volatile oil, and essential oil from fruits	Caryophyllene oxide, trans-caryophyllene (19.17%), sabinene (18.05%), 1,8-cineole (16.13%), α-terpinyl acetate (6.91%), dihydroselarene (6.73%)	*In vitro*	[138]
Antifungal	Volatile extracts from leaves, flowers, and fruits	Alpha-pinene, spathulenol, β-farnesene, sabinene, 1,8-cineole, α-terpinyl acetate, (E)-bicyclogermacrene, manool, (E)-caryophyllene	*In vitro*	[139]
Antioxidant	Ethyl acetate extract of fruits	Flavonoids such as casticin, vitexin, and orientin	*In vitro*	[140]
Fracture healing	Ethanol extract of fruits	Flavonoids	*In vitro*	[141]

(Table 3) cont.....

Effect	Plant Part Used	Key Chemical Compounds	Experimental Model	Refs.
Anti-inflammatory	Methanol extract of aerial parts	Artemetin, casticin, 3,3'-dihydrox- -5,6,7, 4'-tetramethoxyflavone, penduletin, methyl 4-hydroxybenzoate	*In vitro*	[142]

Table 4. Clinical trial of *Vitex.*

Disorder	Formulation	Dosage	Study Design	Patients	Duration	Results	Refs.
Menopausal symptoms	Essential oil from V. agnus-castus (fruits/leaves)	Group 1: Transdermal, oral, and inhalation; Group 2: 1.5% cream/lotion with essential oil	Two clinical trials	23 women (1st study), 52 women (2nd study)	3 months	Improvement in menopausal symptoms	[143]
Primary dysmenorrhea	V. agnus-castus extract	Group 1: Yasmin (0.03 mg ethinyl estradiol + 3 mg drospirenone); Group 2: 4 mg extract tablet daily	Prospective, comparative Doppler study	60 women with dysmenorrhea, 30 healthy controls	3 cycles	Reduced VAS (pain) scores	[144]
Cyclic mastalgia	Fructus agni casti fruit extract	1 tablet daily (Group 1) or 200 mg/day flurbiprofen (Group 2)	Randomized, double-blind, drug-controlled trial	104 premenopausal women	3 months	Comparable effect to flurbiprofen	[145]
Fracture healing	Agnugol® tablet (4 mg V. agnus-castus dried extract)	Various combinations of magnesium oxide and placebo	Double-blind, randomized, placebo-controlled trial	64 women	8 weeks	Enhanced fracture healing	[146]

Dosage: The German Commission E recommended 30–40 mg of dried fruit extract daily, 40 drops of tincture, or 2.6–4.2 mg of dry native extract (standardised to 0.6% caricin). Furthermore, it has been suggested that consuming 3–6 g of dry herb and 1 g of dried fruit daily might help cure irregular menstruation. After two days of treatment with the essential oil of Vitex agnus-castus leaves, no animal death was seen, even at the highest dose (5000 mg/kg). As a result, the LD50 of this essential oil in mice exceeded the 5 g/kg maximum dose [147]. *Adverse Effects:* When this plant is used, there are only minor and temporary side effects. The most frequent side effects include headache, gastrointestinal disturbances, weight gain, acne, dizziness, nausea, intermenstrual hemorrhage or menstrual irregularities, and allergic responses [148]. *Drug Interaction:* Systematic reviews have not identified or documented any medication interactions. Chaste tree may theoretically conflict with dopaminergic antagonists like metoclopramide and bromocriptine. Furthermore, due to their potential effect on ERs, antipsychotic medications should not be used concurrently. Instead, they should be used carefully in conjunction with oral contraceptives and hormone replacement therapy. CYPs 1A2, 2C19, 2D6, and 3A4 were shown to be inhibited by *Vitex agnus-castus* extract; however, *in vivo* tests showed that the effects on CYPs 2C19 and 3A4 were particularly strong. Thus, these herbal dose forms may have an impact on concurrent use with medications that are processed by these enzymes [149].

Pregnancy and Lactation: Because of its progesteronic and oestrogenic properties, *Vitex agnus-castus* should be avoided or forbidden during pregnancy. Until human studies are controlled, it is unknown if the plant is safe to take during pregnancy. During pregnancy planning, *V. agnus-castus* drugs should be administered. Due to probable hormonal effects, it is advised to avoid using the chaste tree while nursing, even if there are no scientific data proving that its compounds move into breast milk. More human investigation and clinical trials are necessary to establish if components of *Vitex agnus-castus* may transit the placenta into the foetus and breast milk, even though its phytoestrogenic and phytoprogesteronic properties make it unlikely to be dangerous for newborns [150].

WILLOW

Biological source: It is obtained from the dried bark and leaves of *Salix nigra,* belonging to the family *Salicaceae*. Traditionally, the genus Populus (poplar) and *Salicaceae* (the Willow and Poplar family), Salix, or willow (Fig. **10**), is amentiferous and prevalent in northern temperate zones. The Salicaceae have currently been expanded to include the majority of Flacourtiaceae's tropical species, which don't make catkins. As a result, the Salicaceae family currently has 1,220 species and 56 genera. The Salicaceae family comprises fast-growing trees and shrubs with broad economic and environmental uses. These plants are employed for basket-making and caning owing to the suppleness of willow twigs. They serve architectural, horticultural, and aesthetic objectives, beautifying landscapes while stabilizing soil to avoid erosion. Additionally, they give resources for lumber, paper, fences, shelter, arrow shafts, fish traps, whistles, nets, and rope. The family also contributes to renewable energy as a source of biomass fuel [151].

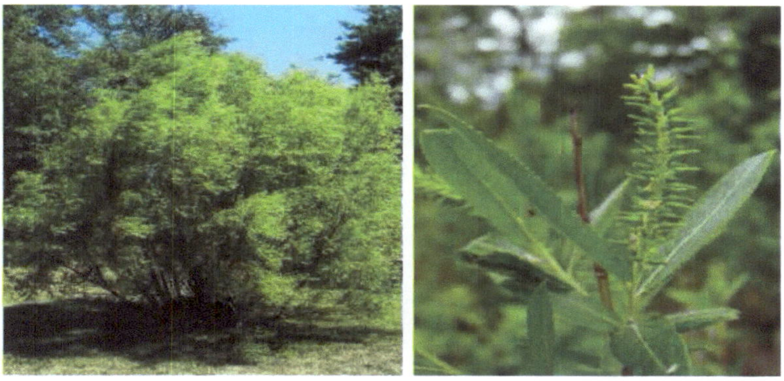

Fig. (10). Willow.

Geographical Source: North America and Africa are home to Salix species. America, Asia, and Europe. Salix species, which may be found in temperate, subtropical, and tropical climates, are trees, shrubs, or prostrate plants that grow quickly and are more tolerant of a variety of climatic circumstances than Populus species [152]. *Chemical Components:* Several phytoconstituents or secondary metabolites of the Salix genus have been identified, including flavonoids, phenolic and nonphenolic glycosides, procyanidins, organic acid derivatives, and organic acids, simple phenolics, sterols and terpenes, lignans, volatiles, and fatty acids. Salix leaves are the primary source of flavonoids, phenolic acids, their derivatives, and phenolic glycosides, while stem bark is the primary source of procyanidins [153].

Traditional Uses

Salix plants have been utilized for medical purposes since ancient times and have been connected to the invention of aspirin and acetylsalicylic acid. These botanicals have long been used to alleviate fever, inflammation, and excruciating musculoskeletal joint pain. A significant physiologically active metabolite of Salix, salicin hydrolyzes in the gastrointestinal system to produce D-glucose and salicyl alcohol. Upon absorption, the latter undergoes oxidation to produce salicylic acid, the active medication that blocks cyclooxygenases. It has been utilised in traditional medicine to treat both acute and persistent fevers. Also used in infection and inflammation. The usage of *S. tetrasperma* Roxb. to treat conditions includes epilepsy, diabetes, fever, rheumatism, piles, swellings, bladder stones, diarrhoea, wounds, earache, coughing, colds, and coughs. Bark from *S. alba L.* has long been used to treat fever, headaches, rheumatism, and the flu [154].

Pharmacological Activity

Anti-microbial Activity of Salix: Multidrug-resistant bacteria are common, and natural resources have been utilised to find novel antibacterial chemicals since they offer a limitless potential for finding new medications, especially to combat these germs. Salix extracts' antimicrobial activity is mostly assessed *via* antibiofilm function tests, broth microdilution techniques, agar well diffusion, and disc diffusion experiments. Microbial growth inhibition zones and percentages, as well as Minimum Inhibitory Concentrations (MICs), demonstrated the strength of Salix species as antimicrobials and predicted their potential as functional foods [155]. *Antifungal Action:* The growth curve research, filter disc test, broth microdilution, and poisoned food methodologies were used to determine the antifungal properties of salix extracts. The effectiveness of the antifungal against Candida was evaluated in various plants like *Guilliermondii Oxysporum, C. glabrata, C. parapsilosis, and Fusarium* [156]. *Antioxidant Activity:* Numerous human illnesses, including cancer, diabetes, ulcers, autoimmune and cardiovascular disorders, viral infections, and inflammation, have been linked to Reactive Oxygen Species (ROS). The polyphenolic content of salix species, including *S. tetrasperma Roxb., S. atrocinerea Brot., S. fragilis L.*, and *S. viminalis* L., demonstrates antioxidant action. Strong *in vitro* and *in vivo* antioxidant activity was shown by the effect of *S. tetrasperma* Roxb. extract on neuropathic pain. Isorhamnetin-3-O-β-D-rutinoside, triandrin, gallocatechin, tremuloidin, aromadendrin, salicin, and chrysoeriol-7-O-glucuronid were among the compounds found in *S. subserrata* Willd. Leaf extracts that showed antioxidant properties against oxidative stress in *Caenorhabditis elegans* [157].

Neuroprotective Function: The neuropharmacological characteristics of Salix species have not been extensively studied. According to one research, *S. tetrasperma* Roxb. leaf extract reduced muscular grip and motility, suggesting skeletal muscle relaxation and CNS depression, which may be caused by flavonoids binding to GABA receptors. Another work from our group demonstrated its neuroprotection in models of neuropathic pain and sciatic nerve damage, reducing inflammation and oxidative stress in the brain stem and sciatic nerve to relieve hyperalgesia and allodynia [158]. *Hepatoprotective Action:* The floral extract of *S. subserrata* Willd. Showed significant hepatoprotective benefits in a model of liver damage caused by carbon tetrachloride (CCl_4), mainly by lowering elevated liver enzymes and the protein levels of two inflammatory biomarkers (NF-κB and TNF-α). Additionally, it had a remarkable ability to reduce lipid peroxidation and showed antioxidant qualities associated with many active ingredients, such as flavonoids like luteolin-7-glucoside, rutin, and quercetin, and phenolic compounds like salignin and catechins. Table **5** shows the clinical trials of willow [159].

Table 5. Clinical trial of willow.

Disease/Activity	Formulation/Dosage	Model	Outcome	Refs.
Anticancer	0.2 and 0.6 ml of 10% w/v extract orally	EACC-induced tumor in mice (*in vivo*)	Tumor growth was reduced, and survival time was extended	[160]
Neuroprotective	200 and 400 mg/kg orally	*In vivo* study on mice	Decreased locomotor activity indicated CNS depressant and muscle relaxant effects.	[161]
Hepatoprotective	150 mg/kg orally	CCl_4-induced liver damage in rats	Lowered liver enzyme levels; reduced TNF-α and NF-κB expression	[162]
Antilipidemic	2.5 or 10 g/kg extract with food orally	High-fat diet (HFD) mice model	Reduced body weight and fat accumulation in the parametrial tissue	[163]

VALERIAN

Biological Source: Valerian, a member of the Valerianaceae family (Fig. **11**). The well-known herb and medicinal plant Valeriana officinalis is used extensively worldwide, particularly in China, Europe, and the Middle East. The *Valerianaceae* family, which is widely distributed across the globe, includes plants (rarely shrubs) with opposing leaves, a sympetalous, spurred corolla, one to four stamens, and an undeveloped, tricarpellate ovary with one functional locule and one apical ovule. The fruit is an achene, and some individuals have a calyx that looks like a pappus. Economic uses include a few species of culinary, medicinal, and essential oil plants, as well as certain cultivated ornamentals (such as Centranthus). Valeriana officinalis is a native of Europe and Asia that has spread to eastern North America. This noble perennial is found in Northern Europe [164].

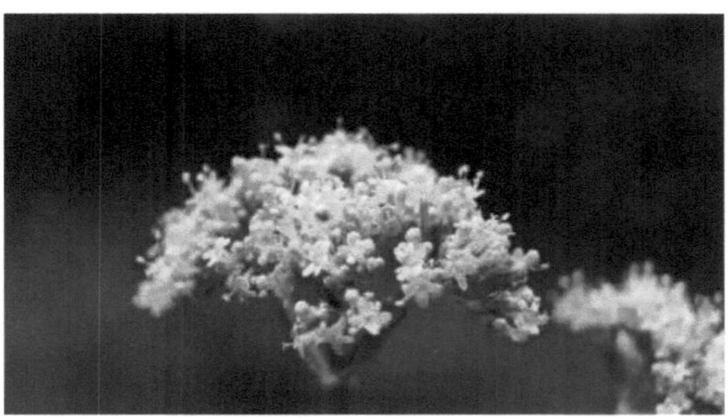

Fig. (11). Valerian.

Chemical Constituents: Essential minerals, including copper (13.1 ppm), manganese (16.8 ppm), and zinc (75.1 ppm), have been discovered to be present in Valerian root [165]. More than 150 distinct chemical components make up valerian, many of which have pharmacological and physiological effects. Depending on the plant's origin, growing environment, processing techniques, and storage circumstances, these chemicals' composition might vary greatly. Manufacturers standardise valerian extracts to guarantee constant quality. The following are important pharmacologically active components: terpenes, alkaloids, organic acids and their derivatives, Valepotriates, and flavones. The calming effects of valerian are mainly attributed to a class of alkaloids called valepotriates. Terpenes are the main class of alkaloids, which are found in trace amounts (0.01–0.05%).

Valerian contains important alkaloids such as actinidine, chatinine, viterianine, alpha-methyl pyrryl ketone, and naphthyridine methyl ketone [166]. Actinidine has special qualities due to its cyclopentapyridine structure, which is also present in Actinidia polygama (silver vine) and valerian essential oil. Notably, actinidine is a psychoactive alkaloid that influences the GABA (gamma-aminobutyric acid) system and functions as a benzodiazepine receptor agonist. It may also draw cats. The soothing effects of valerian may be attributed to this modulation, which has an impact on the central nervous system. Quinolic acid and lysine are used in the biosynthesis of actinidine. The effects of alpha-methyl pyrryl ketone on the central nervous system were investigated in a 1970 study carried out in Germany. Furthermore, naphthyridyl methyl ketone structural analogues were suggested as possible schizophrenia therapies. Despite these discoveries, it is still unknown how exactly valerian alkaloids contribute to its overall therapeutic effect since each of these substances has not been thoroughly investigated separately [167].

Traditional Use of Valerian

In Europe, valerian, which comes from the roots of V. officinalis, is used as a sedative to treat anxious states and sleep disorders brought on by worry. It is often used as a gentler alternative to more potent synthetic sedatives like benzodiazepines because of its moderate sedative and sleep-promoting qualities [168]. Valerian is also used as a smooth-muscle relaxant for cramping in the stomach and intestines and as a tranquillizer for hyper-excitability. Supplements containing dried root or extracts in the form of tablets and soft gelatin capsules are now available [169]. These supplements are widely used; in the US and Europe, an estimated 210 and 125 million doses are marketed each year, respectively. Traditionally, Valerian has been used to treat stress, anxiety, sleeplessness, restlessness, and epilepsy. On the other hand, withdrawal symptoms may result from high dosages. Valerian should not be used by those who have liver illness.

Because some people lack the digestive conversion qualities necessary to properly break down valerian, they may suffer adverse effects, including headaches and sleep terrors, which might cause anxiety [170]. Clinical Trials are discussed in Table **6**.

Table 6. Clinical trial of valerian.

Disease	Formulations	Type of Study	Outcome	Refs.
Insomnia	*Valeriana officinalis* extract	Double-blind, randomized, placebo-controlled studies evaluating the impact of valerian monopreparations on subjects' ability to sleep	Sleep quality improved	[171]
Each ache is caused by tension	Root extract	88 participants with tension-type headache	The current study showed that valerian could lessen the impact of tension-type headaches on daily functioning, disability, and headache severity.	[172]
Women experiencing postmenopausal insomnia	530 mg of concentrated valerian extract	randomized, triple-blind, controlled trial on 100 postmenopausal women aged between 50 and 60.	When menopausal women suffer from sleeplessness, Valerian helps them sleep better.	[173]

Adverse Effects: Excessive use of Valerian can lead to headache, uneasiness, excitability, and cardiac disturbances [174].

SPIRULINA

Biological Source: Spirulina is a blue-green alga obtained from *Spirulina platensis* belonging to the family *Oscillatoriaceae*. For a very long time, humans have been utilising the safe and healthful meal known as spirulina (Fig. **12**). This cyanobacterium is tiny and filamentous. It is manufactured for commercial purposes in huge outdoor ponds under regulated settings. The information that is presently known on the therapeutic potential and uses of spirulina in humans, coupled with clinical data addressing the supplement's safety and adverse effects, is presented here. The chemical makeup of spirulina, which includes vital fatty acids, proteins, carbs, essential amino acids, minerals (particularly iron), vitamins, and colours, may be helpful to health [175]. In this respect, it appears that the three principal bioactive components of spirulina, the protein phycocyanin, γ-linolenic acid, and sulfated polysaccharides, have a considerable influence on enhancing physiological processes. Usually found in tropical and subtropical locations, these warm-water organisms have higher salinity, pH, and carbonate/bicarbonate concentrations. They are non-heterocystous cyanobacteria that are filamentous. Filtration and other physical separation procedures are simply employed to collect their huge filaments, which have a diameter ranging from 3 to 12 μm. In 1827, Turpin isolated spirulina from a freshwater sample [176].

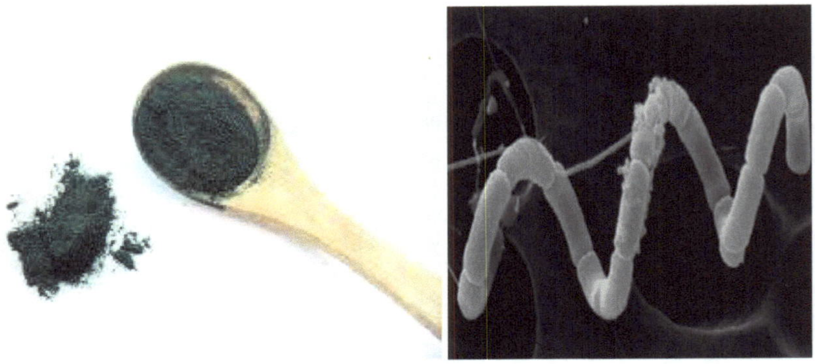

Fig. (12). Spirulina.

Geographical Source: Spirulina is a common organism. Since Turpin first isolated Spirulina species from a freshwater stream in 1827, they have been found in a wide range of habitats, including freshwater, brackish water, marshes, sand, dirt, and the ocean. Spirulina species, for instance, have been isolated from warm waters found in fishponds, power plants, salt pans, thermal springs, tropical oceans up to the North Sea, *etc.* Because of this, the organism seems to be able to adapt to a wide range of environments, filling areas where other bacteria would find it very difficult or impossible to flourish. Prominent instances are alkalophilic S. platensis in many alkaline lakes in Africa and S. maxima colonies in Lake Texcoco, Mexico. Spirulina is kept as a quasi-monoculture in a few of these lakes [177].

Chemical Constituents: Spirulina contains protein, ranging between 55 and 70 percent of the dry weight, which is an exceptionally high percentage of protein. It is a complete protein since it has every necessary amino acid. Polyunsaturated fatty acids make up 1.5–2.0 percent of total lipid, which is high in spirulina. The linolenic acid, arachidonic acid, stearidonic acid, eicosapentaenoic acid, and docosahexaenoic acid are rich in spirulina. Spirulina has vitamin C, vitamin D, vitamin E, and vitamins B_1, B_2, B_3, B_6, and B_{12} [178].

Nutritional Properties of Spirulina: Due to its many medicinal advantages, spirulina is gaining popularity in the health food sector as a functional food and nutraceutical. It was declared the "best food for the future" at the World Food Conference in 1974, and the United Nations calls it the "most ideal food for mankind." Spirulina has been proposed as one of the primary foods that could be grown on long-term space missions in the late 1980s and early 1990s by prestigious space agencies such as the National Aeronautics and Space Administration (NASA) and the European Space Agency (ESA), and the FDA has confirmed that it is "one of the best protein sources". Spirulina is believed to be rich in a variety of substances, such as carbs, protein, β-carotene, γ linolenic acid (GLA), vitamins, minerals, phytonutrients, sulpholipids, and glycolipids. Spirulina adds specific health benefits to functional meals and improves the nutritional content of food items. So far, businesses have solely used dry powdered spirulina for food compositions and value addition; fresh spirulina has not been utilised. A later version of the yoghurt, which included fresh spirulina, demonstrated greater nutritional and health advantages. The spirulina drying process was effectively eliminated by the research, and the quality of the finished product was little affected. Furthermore, the methanolic and aqueous extracts of Spirulina biomass may have nutraceutical advantages. There are marketed items that are supplemented with spirulina due to the enhanced protein content. Bread, biscuits, cakes, cheese, yoghurt, ice cream, infant food, and protein bars for athletes are some of the forms it comes in [179]. Table **7** contains the clinical studies on spirulina.

Table 7. Clinical trials of spirulina.

Disease/Condition	Dose/Formulation	Clinical Trial / *In Vivo* / *In Vitro*	Outcome	Refs.
Chronic Fatigue	3 g/day	*In vivo*	Increased lactobacillus in the gut promotes Vitamin B6 production, aiding in energy release.	[180]
Allergy, Rhinitis, Immunomodulation	Daily Spirulina supplementation for 12 weeks	*In vivo* (Human trial)	Enhanced IgA levels in saliva, suggesting improved mucosal immunity	[181]
Antiviral	Calcium Spirulina and aqueous extract	*In vitro*	Inhibited replication of enveloped viruses like HSV-1, CMV, measles, influenza A, and HIV-1	[182]
Cholesterol and Diabetes Management	4.2 g/day to 15 male volunteers	*In vivo*	Lowered LDL cholesterol and reduced atherogenic risk after 8 weeks	[183]

Dosage: Consuming 1.0–8.0 g of spirulina daily has been shown to provide numerous health advantages. Elderly people should consume no more than 2.0–3.0 g of spirulina per day, whereas children should consume no more than 1.0–2.0 g. It is handy to take spirulina as tablets before, during, or after meals.

Spirulina powder is frequently used to fruit smoothies for breakfast and veggie smoothies for even afternoon meals [184].

WHEATGRASS

Biological Source: It is obtained from the young parts of *Triticum aestivum* belonging to the family *Poaceae.* This plant is the most common in India. However, its origin is still unknown. Among its many nutritional advantages, this plant has been shown to have anti-inflammatory, antibacterial, anti-carcinogenic, immunomodulatory, laxative, astringent, diuretic, antioxidant, and anti-aging properties. It has been shown to be beneficial in the treatment of oedema, atherosclerosis, renal issues, colitis, and acidity [185]. Wheatgrass (Fig. **13**) juice promotes the creation of healthy tissue cells and aids in the production of red blood cells. 23 kg of fresh veggies are equivalent to 100 g of wheatgrass powder. Wheatgrass should ideally be taken 1 hour before eating. This may reduce appetite and enable the body to thoroughly metabolise it without competing with other nutrients. To gain the greatest benefits of the juice, it is advised to drink a lot of water, at least one litre. It's best to take wheatgrass supplements in the middle of the morning or mid-afternoon to get this “green” energy boost [186].

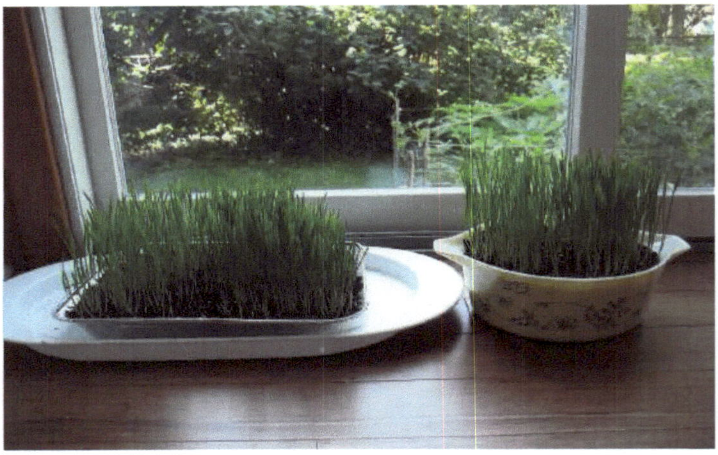

Fig. (13). Wheatgrass.

Pharmacognostical Characteristics: The glabrous, simple, hollow or pithy culms of wheatgrass have leaves that are about 1.2 m tall, flat, narrow, 20–38 cm long, and 1.3 cm wide. The long, thin, dorsally compressed, and somewhat flattened spikes [187]. *Chemical Constituents:* Wheatgrass is a food that is harvested before the plant produces the bloom head. 860 mg of protein, 18.5 mg of chlorophyll, 15 mg of calcium, 38 mg of lysine, 7.5 mg of vitamin C, and a variety of micronutrients, such as B complex vitamins and amino acids, are all present in 3.5

grammes of wheatgrass [188]. Alkaloids, polysaccharides, gum, mucilage, and saponins are some of the phytochemical constituents of wheatgrass. It is shown to have a greater water-soluble extractive value than an alcohol-soluble one. This is because around 70% of wheatgrass is made up of water-soluble chlorophyll [189].

Nutritional Benefits: Wheatgrass is renowned for its possible anti-inflammatory and anti-aging effects. Regular ingestion of wheatgrass leaf extract is considered to boost general health, especially helping the digestive system. It is also believed to be more nutrient-dense than typical veggies like spinach and broccoli. Traditionally, wheatgrass has been advised for a wide variety of health issues, including the common cold, cough, bronchitis, fever, infections, and irritation of the mouth and throat. Additionally, it is utilised to handle numerous skin-related diseases such as hemorrhoids, psoriasis, poison ivy responses, eczema, burns, and is also advised as a supportive therapy in thalassemia [190]. Furthermore, wheatgrass extract had a notable reduction in the abdominal pain and rectal bleeding linked to ulcerative colitis, and other Inflammatory Bowel Diseases (IBD). The authors proposed that wheatgrass's flavonoids, apigenin, and agropyrene, which are anti-inflammatory substances, may have contributed to the reduction of symptoms. Indole, another flavonoid found in wheatgrass, aids in the liver's generation of enzymes and deactivates carcinogens. Vitamins A, C, and E, examples of natural antioxidants, are found in wheatgrass [191]. All of the essential amino acids—primarily arginine, serine, glutamic acid, aspartic acid, and alanine—are present in wheatgrass and aid in supplying the body with an adequate quantity of protein. Wheatgrass also helps to maintain good hair, reduce tooth decay, enhance blood sugar balance, help with digestion, lower high blood pressure, and remove toxins from the body [192]. The clinical trials of Wheatgrass have been discussed in Table **8**.

Table 8. Clinical trials of wheatgrass.

Disease / Condition	Formulation	Clinical Trial / *In Vivo*	Outcome	Refs.
Thalassemia Major (Children)	Wheatgrass tablets: 2–3 tablets/day (ages 1–3), 6 tablets/day (ages 4–8), 8 tablets/day (>8 yrs)	Clinical trial on 40 children	Increased hemoglobin levels, longer interval between transfusions, reduced blood volume needed	[193]
Obesity	Wheatgrass powder: 1 spoon (3g) daily for healthy individuals, 2 spoons for obese patients	*In vitro*	Aids in weight control	[194]
Breast Cancer	Wheatgrass extract	*In-vitro*	Reduces skin toxicity from radiotherapy	[195]

CHLORELLA

Biological Source: It is obtained from the single-celled green algae known as *Chlorella vulgaris,* belonging to the family *Chlorellaceae*. The oldest living things on Earth are microalgae, a diverse group of single- and multicellular microorganisms that have withstood a variety of extreme environmental circumstances. For millennia, both people and animals have relied on them for sustenance. Because it is filled with proteins, minerals, lipids, and other nutrients, chlorella is one type of single-celled algae that has enormous nutritional value. Research has shown that chlorella has a variety of health benefits, from fibromyalgia to hypertension, which has led to a recent surge in interest in chlorella as a nutritional source [196]. The earliest civilizations relied heavily on microalgae. The Chinese employed the blue-green algae Nostoc to survive the famine in the early 2000s, according to reports of its first use. Chlorella (Fig. **14**) is a green, unicellular, freshwater algae that is a member of the Chlorellaceae family. The name comes from the Latin suffix "ella," which means "green," and the word "chloros," which means tiny. Chlorella cells are 2–8 microns thick and lack flagella. Chlorella is made up of Photosynthetic pigments that are green. Thanks to chlorophyll a and chlorophyll b, it has the highest concentration of chlorophyll on the market. Protein makes up 55–60% of chlorella, and 1-4% vitamins and minerals, 9–18% dietary fiber, and chlorophyll. Of the different species found, *Chlorella vulgaris* has been the subject of the greatest investigation to date. *Chlorella vulgaris* was the first algal culture to be reported as being scientifically clean, discovered by M.J. Beijerinck, a Dutch microbiologist, in 1890. In 1919, Otto Warburg published papers on his application of chlorella to plant physiology research [197].

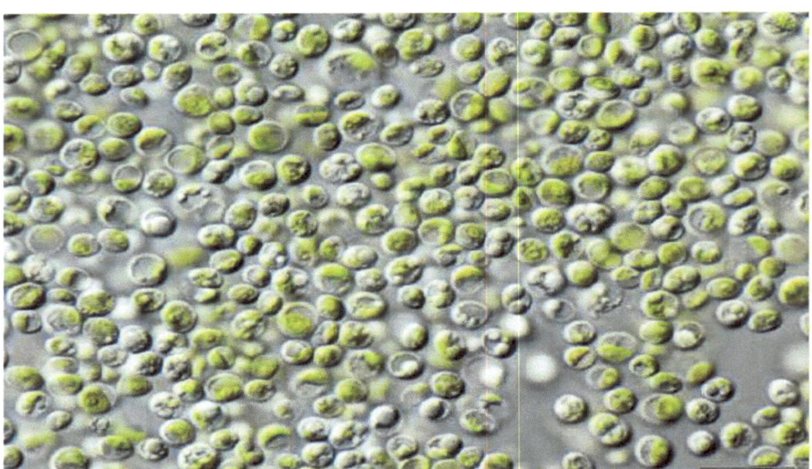

Fig. (14). Chlorella.

Chemical Constituents: It contains 60% of essential amino acids. Since microalgal protein has a low molecular weight, it can be easily digested. Chlorella contains lipids, which include oleic, palmitic, and linolenic acid. Polysaccharides are found to be present in Chlorella. One of the main ingredients of chlorella, β-1,3-glucan, has anti-oxidant and immunostimulatory properties and efficiently lowers blood lipid levels. In addition to glucose, complexes of galactose, mannose, rhamnose, N-acetylglucosamide, and N-acetylgalactosamine are present [198]. It has been demonstrated that these complexes possess immunostimulating qualities. It's a protective effect against the fungus *Candida albicans* and the bacteria Listeria monocytogenes. Chlorella is a major source of chlorophyll, providing health benefits like healing of sores, ulcers, and haemorrhoids, regulating menstruation, and improving diabetes and asthma. Its structure resembles hemin, which forms haemoglobin. Chlorella is a very rich source of vitamins and minerals. A few of Alpha- and beta-carotene, as well as vitamins B_1, B_2, B_3, B_5, B_6, E, and K, are the vitamins that are present in chlorella in significant amounts. Vitamins that are present in trace amounts include folic acid, Vitamin B_{12}, choline, inositol, and biotin [199].

Nutritional Benefits: A substance called lutein, which is produced by chlorella, has been shown to have anti-cataract and macular degeneration prevention and treatment benefits [200]. It has been established that chlorella extracts have antibacterial, antioxidant, anti-inflammatory, and tumor-fighting properties. It has been demonstrated that chlorella improves the immune system, lowers blood pressure and cholesterol, and speeds up wound healing. Moreover, it can benefit individuals who have ulcerative colitis, hypertension, and fibromyalgia by alleviating their symptoms and enhancing their quality of life. Chlorella lowered the levels of Low-Density Lipoprotein (LDL) cholesterol and inhibited aortic atheromatous lesions significantly [201].

Adverse Effects: Certain brands of chlorella tablets can cause nausea, vomiting, and stomach problems. If not properly digested, chlorella is poorly absorbed and can cause digestive problems. It has been demonstrated that taking chlorella tablets can result in acute tubulointerstitial nephritis, which can eventually induce renal failure. Additionally, it has been classified as a mild allergen, and for some individuals, it may have clinical importance [202].

ALFALFA

Biological Source: It is obtained from the legume of *Medicago sativa,* belonging to the family *Papilionoideae*. Alfalfa's (Fig. **15**) high yield, good quality, tolerance to frequent cuttings, and wide range of adaptability make it a valuable feed source for livestock industries worldwide. It can be applied to soil enhancement, pasture, hay, silage, dehydrated goods, and seed production. About 30 million acres are used to raise alfalfa worldwide. While almost seven million hectares are farmed in the United States, more than four million hectares of alfalfa are produced in Canada, either in monoculture or in combination with grasses [203]. Using traditional breeding methods, several alfalfa cultivars with increased salt tolerance have been created. The response of alfalfa plants to salt stress is physiologically and genetically complicated, and salt tolerance is regulated by several genes and includes a variety of biochemical and physiological pathways, making it difficult to genetically improve alfalfa [204].

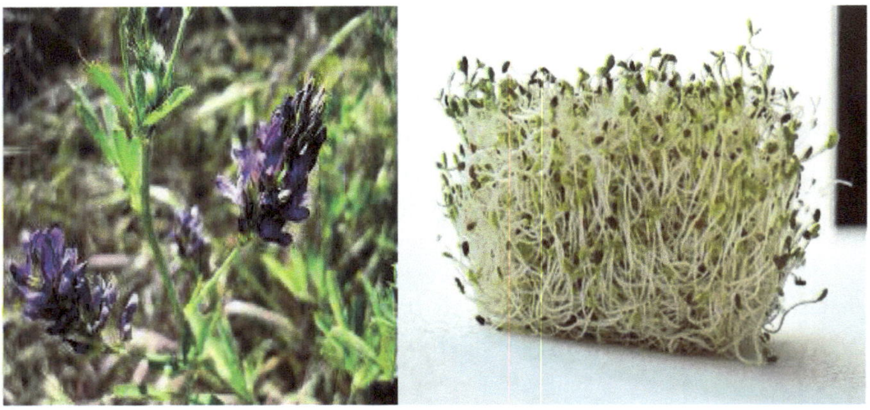

Fig. (15). Alfalfa.

Geographical Source: The plant is native to numerous locations spanning Africa, Asia, and Europe. In Africa, it is found in nations such as Algeria, Libya, Morocco, and Tunisia. In Asia, its presence spans over a wide variety of countries, including Afghanistan, Armenia, Azerbaijan, China, Cyprus, Georgia, Iran, Iraq, Jordan, Kazakhstan, Korea, Kyrgyzstan, Lebanon, Mongolia, Pakistan, Palestine, Russia (Asian portion), Syria, Tajikistan, Turkey, Turkmenistan, and Uzbekistan. In Europe, it grows in Albania, Austria, Belarus, Belgium, Bulgaria, Czechoslovakia, Denmark, Estonia, Finland, the former Yugoslavia, France, Germany, Greece, Hungary, Ireland, Italy, Latvia, Lithuania, Moldova, the Netherlands, Norway, Poland, Portugal, the European part of Russia, Spain, Sweden, Switzerland, and the United Kingdom [205].

Traditional use: Sprouts of Mendeligo sativa were eaten as a salad. In health food stores, its leaves or seeds were also offered as nutritional supplements in the form of pills, capsules, and bulk powdered herb. It has historically been used in Ayurveda and homeopathic medicine to treat obesity, diabetes, inflammation, renal pain, and problems of the central nervous system [206]. Alfalfa sprouts or leaves have also historically been used as an anticancer, anti-rheumatic, cardiotonic, depurative, lactagogue, emmenagogue, antiscorbutic, and to treat boils. It has also been used to treat arthritis, renal issues, and fever [207]. The plant was used as a diuretic and to alleviate renal and vesicular edema in South America [208].

ChemiBMS-HDFH-2025-HT1-7342-1 cal Constituents

- Primary Phytochemicals: carbohydrates, saponins, lignin, tannins, alkaloids, triterpene glycosides, Proteins, carotenoids, sterols, flavones, isoflavonoids, and phytoestrogens (coumestrol).
- Protein-Xanthophyll Extract: Contains 45-60% protein, 9-11% fat, 1-2% simple sugars, polysaccharides, saponins, minerals, coumestrol, isoflavones, L-canavanine, and phytynians [209].
- Phytoestrogenic Compounds: Coumetarol, loliolide, liquiritigenin, isoliquiritigenin [210].
- Bioactive Compounds: Alkaloids, amino acids, coumarins, flavonoids, steroids, volatile components, acids, purines, vitamins, ketones, fructose, pectin, and chlorophyll.
- Minerals and Trace Elements: Iron, calcium, copper, manganese, and zinc [211]. The clinical trials of mendeligo have been discussed in Table **9**.

Table 9. Clinical trials of mendeligo.

Activity	Formulation / Dose	Model	Outcome	Refs.
Antioxidant	Extract from *Medicago sativa* flowers	*In vitro*	Polysaccharides in the extract showed strong antioxidant activity by scavenging hydroxyl and DPPH radicals.	[212]
Antidiabetic	Aqueous ethanol extract of *Medicago sativa*	*In vivo* (rats)	Lowered serum glucose, cholesterol, triglycerides, and LDL; increased HDL; improved pancreatic islet size.	[213]
Reproductive health	Alfalfa ethanolic extract (9, 18, 36 mg/kg for 15 days in female rats)	*In vivo*	Enhanced follicle growth, ovulation, and corpus luteum formation due to estrogen-like properties	[214]
Anti-inflammatory	Ethyl extract from *Medicago sativa* sprouts	*In vitro*	Decreased TNF-α, IL-6, and IL-1β levels post-LPS exposure; improved survival rate	[215]
Dermatological	Cream containing alfalfa leaf extract	*In vitro*	Reduced MDA levels in skin tissue significantly in both low and high dose groups	[216]

(Table 9) cont.....

Activity	Formulation / Dose	Model	Outcome	Refs.
Neuroprotective	Methanol extract of *Medicago sativa*	*In vitro*	Improved memory and provided CNS protection due to triterpene saponins	[217]
Cardioprotective	Ethanolic extract of alfalfa stem	*In vivo*	Restored lipid profile and normalized cardiac and liver enzyme levels	[218]
Hepatoprotective	Aqueous extract of *Medicago sativa*	*In vivo*	Reduced liver damage caused by carbon tetrachloride (CCl_4)	[219]
Anti-anemia	Ethanolic leaf extract	Clinical (102 girls)	Significantly increased hemoglobin levels in anemic adolescent girls	[220]

Dosage: In general, moderate use of Medicago sativa leaves in teas and capsules is regarded as safe and free of serious adverse effects. Large-scale consumption of Medicago sativa seeds and sprouts has been linked to lupus aggravation or the promotion of lupus-like symptoms; this effect is ascribed to the amino acid canavanine [221]. *Pregnancy:* There has been no research on the safety of Medicago sativa during pregnancy or breastfeeding in humans or animals, but herbalists believe it is safe because farmers do not forbid their cattle from eating Medicago sativa during these times. In dairy cows, the Medicago sativa diet reduced fat, raised milk protein, and enhanced milk output [222].

PHYLLANTHUS

Biological Source: Phyllanthus is a genus of plants in the Euphorbiaceae family. One of the biggest genera in the family Phyllanthaceae, *Phyllanthus* (Fig. **16**) comprises eleven sub-genus that include more than seven hundred species that are well-known. These subgenera are worldwide in distribution, with the majority of their distribution occurring in the tropics and subtropics [223]. The most significant species that have been traditionally utilized for the treatment of a variety of human illnesses are those that belong to Formerly, the subgenera Cicca (Now considered a Genus), Kirganelia, and *Phyllanthus*. Over the course of several centuries, numerous Southeast Asian nations, Brazil, India, and China have made use of plants belonging to the genus *Phyllanthus* as ingredients in herbal prescriptions [224]. Extracts from *Phyllanthus amarus* (*P. amarus*) have been shown to have strong antioxidant properties and may prevent the development of bacteria. In the treatment of conditions like diarrhoea, dysentery, dropsy, runny nose, wintertime common colds, blennorrhagia, colic, indigestion, alternating fevers, hepatitis, and malaria, this is very important [225]. *Phyllanthus niruri* L., often referred to as *P. niruri*, has a long history of use in traditional and folk medicine for treating a variety of illnesses. Asthma, joint pain, appetite loss, constipation, injuries, corneal opacity, conjunctivitis, diabetes mellitus, dropsy, gout, gonorrhoeal infections in both men and women, inflammatory diseases, skin itching, liver diseases, kidney stones or failures, leucorrhea, vaginitis, menorrhagia, irregular menstruation in women, obesity, scabies, stomach aches, tumours, typhoid fever, urinogenital system disorders, viral infections, and many more are among these conditions [226].

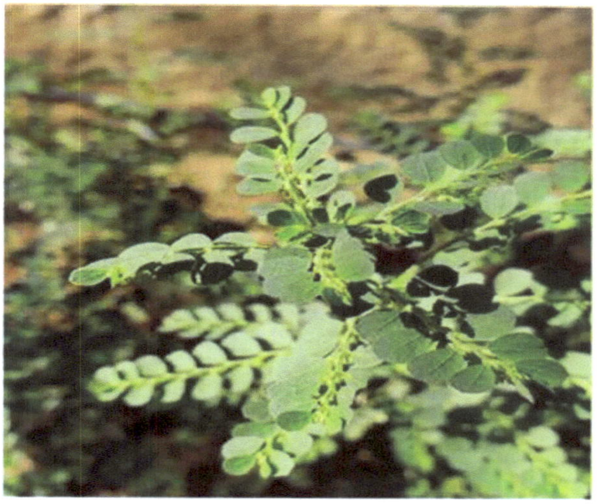

Fig. (16). *Phyllanthus.*

Geographical Source: About 6500 species are found in the *Phyllanthus* genus, which belongs to the Euphorbiaceae family. Out of these, 200 are found in the United States, 100 are found in Africa, 70 are found in Madagascar, and the remaining species are found in Asia and Australasia [227]. North, Central, and South America are the natural habitats of a great number of species belonging to this family. The word "*Phyllanthus*" literally translates to "leaf and flower" because the flower and the fruit appear to merge into a single entity with the leaf [228]. Webster's revision of the taxonomic classification of this genus includes other closely related species, such as *P. amarus*, which were placed under the sub-section Swartiziani of the section *Phyllanthus*. Following an examination of the morphology and geographical distribution of *P. amarus*, the nomenclature, taxonomic distinctness, and near relatives of this species were discussed at great length. It is believed to be linked to *P. abnormis*, which is exclusive to sandy regions in the southern states of the United States, including Texas and Florida. Therefore, it is quite probable that *P. amarus* evolved in the Caribbean region as a species that is a vicarious counterpart to *P. abnormis*, which is native to the southern United States, and that it has spread across the tropics through the use of trading vessels. *P. amarus* is found in a broad range of locations around the globe, including all tropical and subtropical climates. In the course of paleobotanical research, the precise geographical origin of this plant has not been discovered. It is native to the tropical rainforests of the Amazon as well as other tropical nations such as India, China, the Bahamas, and the Philippines [229, 230]. *P. amarus* is a widespread pantropical weed that thrives in locations that are damp, shaded, and provide plenty of sunlight. The *Phyllanthus amarus* species is believed to be the most generally occurring *Phyllanthus* species in India [231].

Chemical Constituents: Numerous secondary metabolites, including alkaloids, terpenoids, glycosides, flavonoids, tannins, and sapogenins, were found in the first study of the phytochemical characteristics of Phyllanthus species [232, 233]. Because of their high tannin content, Phyllanthus plants are mostly made up of phenolic chemicals, especially tannins. The fruits of *P. emblica* L. were shown to have over 100 phenolic components with a broad spectrum of biological activity using high-performance liquid chromatography-mass spectrometry [234]. Over 81 distinct compounds were extracted from Phyllanthus species between 2016 and 2018, with diterpenoids, triterpenoids, flavonoids, and phenylpropanoids accounting for the majority of these compounds [235].

Nutritional Properties: It has been discovered that the nutritional and medicinal properties of plants are due to the chemical features of the plants themselves [236]. The leaves of *P. niruri* had a higher percentage of dry matter, which was 91.06%. It has been shown by proximate analysis that the leaves contain a significant quantity of glucose and energy, as well as protein, crude fibre, moderate fat, and a small amount of fat and ash. There is evidence that feeds fibres enhance the body's ability to absorb dietary nutrients while simultaneously reducing the body's ability to absorb cholesterol. In addition to their role as enzymes, proteins are essential for the creation and repair of physiological tissues. The leaf contained a crude protein content of 14.74 percent, which was higher than the majority of medicinal plants [237]. The leaf is abundant in potassium (K), phosphorus (P), and a reasonable level of calcium (Ca), magnesium (Mg), and sodium (Na), but it is deficient in copper (Cu), iron (Fe), zinc (Zn), and manganese (Mn). In terms of the mineral and vitamin content, the leaf has a moderate level of sodium (Na). The high quantities of potassium, magnesium, and phosphate ions found in the leaf of the plant may be responsible for the traditional usage of the plant to avoid oedema, renal difficulties, and oliguria [238]. These ions may serve the goal of maintaining osmotic pressure, water balance, and pH in the body. Table **10** shows the clinical trials of *Emblica officinalis* that have been reported in the literature.

Table 10. Clinical trials of *Emblica officinalis*.

Disease / Activity	Dose	Model	Outcome	Refs.
Antiparasitic	250–1000 µg/mL	*In vitro*	Dried fruits of *Emblica officinalis* (syn. *Phyllanthus emblica*) showed significant antitrypanosomal effects. At 250 µg/mL, a notable reduction in trypanosomes was observed, with complete elimination in 5 hours.	[239]
Cardiovascular Protection	10 µg/mL	*In vivo*	A 7:3 ethanolic blend of *P. emblica* fruit and *Alpinia galanga* rhizome extracts showed synergistic antioxidant activity in endothelial cells (ECV304), increased cell viability, and inhibited lipid peroxidation induced by H_2O_2.	[240]
Anticancer	3.13 µg/mL	*In vitro*	*Phyllanthus amarus* extract showed strong anti-tumor properties, enhanced the effect of 5-fluorouracil (5-FU), induced G2/M cell cycle arrest, and influenced nucleotide metabolism in HepG2 cancer cells.	[241]
Anti-aging / Skin Protection	2.0 µg/mL	*In vitro*	*Phyllanthus orbicularis* K. aqueous extract demonstrated effective UVA and UVB photoprotection, acting as a natural sunscreen and helping prevent genetic and DNA damage from sunlight exposure.	[242]

Dosage: Due to the fact that it has the ability to cleanse the blood, taking Bhumi Amla in the form of tablets or capsules twice a day might be beneficial in the treatment of skin conditions. It is possible that consuming Bhumi Amla powder in conjunction with water will not only help prevent hair loss but also encourage the development of new hair [243].

LINGZHI MUSHROOM

Biological Source: The Lingzhi mushroom, an oriental fungus also known as *Ganoderma lucidum*, Reishi (*Ganoderma lucidum*). As per the Chinese terminology, the term Lingzhi (Fig. **17**) is a blend of spiritual power and the essence of immortality. It is also regarded as the "herb of spiritual power," and it is a symbol of prosperity, good health, divine power, and longevity. G. lucidum is superior to other cultivated mushrooms when compared to them because its medicinal significance is even greater than its nutritional value [244]. Powders, supplements, and tea are some of the ways that *commercial G. lucidum* products can be obtained. Other forms are also available. Mycelia, spores, and the fruiting body of the mushroom are the parts that are responsible for creating these organisms. The specific applications and health benefits of Lingzhi encompass blood glucose regulation, immune system modulation, protection of the liver, bacteriostasis, and several other health benefits. Traditional use, anecdotal evidence, and cultural convention are the main sources of evidence supporting the many opinions that have evolved regarding the health benefits of *G. lucidum*. Recent research, however, has furnished scientific proof to support some of the long-standing claims that Lingzhi is good for medical health [245].

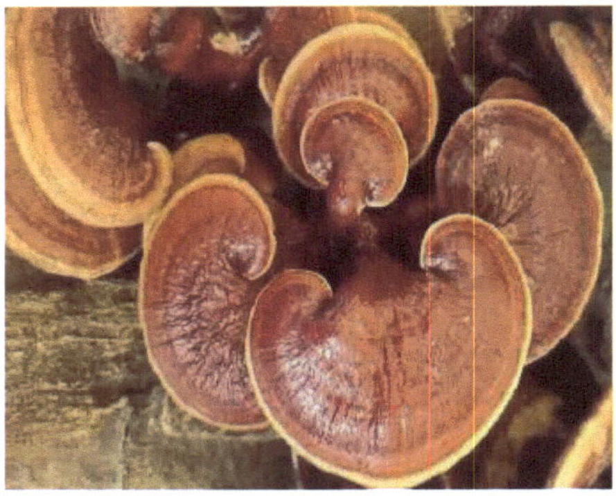

Fig. (17). Lingzhi.

Geographical Source: As a result of the mushroom's erratic distribution in the wild and the growing demand for *G. lucidum* as a therapeutic herb, there have been attempts to cultivate the fungus [246]. Individual species of the Ganoderma genus require distinct environmental conditions to flourish and be cultivated. To add insult to injury, several varieties are preferred in various geographical places. In South China, for instance, the black *G. lucidum* variety is the most popular, but in Japan, the red *G. lucidum* variety is the most appreciated. *G. lucidum* can flourish in environments that are hot and humid, and the subtropical parts of the Orient are home to a large number of diverse wild forms. A significant amount of the mushroom has been obtained by the cultivation of *G. lucidum* ever since the early 1970s. Utilizing substrates such as grain, sawdust, and wood logs, it has been possible to successfully cultivate *G. lucidum* in an artificial environment [247].

Chemical Constituents: There are various types of bioactive compounds that may be found in mushrooms. Some examples of these substances are terpenoids, steroids, phenols, nucleotides and their derivatives, glycoproteins, and polysaccharides. Besides the inclusion of all the amino acids necessary, proteins of mushrooms are exceptionally rich in lysine and leucine. The low level of total fat of mushrooms and the high ratio of polyunsaturated fatty acids to the total fatty acids of mushrooms are both regarded as major factors in the health benefits of mushrooms [248]. Three substances in G. lucidum are physiologically active and are vital to the physiology: polysaccharides, peptidoglycans, and triterpenes. Variation exists in the amount and percentage of each of the components that could be present in natural and commercial goods. Varied between undetectable and 7.8%, and varied between 1.1–5.8% for the number of triterpenes and polysaccharides, respectively, when eleven commercial Lingzhi products bought in Hong Kong markets were analysed for the two principal active components, triterpenes and polysaccharides. The samples were picked randomly. There are various reasons why deviations of this sort may arise, such as modifications in the species or strains of mushrooms utilised and variations in the production methods [249].

Nutritional Properties: Water makes up around 90% of the weight of the majority of mushrooms. Two to eight percent fat, three to twenty-eight percent carbohydrate, three to thirty-two percent fibre, eight to ten percent ash, and a few vitamins and minerals make up the remaining ten percent. Potassium, calcium, phosphorus, magnesium, selenium, iron, zinc, and copper make up the majority of the mineral makeup. G. lucidum was discovered to contain 1.8% ash, 26–28% carbohydrates, 3–5% crude fat, 59% crude fibre, and 7–8% crude protein among its non-volatile components. This was discovered *via* a conducted study [250]. The clinical trials of Lingzhi have been discussed in Table **11**.

Table 11. Clinical trials of lingzhi.

Disease / Activity	Dose	Study Type	Outcome	Refs.
Immune System Support	10 capsules/day	*In vitro*	The fungus enhanced lymphocyte function. In athletes under stress, it helped improve immune response.	[251]
Anti-Cancer	0.8, 3.2, or 12.8 mg/mL	*In vitro* and *in vivo*	*Ganoderma lucidum* polysaccharides (GLP) showed anticancer activity through immune boosting, cell growth inhibition, apoptosis promotion, and prevention of metastasis and angiogenesis.	[252]
Anti-Depressant	1,800 mg	*In vivo*	Polysaccharide extract (Ganopoly) was found to be effective and safe for treating neurasthenia in Chinese patients.	[253]
Antioxidant	250 mg/kg body weight	*In vivo*	Ethanol extract of *G. lucidum* reduced cardiotoxic effects of adriamycin by lowering lipid peroxidation and increasing antioxidant enzyme levels in heart tissues.	[254]
Hypoglycemic Effect	50–200 mg/kg	*In vivo*	Pre-treatment with GL-PS for 10 days showed blood sugar-lowering effects by protecting pancreatic β-cells from damage caused by alloxan.	[255]

Dosage: Usually, a dried extract of the mushroom is used. In the above-mentioned cases, the dose is approximately 10 times less than that of the mushroom itself, which is consumed [255].

SAW PALMETTO

Biological Source: Saw palmetto is obtained from the partially dried ripe fruit of *Sereno repens* or *Sabal serrulatum,* belonging to the family *Arecaceae*. The symptoms of benign prostatic hyperplasia may be treated with saw palmetto, a natural treatment. The active component is found in the fruit of the American dwarf palm tree. Studies have shown that saw palmetto (Fig. **18**) may help reduce the symptoms of benign prostatic hyperplasia. Saw palmetto is less expensive and better tolerated than medications like finasteride, yet it seems to be as effective [256]. There are no known drug interactions with saw palmetto, and the few side effects that have been reported are minor. Information on its long-term usage is lacking. The herbal remedy has also been used to treat chronic prostatitis, although its efficacy has not yet been shown [257].

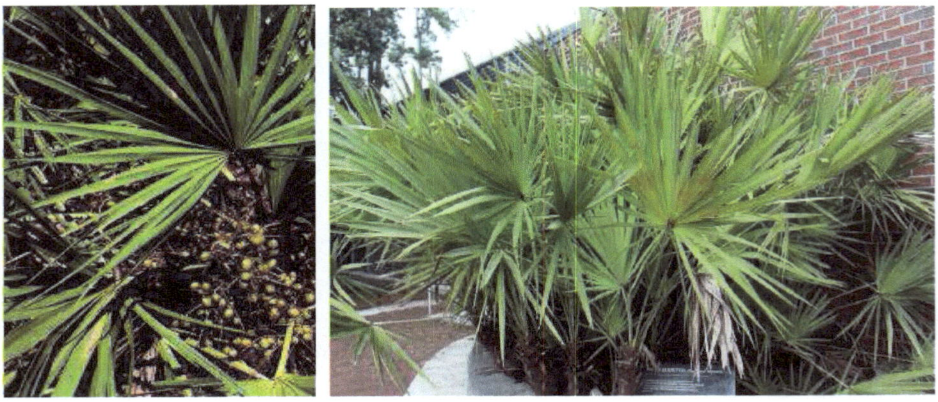

Fig. (18). Saw palmetto.

Geographical Source: Saw palmetto, or *Serenoa repens* or *Sabal serrulatum*, is a herb employed to treat benign prostatic hyperplasia (BPH) in the US. It is derived from the partially dried ripe fruit of the American dwarf palm tree, indigenous to coastal areas. Saw palmetto is utilized in 50% of BPH treatment in Italy and 90% in Germany. The therapeutic component of the plant is the free fatty acids and sterols present in the berry. The extraction process involves a solvent, and the solvent used determines the final product formulation. The most commonly researched formulation is Permixon, which employs hexane, but others utilize ethanol, methanol, and liquid carbon dioxide. Saw palmetto has been historically taken with nettle root and pumpkin seeds [258].

Chemical Constituents: A diverse range of phytosterols and fatty acids are among the many chemical components found in saw palmetto extract. Among the phytosterols found are delta5-avenasterol, delta7-avenasterol, delta7-stigmasterol, cholesterol, campesterol, stigmasterol, and β-sitosterol. About 59.4% of the total sterol content is made up of β-sitosterol, the most prevalent sterol. The extract's total sterol content is typically 1864 mg/kg. The fatty acid profile comprises long-chain acids like palmitic, stearic, oleic, and linoleic as well as short-chain acids like caprylic, capric, and lauric. With 17.6% of the total fatty acids being short-chain acids, lauric acid is the most abundant, while oleic acid makes up 49.1% of the composition. The extract's other physical and chemical characteristics, such as its levels of free and total fatty acids, peroxide, iodine, and saponification, have all been examined. Notably, the extract's unique biochemical profile is enhanced by the presence of up to 90% free fatty acids and the lack of tocopherols [259]. The clinical trials of saw palmetto have been discussed in Table **12**.

Table 12. Clinical trials of saw palmetto.

Disease	Dose	Clinical Trial/*In Vivo*	Outcome	Refs.
Benign prostatic hyperplasia with lower urinary tract symptoms	160 mg twice daily or placebo for 30 days.	18 randomized clinical trials involving more than 2,900 men with symptomatic BPH	A study showed a mild to moderate improvement in symptom score and urinary flow without decreasing prostate size.	[260]
Benign prostate hyperplasia and androgen deficiency	12-week double-blind treatment with 500 mg doses of β-sitostero- -enriched saw palmetto oil, conventional saw palmetto oil, and placebo orally in the form of capsules (n = 33 in each group).	Ninety-nine male subjects aged 40–65 years, having mild-t- -moderate BPH symptoms	Study demonstrates that β-sitosterol-enriched saw palmetto oil is more effective than conventional oil in treating BPH and androgen deficiency, improving quality of life.	[261]

Contraindication: The main adverse consequence that arises from Saw palmetto can be taken with food to reduce minor gastrointestinal upset in adults. The saw palmetto is thought to be extremely safe, despite the lack of rigorous toxicological research. Rats and dogs given 2 g per kg of saw palmetto daily for six months showed no carcinogenic or teratogenic effects, and this dosage was well tolerated, according to one study. Human clinical trials have not revealed any changes in laboratory markers that are clinically significant. Because saw palmetto lowers PSA levels, there has been some worry that it could conceal prostate cancer. However, this effect on PSA levels was not shown in a randomized study with over 1,000 individuals [262].

Dosage: According to clinical research, saw palmetto may be successfully treated using a lipophilic extract that contains 80–90% of the volatile oil. A six-month trial did not find a higher level of effectiveness at a daily dosage of 480 mg. Because teas don't contain volatile oils, they aren't thought to be effective. One to two grams of whole berries can be consumed each day. Because saw palmetto is not standardized in the US, different dosages may be advised. There are no known medication interactions with saw palmetto, and common herbal products can differ from those used in clinical studies [263].

SUMMARY

The role of nutraceuticals in the prevention and treatment of disease is greatly acknowledged in this chapter. Dietary supplements and nutraceutical doses for optimal health maintenance and therapeutic purposes are also captured for herbs. Nutraceutical chemical classes, individual profiles of nutraceuticals, and their clinical application are also dealt with. Herbs for liver care, brain health, anti-inflammatory, antidiabetic, antioxidant, antihypertensive, stomach ulcer, immunomodulator, diuretic, and antipyretic were extensively discussed. Superfoods like chlorella, wheatgrass, spirulina, milk thistle, turmeric, and Lingzhi mushroom were also discussed. Ayurvedic nutraceuticals like Andrographis, ashwagandha, bacopa, boswellia, fenugreek, garlic, ginger, turmeric, tribulus, and vitex were included in this chapter. Individual herb source, geographical occurrence, morphology, chemical constituents, adulterants, traditional use, pharmacological use, and clinical studies were included for most of the drugs in this chapter. Dosage form, interaction, adverse reaction, and indication to use during pregnancy and lactation are also included for some herbs. The overall spectrum of the herbs in the chapter represents most of the nutraceuticals that are in clinical use.

EXERCISE

Part 1: Short Answer Questions

1. What is the primary active compound in Turmeric responsible for its anti-inflammatory effects?
2. Which essential mineral, crucial for thyroid function, is abundantly found in Kelp?

3. Milk Thistle (*Silybum marianum*) is most renowned for its protective effects on which organ?
4. What is the common name for *Vitex agnus−castus*, and what is its primary use in women's health?
5. The bark of the Willow tree contains salicin, a precursor to which common over-the-counter drug?[1]
6. *Valeriana officinalis* is most commonly used to address what two health concerns?
7. Saw Palmetto is primarily used to support the health of which gland in men?
8. What type of microorganism is Spirulina?
9. Lingzhi Mushroom (*Ganoderma lucidum*) is classified as a type of substance that helps the body adapt to stress.
10. Which part of the grape plant is used to make Grape Seed Extract?
11. Psyllium husk is a rich source of what type of fiber?
12. Which herb is famously associated with the management of mild to moderate depression?
13. What is the main safety concern associated with the consumption of Alfalfa sprouts?
14. *Tribulus terrestris* is traditionally used to support what aspect of health?[7]
15. What green pigment, structurally similar to haemoglobin, is found in high concentrations in Wheatgrass and Chlorella?

Part 2: Mid-Length Answer Questions

1. Explain the primary mechanism by which Hawthorn (*Crataegus species*) exerts its beneficial effects on the cardiovascular system.
2. Describe how Psyllium husk can be effective for both constipation and diarrhoea.
3. What are proanthocyanidins, found in Grape Seed Extract, and why are they considered potent nutraceuticals?
4. Explain the mechanism through which St. John's Wort (*Hypericum perforatum*) can cause significant drug interactions. Name one class of drugs it commonly interacts with.
5. Describe the role of the active complex, silymarin, in protecting the liver. What are its proposed mechanisms of action?
6. How does Valerian root influence the GABAergic system to promote relaxation and sleep?
7. Explain the difference between Spirulina and Chlorella in terms of their cell wall structure and how this impacts their digestion and processing.
8. What are phytoestrogens? Discuss how the phytoestrogenic compounds in Alfalfa might be beneficial and also outline potential concerns.

9. Describe the traditional use of Phyllanthus species in Ayurvedic medicine, specifically concerning the liver and kidneys.
10. How is Saw Palmetto believed to work in managing the symptoms of Benign Prostatic Hyperplasia (BPH)? Name the key enzyme it is thought to inhibit.
11. Explain why Turmeric is often formulated with black pepper extract (piperine) in nutraceutical supplements.
12. Describe how *Vitex agnus-castus* is thought to regulate the female hormonal cycle, specifically mentioning its effect on the pituitary gland and prolactin levels.

Part 3: Long Answer Questions

1. Compare and contrast the nutraceutical applications, primary active compounds, and mechanisms of action for Willow bark and Turmeric as anti-inflammatory agents. Discuss their respective safety profiles and potential side effects.
2. Lingzhi Mushroom (*Ganoderma lucidum*) is known as an "adaptogen."[10] Define what an adaptogen is. Elaborate on the various therapeutic properties of Lingzhi, including its effects on the immune system, stress response, and cardiovascular health, referencing its key bioactive compounds like polysaccharides and triterpenes.
3. Discuss the use of microalgae (Spirulina and Chlorella) and cereal grasses (Wheatgrass) as nutraceuticals. In your answer, evaluate their nutritional profiles, proposed health benefits (*e.g.*, detoxification, antioxidant effects), and potential risks, such as contamination with heavy metals or bacterial toxins.
4. A patient is taking Warfarin (an anticoagulant), a statin for cholesterol, and an oral contraceptive. From the provided list of herbs, identify at least three herbs that would be strongly contraindicated for this patient. For each herb you identify, explain the specific mechanism of interaction with the patient's medications and the potential adverse outcomes.

Part 4: Case Studies

Case 1: *A 62-year-old male presents with symptoms of Benign Prostatic Hyperplasia (BPH), including nocturia (waking up at night to urinate), a weak urinary stream, and a feeling of incomplete bladder emptying. He is hesitant to start pharmaceutical treatment and asks about herbal options.*

- **Task:** Identify the most appropriate herb from the list for his condition. Justify your choice by explaining its mechanism of action. Outline the expected benefits and any important safety information or contraindications you would provide to the patient.

Case 2: *A 48-year-old woman is entering perimenopause. She reports experiencing irregular menstrual cycles, hot flashes, night sweats, and increased irritability. She is looking for a non-hormonal, natural approach to manage these fluctuations.*

- **Task:** Based on the list, recommend and justify the use of one or more herbs to help manage her symptoms. Explain how the chosen herb(s) could address her specific complaints (*e.g.*, hormonal regulation, nervous system support).

Case 3: *A 35-year-old competitive athlete is looking for natural supplements to improve recovery, reduce exercise-induced inflammation, and support overall vitality. They are currently healthy with no underlying conditions.*

- **Task:** Propose a combination of at least two nutraceuticals from the list that could be beneficial. For each one, explain its specific role in supporting the athlete's goals (*e.g.*, anti-inflammatory, antioxidant, nutrient density). Discuss the proper context of use (*e.g.*, timing, form).

Case 4: *A 50-year-old individual has recently been told they have "fatty liver" (non-alcoholic fatty liver disease) and borderline high cholesterol. They are making dietary and lifestyle changes, but want to incorporate an herbal supplement to support liver health and function.*

- **Task:** Recommend the most suitable herb for liver support from the list. Explain its hepatoprotective mechanisms. Additionally, suggest a second herb from the list that could help with their digestive health and cholesterol management, explaining its mechanism as well.

Case 5: *A 28-year-old graduate student complains of persistent low mood, lack of motivation, and feelings of sadness for the past three months, which he describes as "a case of the blues he can't shake." He also has trouble sleeping. His symptoms are affecting his studies. He is not on any other medication.*

- **Task:** Identify an appropriate herbal intervention from the list for his mood symptoms. Discuss the evidence for its use, its proposed mechanism of action, and the average timeframe for seeing benefits. Crucially, what are the most important warnings and potential interactions you must counsel him on before he begins taking it? Suggest another herb from the list that could be used specifically for his sleep difficulties.

REFERENCES

[1] Bommakanti V, Ajikumar AP, Sivi CM, *et al.* An overview of herbal nutraceuticals, their extraction, formulation, therapeutic effects and potential toxicity. Separations 2023; 10: 10. [http://dx.doi.org/10.3390/SEPARATIONS10030177]

[2] Barnes J. Nutraceuticals-Lisa Rapport, Brian Lockwood, Published by Pharmaceutical Press, 2002, London, 184 pp, ISBN 0 85369 503 2, HB@ $29-95 (UK). Complement Ther Med 2002; 4(10): 241. [http://dx.doi.org/10.1016/S0965-2299(02)00083-3]

[3] Ling S, Nheu L, Dai A, Guo Z, Komesaroff P. Effects of four medicinal herbs on human vascular endothelial cells in culture. Int J Cardiol 2008; 128(3): 350-8. [http://dx.doi.org/10.1016/j.ijcard.2007.05.111] [PMID: 17692965]

[4] Rigelsky JM, Sweet BV. Hawthorn: Pharmacology and therapeutic uses. Am J Health Syst Pharm 2002; 59(5): 417-22. [http://dx.doi.org/10.1093/ajhp/59.5.417] [PMID: 11887407]

[5] Miller AL. Botanical influences on cardiovascular disease. Alternative medicine review: a journal of clinical therapeutic. 1998; 3(6): 422-31.

[6] Hobbs C, Foster S. Hawthorn-A Literature Review. HerbalGram 1990; 22: 19-33.

[7] Upton R, Petrone C. Hawthorn leaf with flower. Santa Cruz: American Herbal Pharmacopoeia 1999.

[8] Tauchert M, Gildor A, Lipinski J. High-Dose crataegus (hawthorn) extract WS 1442 for the treatment of NYHA class II heart failure patients. Herz 1999; 24(6): 465-74. [http://dx.doi.org/10.1007/BF03044432] [PMID: 10546150]

[9] Eichstadt H, Bader M. Danne 0., Kaiser W., Stein U., Felix R., Crataegus-Extrakt hilft den Patienten mit NYHA-II Herzinsuffizienz.(Hawthorn extract helps patients with NYHA stage II heart failure). Therapiewoche 1989; 39: 3288-96.

[10] Bödigheimer K, Chase D. Effectiveness of hawthorn extract at a dosage of 3 x 100 mg per day. Multicentre double-blind trial with 85 NYHA stage II heart failure patients. Munch Med Wochenschr 1994; 136.

[11] Eiff MV, Brunner H, Haegeli A, *et al.* Hawthorn/passion flower extract and improvement in physical exercise capacity of patients with dyspnoea class II of the NYHA functional classification. Acta Ther 1994; 20(1): 47.

[12] Robbers JE, Tyler VE. Tyler's herbs of choice The therapeutic use of phytomedicinals 1999.

[13] Anderson LA, Newall CA, Phillipson JD. Herbal Medicines: A guide for health care professionals. Pharmaceutical Press 1996.

[14] Hahn F, Klinkhammer F, Oberdorf A. [Preparation and pharmacological research on a new therapeutic agent from Crataegus oxyacantha]. Arzneimittelforschung 1960; 10: 825-9. [PMID: 13710559]

[15] Brinker F. Herb contraindications and drug interactions Edn2. Sandy, OR: Eclectic Medical 1998.

[16] McGuffin M, Ed. Botanical safety handbook. CRC Press 1997.

[17] Family Physician A, Dahmer S, Scott E. Health Effects of Hawthorn. Am Fam Physician 2010; 81: 465-8.

[18] Nowshehri JA, Bhat ZA, Shah MY. Pharmacognostic standardisation and phytochemical evaluation on the seeds of two Vitis vinefera L. varieties grown in Kashmir Valley, India. Pharmacogn J 2016; 8(5): 465-70. [http://dx.doi.org/10.5530/pj.2016.5.9]

[19] Vayupharp B, Laksanalamai V. Recovery of antioxidants from grape seeds and its application in fried food. [http://dx.doi.org/10.4172/2157-7110.1000152]

[20] Kar P, Laight D, Shaw KM, Cummings MH. Flavonoid-rich grapeseed extracts: a new approach in high cardiovascular risk patients? Int J Clin Pract 2006; 60(11): 1484-92. [http://dx.doi.org/10.1111/j.1742-1241.2006.01038.x] [PMID: 17073843]

[21] El-Hawary S, El-Fouly K, El Gohary HM, Meselhy KM, Slem A, Talaat Z. Phytochemical and Biological Investigation of Vitis vinifera L.(Flame cultivar), Family Vitaceae Cultivated in Egypt. Nat Sci 2012; 10(10): 48-59.

[22] Medouni-Adrar S, Boulekbache-Makhlouf L, Cadot Y, *et al.* Optimization of the recovery of phenolic compounds from Algerian grape by-products. Ind Crops Prod 2015; 77: 123-32. [http://dx.doi.org/10.1016/j.indcrop.2015.08.039]

[23] Shinagawa FB, Santana FC, Torres LRO, Mancini-Filho J. Grape seed oil: a potential functional food? Food Sci Technol (Campinas) 2015; 35(3): 399-406. [http://dx.doi.org/10.1590/1678-457X.6826]

[24] Hernández-Jiménez A, Gómez-Plaza E, Martínez-Cutillas A, Kennedy JA. Grape skin and seed proanthocyanidins from Monastrell x Syrah grapes. J Agric Food Chem 2009; 57(22): 10798-803. [http://dx.doi.org/10.1021/jf903465p] [PMID: 19856914]

[25] Monteleone E, Condelli N, Dinnella C, Bertuccioli M. Prediction of perceived astringency induced by phenolic compounds. Food Qual Prefer 2004; 15(7-8): 761-9. [http://dx.doi.org/10.1016/j.foodqual.2004.06.002]

[26] Garavaglia J, Markoski MM, Oliveira A, Marcadenti A. Grape seed oil compounds: Biological and chemical actions for health. Nutrition and metabolic insights. 2016 Jan; 9:NMI-S32910.

[27] Xia EQ, Deng GF, Guo YJ, Li HB. Biological activities of polyphenols from grapes. Int J Mol Sci 2010; 11(2): 622-46. [http://dx.doi.org/10.3390/ijms11020622] [PMID: 20386657]

[28] Freedman JE, Parker C III, Li L, *et al.* Select flavonoids and whole juice from purple grapes inhibit platelet function and enhance nitric oxide release. Circulation 2001; 103(23): 2792-8. [http://dx.doi.org/10.1161/01.CIR.103.23.2792] [PMID: 11401934]

[29] Khurana S, Venkataraman K, Hollingsworth A, Piche M, Tai T. Polyphenols: benefits to the cardiovascular system in health and in aging. Nutrients 2013; 5(10): 3779-827. [http://dx.doi.org/10.3390/nu5103779] [PMID: 24077237]

[30] Soobrattee MA, Neergheen VS, Luximon-Ramma A, Aruoma OI, Bahorun T. Phenolics as potential antioxidant therapeutic agents: mechanism and actions. Mutat Res 2005; 579(1-2): 200-13. [PMID: 16126236]

[31] Cetin A, Kaynar L, Koçyiğit I, *et al.* The effect of grape seed extract on radiation-induced oxidative stress in the rat liver. Turk J Gastroenterol 2008; 19(2): 92-8. [PMID: 19110663]

[32] Olas B, Wachowicz B, Stochmal A, Oleszek W. The polyphenol-rich extract from grape seeds inhibits platelet signaling pathways triggered by both proteolytic and non-proteolytic agonists. Platelets 2012; 23(4): 282-9. [http://dx.doi.org/10.3109/09537104.2011.618562] [PMID: 21958130]

[33] Santangelo C, Varì R, Scazzocchio B, Di Benedetto R, Filesi C, Masella R. Polyphenols, intracellular signalling and inflammation. Ann Ist Super Sanita 2007; 43(4): 394-405. [PMID: 18209273]

[34] Huang S, Yang N, Liu Y, *et al.* Grape seed proanthocyanidins inhibit colon cancer-induced angiogenesis through suppressing the expression of VEGF and Angl. Int J Mol Med 2012; 30(6): 1410-6. [http://dx.doi.org/10.3892/ijmm.2012.1147] [PMID: 23026853]

[35] Engelbrecht AM, Mattheyse M, Ellis B, *et al.* Proanthocyanidin from grape seeds inactivates the PI3-

kinase/PKB pathway and induces apoptosis in a colon cancer cell line. Cancer Lett 2007; 258(1): 144-53.
[http://dx.doi.org/10.1016/j.canlet.2007.08.020] [PMID: 17923279]

[36] Li AN, Li S, Zhang YJ, Xu XR, Chen YM, Li HB. Resources and biological activities of natural polyphenols. Nutrients 2014; 6(12): 6020-47.
[http://dx.doi.org/10.3390/nu6126020] [PMID: 25533011]

[37] Cheah KY, Howarth GS, Bindon KA, Kennedy JA, Bastian SEP. Low molecular weight procyanidins from grape seeds enhance the impact of 5-Fluorouracil chemotherapy on Caco-2 human colon cancer cells. PLoS One 2014; 9(6): e98921.
[http://dx.doi.org/10.1371/journal.pone.0098921] [PMID: 24905821]

[38] Lacatusu I, Badea N, Badea G, *et al.* Lipid nanocarriers based on natural oils with high activity against oxygen free radicals and tumor cell proliferation. Mater Sci Eng C 2015; 56: 88-94.
[http://dx.doi.org/10.1016/j.msec.2015.06.019] [PMID: 26249569]

[39] Liu RH. Potential synergy of phytochemicals in cancer prevention: mechanism of action. J Nutr 2004; 134(12) (Suppl.): 3479S-85S.
[http://dx.doi.org/10.1093/jn/134.12.3479S] [PMID: 15570057]

[40] Husein AI, Ali-Shtayeh MS, Jondi WJ, Zatar NAA, Abu-Reidah IM, Jamous RM. *In vitro* antioxidant and antitumor activities of six selected plants used in the Traditional Arabic Palestinian herbal medicine. Pharm Biol 2014; 52(10): 1249-55.
[http://dx.doi.org/10.3109/13880209.2014.886274] [PMID: 24863277]

[41] Baydar NG, Sagdic O, Ozkan G, Cetin S. Determination of antibacterial effects and total phenolic contents of grape (*Vitis vinifera* L.) seed extracts. Int J Food Sci Technol 2006; 41(7): 799-804.
[http://dx.doi.org/10.1111/j.1365-2621.2005.01095.x]

[42] Subramanian M, Goswami M, Chakraborty S, Jawali N. Resveratrol induced inhibition of *Escherichia coli* proceeds *via* membrane oxidation and independent of diffusible reactive oxygen species generation. Redox Biol 2014; 2: 865-72.
[http://dx.doi.org/10.1016/j.redox.2014.06.007] [PMID: 25009788]

[43] Bokov DO B, Potanina OG P, Nikulin AV N, *et al.* Modern approaches to the analysis of kelp (Laminaria sp.) as pharmacopoeial herbal drugs and food products. Pharmacogn J 2020; 12(4): 929-37.
[http://dx.doi.org/10.5530/pj.2020.12.132]

[44] Kadam SU, Tiwari BK, O'Donnell CP. Extraction, structure and biofunctional activities of laminarin from brown algae. Int J Food Sci Technol 2015; 50(1): 24-31.
[http://dx.doi.org/10.1111/ijfs.12692]

[45] Ulbricht C, Basch E, Boon H, *et al.* Seaweed, kelp, bladderwrack (*Fucus vesiculosus*): an evidence-based systematic review by the natural standard research collaboration. Altern Complement Ther 2013; 19(4): 217-30.
[http://dx.doi.org/10.1089/act.2013.19401]

[46] Edwards SE, da Costa Rocha I, Williamson EM, Heinrich M. Bladderwrack; Kelp. Phytopharmacy: An evidence-based guide to herbal medicinal products. 2015; 27: 62.

[47] Rainone F. Milk thistle. Am Fam Physician 2005; 72(7): 1285-8.
[PMID: 16225032]

[48] Hobbs C. Milk thistle: The liver herb. Botanica Press 1987.

[49] Karkanis A, Bilalis D, Efthimiadou A. Cultivation of milk thistle (Silybum marianum L. Gaertn.), a medicinal weed. Ind Crops Prod 2011; 34: 825-30.
[http://dx.doi.org/10.1016/J.INDCROP.2011.03.027]

[50] Foster S. Milk thistle: Silybum marianum. American Botanical Council 1991.

[51] Goeden RD. The Palearctic insect fauna of milk thistle, Silybum marianum, as a source of biological

control agents for California. Environ Entomol 1976; 5(2): 345-53. [http://dx.doi.org/10.1093/ee/5.2.345]

[52] Khan MA, Abbasi BH, Ahmed N, Ali H. Effects of light regimes on *in vitro* seed germination and silymarin content in Silybum marianum. Ind Crops Prod 2013; 46: 105-10. [http://dx.doi.org/10.1016/j.indcrop.2012.12.035]

[53] Kumar T, Larokar YK, Iyer SK, Kumar A, Tripathi DK. Phytochemistry and pharmacological activities of Silybum marianum: a review. Int J Pharm Phytopharmacol Res 2011; 1(3): 124-33.

[54] Flora K, Hahn M, Rosen H, Benner K. Milk thistle (Silybum marianum) for the therapy of liver disease. Am J Gastroenterol 1998; 93(2): 139-43. [http://dx.doi.org/10.1111/j.1572-0241.1998.00139.x] [PMID: 9468229]

[55] Pelter A, Hänsel R. The structure of silybin (silybum substance E6), the first flavonolignan. Tetrahedron Lett 1968; 9(25): 2911-6. [C1]. [http://dx.doi.org/10.1016/S0040-4039(00)89610-0]

[56] Pelter A, Hänsel R. Struktur des silybins: I. Abbauversuche. Chem Ber 1975; 108(3): 790-802. [http://dx.doi.org/10.1002/cber.19751080312]

[57] Wagner H, Seligmann O, Seitz M, Abraham D, Sonnenbichler J. Notizen: Silydianin und Silychristin, zwei isomere Silymarine aus Silybum marianum L. Gaertn. (Mariendistel) / Silydianin and Silychristin, two Isomeric Silymarins from Silybum marianum L. Gaertn. (milk thistle). Z Naturforsch B J Chem Sci 1976; 31(6): 876-84. [http://dx.doi.org/10.1515/znb-1976-0630]

[58] Arnone A, Merlini L, Zanarotti A. Constituents of Silybum marianum. Structure of isosilybin and stereochemistry of silybin. J Chem Soc Chem Commun 1979; (16): 696-7. [http://dx.doi.org/10.1039/c39790000696]

[59] Kaloga M. Isosilychristin, ein neues Flayonolignan aus Silybum marianum L. Gaertn. / Isosilychristin, a New Flavonolignan from Silybum marianum L.Gaertn. Z Naturforsch B J Chem Sci 1981; 36(2): 262-5. [http://dx.doi.org/10.1515/znb-1981-0225]

[60] Szilági I, Tétényi P, Antus S, *et al.* [Structure of silandrin and silymonin, two new flavanolignans from a white blooming Silybum marianum variety]. Planta Med 1981; 43(2): 121-7. [http://dx.doi.org/10.1055/s-2007-971488] [PMID: 17402024]

[61] Fiebig M, Wagner H. [New antihepatotoxic effects of flavonolignans of a white flowering variety of Silybum]. Planta Med 1984; 50(4): 310-3. [http://dx.doi.org/10.1055/s-2007-969717] [PMID: 6095354]

[62] Kurkin VA, Zapesochnaya GG, Volotsueva AV, Avdeeva EV, Pimenov KS. Flavolignans of Silybum marianum fruit. Chem Nat Compd 2001; 37(4): 315-7. [http://dx.doi.org/10.1023/A:1013706115045]

[63] Lee DY, Liu YZ. New flavonolignans isolated from the seeds of Silybum marianum. 2003.

[64] Samu Z, Nyiredy S, Baitz-Gács E, *et al.* Structure elucidation and antioxidant activity of (-)-isosilandrin isolated from Silybum marianum L. Chem Biodivers 2004; 1(11): 1668-77. [http://dx.doi.org/10.1002/cbdv.200490125] [PMID: 17191807]

[65] Zhu HJ, Brinda BJ, Chavin KD, Bernstein HJ, Patrick KS, Markowitz JS. An assessment of pharmacokinetics and antioxidant activity of free silymarin flavonolignans in healthy volunteers: a dose escalation study. Drug Metab Dispos 2013; 41(9): 1679-85. [http://dx.doi.org/10.1124/dmd.113.052423] [PMID: 23835761]

[66] Di Pierro F, Putignano P, Montesi L, Moscatiello S, Marchesini Reggiani G, Villanova N. Preliminary study about the possible glycemic clinical advantage in using a fixed combination of Berberis aristata and Silybum marianum standardized extracts *versus* only Berberis aristata in patients with type 2 diabetes. Clin Pharmacol 2013; 5: 167-74.

[http://dx.doi.org/10.2147/CPAA.S54308] [PMID: 24277991]

[67] Valentová K, Vidlář A, Zatloukalová M, *et al.* Biosafety and antioxidant effects of a beverage containing silymarin and arginine. A pilot, human intervention cross-over trial. Food Chem Toxicol 2013; 56: 178-83.
[http://dx.doi.org/10.1016/j.fct.2013.02.023] [PMID: 23439479]

[68] Kawaguchi-Suzuki M, Frye RF, Zhu HJ, *et al.* The effects of milk thistle (Silybum marianum) on human cytochrome P450 activity. Drug Metab Dispos 2014; 42(10): 1611-6.
[http://dx.doi.org/10.1124/dmd.114.057232] [PMID: 25028567]

[69] Hawke RL, Schrieber SJ, Soule TA, *et al.* Silymarin ascending multiple oral dosing phase I study in noncirrhotic patients with chronic hepatitis C. J Clin Pharmacol 2010; 50(4): 434-49.
[http://dx.doi.org/10.1177/0091270009347475] [PMID: 19841158]

[70] Malaguarnera G, Bertino G, Chisari G, *et al.* Silybin supplementation during HCV therapy with pegylated interferon-α plus ribavirin reduces depression and anxiety and increases work ability. BMC Psychiatry 2016; 16(1): 398.
[http://dx.doi.org/10.1186/s12888-016-1115-z] [PMID: 27842532]

[71] Biermer M, Schlosser B, Fülöp B, *et al.* High-dose silibinin rescue treatment for HCV-infected patients showing suboptimal virologic response to standard combination therapy. J Viral Hepat 2012; 19(8): 547-53.
[http://dx.doi.org/10.1111/j.1365-2893.2011.01572.x] [PMID: 22762138]

[72] Fried MW, Navarro VJ, Afdhal N, *et al.* Effect of silymarin (milk thistle) on liver disease in patients with chronic hepatitis C unsuccessfully treated with interferon therapy: a randomized controlled trial. JAMA 2012; 308(3): 274-82.
[http://dx.doi.org/10.1001/jama.2012.8265] [PMID: 22797645]

[73] Zhong S, Fan Y, Yan Q, *et al.* The therapeutic effect of silymarin in the treatment of nonalcoholic fatty disease. Medicine (Baltimore) 2017; 96(49): e9061.
[http://dx.doi.org/10.1097/MD.0000000000009061] [PMID: 29245314]

[74] El-Kamary SS, Shardell MD, Abdel-Hamid M, *et al.* A randomized controlled trial to assess the safety and efficacy of silymarin on symptoms, signs and biomarkers of acute hepatitis. Phytomedicine 2009; 16(5): 391-400.
[http://dx.doi.org/10.1016/j.phymed.2009.02.002] [PMID: 19303273]

[75] Loguercio C, Andreone P, Brisc C, *et al.* Silybin combined with phosphatidylcholine and vitamin E in patients with nonalcoholic fatty liver disease: A randomized controlled trial. Free Radic Biol Med 2012; 52(9): 1658-65.
[http://dx.doi.org/10.1016/j.freeradbiomed.2012.02.008] [PMID: 22343419]

[76] Bakhshaee M, Jabbari F, Hoseini S, *et al.* Effect of silymarin in the treatment of allergic rhinitis. Otolaryngol Head Neck Surg 2011; 145(6): 904-9.
[http://dx.doi.org/10.1177/0194599811423504] [PMID: 21952357]

[77] Marjani M, Baghaei P, Kazempour Dizaji M, *et al.* Evaluation of hepatoprotective effect of silymarin among under-treated tuberculosis patients: a randomized clinical trial. Iran J Pharm Res 2016; 15(1): 247-52.
[PMID: 27610165]

[78] Hussain SA, Mortada AH, Jasim NA, Gorial FI. Silibinin improves the effects of methotrexate in patients with active rheumatoid arthritis: pilot clinical study. Oman Med J 2016; 31(4): 263-9.
[http://dx.doi.org/10.5001/omj.2016.52] [PMID: 27403238]

[79] Hussain SA, Jassim NA, Numan IT, Al-Khalifa II, Abdullah TA. Anti-inflammatory activity of silymarin in patients with knee osteoarthritis. A comparative study with piroxicam and meloxicam. Saudi Med J 2009; 30(1): 98-103.
[PMID: 19139781]

[80] Arora P, Sarkar R, Garg V, Sonthalia S, Gokhale N. Melasma update. Indian Dermatol Online J 2014; 5(4): 426-35.
[http://dx.doi.org/10.4103/2229-5178.142484] [PMID: 25396123]

[81] Elyasi S, Hosseini S, Niazi Moghadam MR, Aledavood SA, Karimi G. Effect of oral silymarin administration on prevention of radiotherapy-induced mucositis: A randomized, double-blinded, placebo-controlled clinical trial. Phytother Res 2016; 30(11): 1879-85.
[http://dx.doi.org/10.1002/ptr.5704] [PMID: 27555604]

[82] Becker-Schiebe M, Mengs U, Schaefer M, Bulitta M, Hoffmann W. Topical use of a silymarin-based preparation to prevent radiodermatitis : results of a prospective study in breast cancer patients. Strahlenther Onkol 2011; 187(8): 485-91.
[http://dx.doi.org/10.1007/s00066-011-2204-z] [PMID: 21786113]

[83] Hung JH, Chu CJ, Sung PL, *et al.* Lamivudine therapy in the treatment of chronic hepatitis B with acute exacerbation during pregnancy. J Chin Med Assoc 2008; 71(3): 155-8.
[http://dx.doi.org/10.1016/S1726-4901(08)70009-1] [PMID: 18364269]

[84] Desai A, Shidhaye S, Kadam VJ. Possible use of psyllium husk as a release retardant. Indian J Pharm Sci 2007; 69(2).

[85] Singh B. Psyllium as therapeutic and drug delivery agent. Int J Pharm 2007; 334(1-2): 1-14.
[http://dx.doi.org/10.1016/j.ijpharm.2007.01.028] [PMID: 17329047]

[86] Shah AR, Sharma P, Longvah T, *et al.* Nutritional composition and health benefits of psyllium (Plantago ovata) husk and seed. Nutr Today 2020; 55(6): 313-21.
[http://dx.doi.org/10.1097/NT.0000000000000450]

[87] Belorio M, Gómez M. Psyllium: a useful functional ingredient in food systems. Crit Rev Food Sci Nutr 2022; 62(2): 527-38.
[http://dx.doi.org/10.1080/10408398.2020.1822276] [PMID: 32951436]

[88] Verma A, Mogra R. Psyllium (Plantago ovata) husk: a wonder food for good health. Int J Sci Res 2013; 4(9): 1581-5. [N].

[89] Mehmood MH, Aziz N, Ghayur MN, Gilani AH. Pharmacological basis for the medicinal use of psyllium husk (Ispaghula) in constipation and diarrhea. Dig Dis Sci 2011; 56(5): 1460-71.
[http://dx.doi.org/10.1007/s10620-010-1466-0] [PMID: 21082352]

[90] Jalanka J, Major G, Murray K, *et al.* The effect of psyllium husk on intestinal microbiota in constipated patients and healthy controls. Int J Mol Sci 2019; 20(2): 433.
[http://dx.doi.org/10.3390/ijms20020433] [PMID: 30669509]

[91] Edwards SE, da Costa Rocha I, Williamson EM, Heinrich M. Ispaghula Husk, Psyllium Husk. Phytopharmacy: An Evidence-Based Guide to Herbal Medicinal Products. 2015 Apr 27:222.

[92] Linde K, Berner MM, Kriston L. St John's wort for major depression. Cochrane database of systematic reviews. 2008(4).
[http://dx.doi.org/10.1002/14651858.CD000448.pub3]

[93] Di Carlo G, Borrelli F, Ernst E, Izzo AA. St John's wort: Prozac from the plant kingdom. Trends Pharmacol Sci 2001; 22(6): 292-7.
[http://dx.doi.org/10.1016/S0165-6147(00)01716-8] [PMID: 11395157]

[94] Simmen U, Higelin J, Berger-Büter K, Schaffner W, Lundstrom K. Neurochemical studies with St. John's wort *in vitro*.. Pharmacopsychiatry 2001; 34(Supp. 1): 137-42.

[95] Frommenwiler DA, Reich E, Sudberg S, Sharaf MHM, Bzhelyansky A, Lucas B. John's wort *versus* counterfeit St. John's wort: an HPTLC study. J AOAC Int 2016; 99(5): 1204-12.
[http://dx.doi.org/10.5740/jaoacint.16-0170] [PMID: 27343017]

[96] Ernst E. Second thoughts about safety of St John's wort. Lancet 1999; 354(9195): 2014-6.
[http://dx.doi.org/10.1016/S0140-6736(99)00418-3] [PMID: 10636361]

[97] Hippius H. St John's Wort (Hypericum perforatum)--a herbal antidepressant. Curr Med Res Opin 1998; 14(3): 171-84.
[http://dx.doi.org/10.1185/03007999809113357] [PMID: 9787983]

[98] Yue QY, Bergquist C, Gerdén B. Safety of St John's wort (Hypericum perforatum). Lancet 2000; 355(9203): 576-7.
[http://dx.doi.org/10.1016/S0140-6736(05)73227-X] [PMID: 10683030]

[99] Bilia AR, Gallori S, Vincieri FF. St. John's wort and depression. Life Sci 2002; 70(26): 3077-96.
[http://dx.doi.org/10.1016/S0024-3205(02)01566-7] [PMID: 12008092]

[100] Affuf A, Karpenko JN, Gulyaev DK, Molokhova EI, Blinova OL, Gileva AA, Belonogova VD. Phytochemical study of Tribulus terrestris L. Фармация и фармакология. 2019; 7(6 (eng)): 346-55.

[101] Chhatre S, Nesari T, Kanchan D, Somani G, Sathaye S. Phytopharmacological overview of Tribulus terrestris. Pharmacogn Rev 2014; 8(15): 45-51.
[http://dx.doi.org/10.4103/0973-7847.125530] [PMID: 24600195]

[102] Van Wyk BE, Wink M. Medicinal Plants of the world: chemical constituents, traditional and modern medicinal uses. 2017.

[103] Jayanthy A, Deepak M, Remashree AB. Pharmacognostic characterization and comparison of fruits of Tribulus terrestris L. and Pedalium murex L. 2017.

[104] Semerdjieva IB, Zheljazkov VD. Chemical constituents, biological properties, and uses of Tribulus terrestris: A review 2019.
[http://dx.doi.org/10.1177/1934578X19868394]

[105] Kamenov Z, Fileva S, Kalinov K, Jannini EA. Evaluation of the efficacy and safety of Tribulus terrestris in male sexual dysfunction—A prospective, randomized, double-blind, placebo-controlled clinical trial. Maturitas 2017; 99: 20-6.
[http://dx.doi.org/10.1016/j.maturitas.2017.01.011] [PMID: 28364864]

[106] Santos CA Jr, Reis LO, Destro-Saade R, Luiza-Reis A, Fregonesi A. Tribulus terrestris *versus* placebo in the treatment of erectile dysfunction: A prospective, randomized, double blind study. Actas Urol Esp 2014; 38(4): 244-8.
[http://dx.doi.org/10.1016/j.acuro.2013.09.014] [PMID: 24630840]

[107] Samy MN, Bishr MM, Ahmed AA, Kamel MS. Tribulin, a New Steroidal Saponin from the Aerial parts of *Tribulus terrestris.* Research Journal of Pharmacognosy and Phytochemistry 2012; 4(5): 237-9.

[108] Ştefănescu R, Tero-Vescan A, Negroiu A, Aurică E, Vari CE. A comprehensive review of the phytochemical, pharmacological, and toxicological properties of Tribulus terrestris L. Biomolecules 2020; 10(5): 752.
[http://dx.doi.org/10.3390/biom10050752] [PMID: 32408715]

[109] Prasad S, Aggarwal BB. Turmeric, the golden spice. Herbal Medicine: Biomolecular and Clinical Aspects. 2nd edition. 2011.
[http://dx.doi.org/10.1201/b10787-14]

[110] Verma RK, Kumari P, Maurya RK, Kumar V, Verma RB, Singh RK. Medicinal properties of turmeric (Curcuma longa L.): A review. Int J Chem Stud 2018; 6(4): 1354-7.

[111] Priyadarsini K. The chemistry of curcumin: from extraction to therapeutic agent. Molecules 2014; 19(12): 20091-112.
[http://dx.doi.org/10.3390/molecules191220091] [PMID: 25470276]

[112] Strimpakos AS, Sharma RA. Curcumin: preventive and therapeutic properties in laboratory studies and clinical trials. Antioxid Redox Signal 2008; 10(3): 511-46.
[http://dx.doi.org/10.1089/ars.2007.1769] [PMID: 18370854]

[113] Vogel HA, Pelletier J. Curcumin-biological and medicinal properties. J Pharm (Cairo) 1815; 2(50):

24-9.

[114] Lampe V, Milobedzka J. Studien über Curcumin. Ber Dtsch Chem Ges 1913; 46(2): 2235-40. [http://dx.doi.org/10.1002/cber.191304602149]

[115] Niederau C, Göpfert E. The effect of chelidonium and turmeric root extract on upper abdominal pain due to functional disorders of the biliary system 1999.

[116] Abidi A, Gupta S, Agarwal M, Bhalla HL, Saluja M. Evaluation of efficacy of curcumin as an add-on therapy in patients of bronchial asthma. J Clin Diagn Res 2014; 8(8): HC19-24. [http://dx.doi.org/10.7860/JCDR/2014/9273.4705] [PMID: 25302215]

[117] Chaudhari AU, Karhadkar VM, Waghmare PF, Jamkhande AS. Comparative evaluation of turmeric and chlorhexidine gluconate mouthwash in prevention of plaque formation and gingivitis: a clinical and microbiological study. J Contemp Dent Pract 2011; 12(4): 221-4. [http://dx.doi.org/10.5005/jp-journals-10024-1038] [PMID: 22186854]

[118] Kunnumakkara AB, Bordoloi D, Padmavathi G, *et al.* Curcumin, the golden nutraceutical: multitargeting for multiple chronic diseases. Br J Pharmacol 2017; 174(11): 1325-48. [http://dx.doi.org/10.1111/bph.13621] [PMID: 27638428]

[119] Kurd SK, Smith N, VanVoorhees A, *et al.* Oral curcumin in the treatment of moderate to severe psoriasis vulgaris: A prospective clinical trial. J Am Acad Dermatol 2008; 58(4): 625-31. [http://dx.doi.org/10.1016/j.jaad.2007.12.035] [PMID: 18249471]

[120] Ryan JL, Heckler CE, Ling M, *et al.* Curcumin for radiation dermatitis: a randomized, double-blind, placebo-controlled clinical trial of thirty breast cancer patients. Radiat Res 2013; 180(1): 34-43. [http://dx.doi.org/10.1667/RR3255.1] [PMID: 23745991]

[121] Adhvaryu MR, Reddy NM, Vakharia BC. Prevention of hepatotoxicity due to anti tuberculosis treatment: A novel integrative approach. World J Gastroenterol 2008; 14(30): 4753-62. [http://dx.doi.org/10.3748/wjg.14.4753] [PMID: 18720535]

[122] Golombick T, Diamond TH, Badmaev V, Manoharan A, Ramakrishna R. The potential role of curcumin in patients with monoclonal gammopathy of undefined significance--its effect on paraproteinemia and the urinary N-telopeptide of type I collagen bone turnover marker. Clin Cancer Res 2009; 15(18): 5917-22. [http://dx.doi.org/10.1158/1078-0432.CCR-08-2217] [PMID: 19737963]

[123] Jäger R, Lowery RP, Calvanese AV, Joy JM, Purpura M, Wilson JM. Comparative absorption of curcumin formulations. Nutr J 2014; 13(1): 11. [http://dx.doi.org/10.1186/1475-2891-13-11] [PMID: 24461029]

[124] Panahi Y, Saadat A, Beiraghdar F, Sahebkar A. Adjuvant therapy with bioavailability-boosted curcuminoids suppresses systemic inflammation and improves quality of life in patients with solid tumors: a randomized double-blind placebo-controlled trial. Phytother Res 2014; 28(10): 1461-7. [http://dx.doi.org/10.1002/ptr.5149] [PMID: 24648302]

[125] Steigerwalt R, Nebbioso M, Appendino G, *et al.* Meriva®, a lecithinized curcumin delivery system, in diabetic microangiopathy and retinopathy. Panminerva Med 2012; 54(1) (Suppl. 4): 11-6. [PMID: 23241930]

[126] Belcaro G, Cesarone MR, Dugall M, *et al.* Efficacy and safety of Meriva®, a curcumin-phosphatidylcholine complex, during extended administration in osteoarthritis patients. Altern Med Rev 2010; 15(4): 337-44. [PMID: 21194249]

[127] Kakkar V, Kaur IP. Evaluating potential of curcumin loaded solid lipid nanoparticles in aluminium induced behavioural, biochemical and histopathological alterations in mice brain. Food Chem Toxicol 2011; 49(11): 2906-13. [http://dx.doi.org/10.1016/j.fct.2011.08.006] [PMID: 21889563]

[128] Burgos-Morón E, Calderón-Montaño JM, Salvador J, Robles A, López-Lázaro M. The dark side of

curcumin. Int J Cancer 2010; 126(7): 1771-5.
[http://dx.doi.org/10.1002/ijc.24967] [PMID: 19830693]

[129] Webster DE, He Y, Chen SN, Pauli GF, Farnsworth NR, Wang ZJ. Opioidergic mechanisms underlying the actions of Vitex agnus-castus L. Biochem Pharmacol 2011; 81(1): 170-7. [http://dx.doi.org/10.1016/j.bcp.2010.09.013] [PMID: 20854795]

[130] Hu Y, Hou TT, Xin HL, *et al.* Estrogen-like activity of volatile components from Vitex rotundifolia L. Indian J Med Res 2007; 126(1): 68-72. [PMID: 17890827]

[131] Manivannan S, Bhuvaneswari S, Akshay M, Tharani G, Benasir D, Madhavi P. Evaluation of anti-arthritic potential of vitex agnus-castus in freund's complete adjuvant induced arthritic albino rats.

[132] Bornhorst HL. Growing native Hawaiian plants: a how-to guide for the gardener. Bess Press 2005.

[133] Ono M, Yamasaki T, Konoshita M, *et al.* Five new diterpenoids, viteagnusins A--E, from the fruit of Vitex agnus-castus. Chem Pharm Bull (Tokyo) 2008; 56(11): 1621-4. [http://dx.doi.org/10.1248/cpb.56.1621] [PMID: 18981619]

[134] Dugoua JJ, Seely D, Perri D, Koren G, Mills E. Safety and efficacy of chastetree (Vitex agnus-castus) during pregnancy and lactation. J Popul Ther Clin Pharmacol 2008; 15(1): e74-9. [PMID: 18204102]

[135] Khalilzadeh E, Vafaei Saiah G, Hasannejad H, *et al.* Antinociceptive effects, acute toxicity and chemical composition of Vitex agnus-castus essential oil. Avicenna J Phytomed 2015; 5(3): 218-30. [PMID: 26101755]

[136] Mancho P, Edwards QT. Chaste tree for premenstrual syndrome. An evolving therapy in the United States. Adv Nurse Pract 2005; 13(5): 43-44, 46. [PMID: 15898315]

[137] Arokiyaraj S, Perinbam K, Agastian P, Kumar RM. Phytochemical analysis and antibacterial activity of *Vitex agnus-castus*. International Journal of Green Pharmacy 2009; 3(2): 162. [http://dx.doi.org/10.4103/0973-8258.54912]

[138] Alamoudi MO, Bakrshoom YF. Vitex agnus castus and some female disorders: A review. Agric Rev (Karnal) 2021; 42(Of): 209-14. [http://dx.doi.org/10.18805/ag.R-170]

[139] Maltaş E, Uysal A, Yıldız S, Durak Y. Evaluation of antioxidant and antimicrobial activity of Vitex agnus castus L. 2010; 19(12b): 3094-3099.

[140] Marongiu B, Piras A, Porcedda S, *et al.* Extraction, separation and isolation of volatiles from *Vitex agnus-castus* L. (Verbenaceae) wild species of Sardinia, Italy, by supercritical CO $_2$. Nat Prod Res 2010; 24(6): 569-79. [http://dx.doi.org/10.1080/14786410902899915] [PMID: 20397107]

[141] Hajdú Z, Hohmann J, Forgo P, *et al.* Diterpenoids and flavonoids from the fruits of *Vitex agnus-castus* and antioxidant activity of the fruit extracts and their constituents. Phytother Res 2007; 21(4): 391-4. [http://dx.doi.org/10.1002/ptr.2021] [PMID: 17262892]

[142] Oztürk A, Ilman AA, Sağlam H, *et al.* The effects of phytoestrogens on fracture healing: experimental research in New Zealand white rabbits. Ulus Travma Acil Cerrahi Derg 2008; 14(1): 21-7. [PMID: 18306063]

[143] Lee H, Jung KH, Lee H, Park S, Choi W, Bae H. Casticin, an active compound isolated from Vitex Fructus, ameliorates the cigarette smoke-induced acute lung inflammatory response in a murine model. Int Immunopharmacol 2015; 28(2): 1097-101. [http://dx.doi.org/10.1016/j.intimp.2015.07.041] [PMID: 26321116]

[144] Chopin Lucks B. Vitex agnus castus essential oil and menopausal balance: a research update [Complementary Therapies in Nursing and Midwifery 8 (2003) 148–154]. Complement Ther Nurs

Midwifery 2003; 9(3): 157-60.
[http://dx.doi.org/10.1016/S1353-6117(03)00020-9] [PMID: 12852933]

[145] Aksoy AN, Gözükara I, Kabil Kucur S. Evaluation of the efficacy of *F ructus agni casti* in women with severe primary dysmenorrhea: A prospective comparative D oppler study. J Obstet Gynaecol Res 2014; 40(3): 779-84.
[http://dx.doi.org/10.1111/jog.12221] [PMID: 24245554]

[146] Dinç T, Coşkun F. Comparison of fructus agni casti and flurbiprofen in the treatment of cyclic mastalgia in premenopausal women. Ulus Cerrahi Derg 2014; 30(1): 34-8.
[http://dx.doi.org/10.5152/UCD.2014.2409] [PMID: 25931888]

[147] Eftekhari MH, Rostami ZH, Emami MJ, Tabatabaee HR. Effects of "vitex agnus castus" extract and magnesium supplementation, alone and in combination, on osteogenic and angiogenic factors and fracture healing in women with long bone fracture. Journal of research in medical sciences: the official journal of Isfahan University of Medical Sciences 2014; 19(1): 1.

[148] Vedula GS, Isukapatla T, Ketha A. Protective effect of Vitex altissima Lf bark extract on cisplatin-induced renal injury in Wistar rats. Plant Sci Today 2022; 9(3): 642-9.

[149] Ho SHY, Singh M, Holloway AC, Crankshaw DJ. The effects of commercial preparations of herbal supplements commonly used by women on the biotransformation of fluorogenic substrates by human cytochromes P450. Phytother Res 2011; 25(7): 983-9.
[http://dx.doi.org/10.1002/ptr.3371] [PMID: 21213356]

[150] Daniele C, Thompson Coon J, Pittler MH, Ernst E. Vitex agnus castus. Drug Saf 2005; 28(4): 319-32.
[http://dx.doi.org/10.2165/00002018-200528040-00004] [PMID: 15783241]

[151] Greer E, Pezeshki SR, Shields FD Jr. Influences of cutting diameter and soil moisture on growth and survival of black willow, *salix nigra*. J Soil Water Conserv 2006; 61(5): 311-23.
[http://dx.doi.org/10.1080/00224561.2006.12435901]

[152] Roqueiro G, Maldonado S, Ríos MC, Maroder H. Fluctuation of oxidative stress indicators in Salix nigra seeds during priming. J Exp Bot 2012; 63(10): 3631-42.
[http://dx.doi.org/10.1093/jxb/ers030] [PMID: 22419741]

[153] Renninger H, Kyaw TY, Siegert CM, Rousseau RJ. Water use efficiency, leaf physiology, and productivity of black willow (Salix nigra Marshall) for short rotation bioenergy production in the southern U.S. Biomass Bioenergy 2024; 183: 107135.
[http://dx.doi.org/10.1016/j.biombioe.2024.107135]

[154] Tawfeek N, Mahmoud MF, Hamdan DI, *et al.* Phytochemistry, pharmacology and medicinal uses of plants of the genus salix: An updated review. Front Pharmacol 2021; 12: 593856.
[http://dx.doi.org/10.3389/fphar.2021.593856]

[155] Mostafa I, Abbas HA, Ashour ML, *et al.* Polyphenols from Salix tetrasperma impair virulence and inhibit quorum sensing of Pseudomonas aeruginosa. Molecules 2020; 25(6): 1341.
[http://dx.doi.org/10.3390/molecules25061341] [PMID: 32187997]

[156] Sati S, Singh H, Badoni P, Sati M. Screening of fungicidal activity of Salix and Triumfetta species of Garhwal Himalaya. Am J Phytomed Clin Ther 2013; 1(5): 486-9.

[157] Ramos PAB, Moreirinha C, Silva S, *et al.* The health-promoting potential of Salix spp. bark polar extracts: Key insights on phenolic composition and *in vitro* bioactivity and biocompatibility. Antioxidants 2019; 8(12): 609.
[http://dx.doi.org/10.3390/antiox8120609] [PMID: 31801290]

[158] Hossain MM, Biva IJ, Jahangir R, Vhuiyan MM. Central nervous system depressant and analgesic activity of Aphanamixis polystachya (Wall.) Parker leaf extract in mice. Afr J Pharm Pharmacol 2009; 3(5): 282-6.

[159] Wahid A, Hamed AN, Eltahir HM, Abouzied MM. Hepatoprotective activity of ethanolic extract of Salix subserrata against CCl4-induced chronic hepatotoxicity in rats. BMC Complement Altern Med

2016; 16(1): 263.
[http://dx.doi.org/10.1186/s12906-016-1238-2] [PMID: 27473536]

[160] El-Shemy HA, Aboul-Enein AM, Aboul-Enein KM, Fujita K. Willow leaves' extracts contain anti-tumor agents effective against three cell types. PLoS One 2007; 2(1): e178.
[http://dx.doi.org/10.1371/journal.pone.0000178] [PMID: 17264881]

[161] Virupaksha JH, Nadendla RR, Kumar MS, Kavya S. Effect of Salix tetrasperma Roxburgh leaf extracts on central nervous system activities. Res J Pharm Biol Chem Sci 2016; 7(4): 2060-4.

[162] Wahid A, Hamed AN, Eltahir HM, Abouzied MM. Hepatoprotective activity of ethanolic extract of Salix subserrata against CCl 4-induced chronic hepatotoxicity in rats. BMC complementary and alternative medicine. 2016 Dec;16:1-0. Liu KY, Liu HJ, Zhou B, Han LK. Studies on chemical constituents from Salix babylonica L. and their stimulating lipolysis activity. J Fudan Uni 2008; 4: 022.

[163] Kiplang A, Rono C. Isolation and characterization of active antihyperglycemic component of urtica dioica leaves (doctoral dissertation) available from: http://erepository.uoeld.ac.ke/xmlui/handle/123456789/108

[164] Pilerood SA, Prakash J. Nutritional and medicinal properties of valerian (Valeriana officinalis) herb: A review. Int J Food Sci Nutr Diet 2013; 1(1): 25-33.

[165] Patočka J, Jakl J. Biomedically relevant chemical constituents of Valeriana officinalis. J Appl Biomed 2010; 8(1): 11-8.
[http://dx.doi.org/10.2478/v10136-009-0002-z]

[166] Wang S, Zeng Y, Li Y, *et al.* Chemical constituents from Valeriana officinalis L. var. Iatifolia Miq. and their chemotaxonomic significance. Biochem Syst Ecol 2020; 90: 104041.
[http://dx.doi.org/10.1016/J.BSE.2020.104041]

[167] Dyayiya NA, Oyemitan IA, Matewu R, *et al.* Chemical analysis and biological potential of *Valerian root* as used by herbal practitioners in the Eastern Cape Province, South Africa. Afr J Tradit Complement Altern Med 2016; 13(1): 114-22.
[http://dx.doi.org/10.4314/ajtcam.v13i1.16]

[168] Miyasaka LS, Atallah ÁN, Soares B. Valerian for anxiety disorders. Cochrane Database of Systematic Reviews. 2006(4).
[http://dx.doi.org/10.1002/14651858.CD004515.pub2]

[169] Bent S, Padula A, Moore D, Patterson M, Mehling W. Valerian for sleep: a systematic review and meta-analysis. Am J Med 2006; 119(12): 1005-12.
[http://dx.doi.org/10.1016/j.amjmed.2006.02.026] [PMID: 17145239]

[170] Spinella M. Herbal medicines and epilepsy: the potential for benefit and adverse effects. Epilepsy Behav 2001; 2(6): 524-32.
[http://dx.doi.org/10.1006/ebeh.2001.0281] [PMID: 12609386]

[171] Stevinson C, Ernst E. Valerian for insomnia: a systematic review of randomized clinical trials. Sleep Med 2000; 1(2): 91-9.
[http://dx.doi.org/10.1016/S1389-9457(99)00015-5] [PMID: 10767649]

[172] Azizi H, Shojaii A, Hashem-Dabaghian F, *et al.* Effects of *Valeriana officinalis* (Valerian) on tension-type headache: A randomized, placebo-controlled, double-blind clinical trial. Avicenna J Phytomed 2020; 10(3): 297-304.
[PMID: 32523884]

[173] Taavoni S, Ekbatani N, Kashaniyan M, Haghani H. Effect of valerian on sleep quality in postmenopausal women. Menopause 2011; 18(9): 951-5.
[http://dx.doi.org/10.1097/gme.0b013e31820e9acf] [PMID: 21775910]

[174] Caron MF, Riedlinger JE. Valerian: a practical review for clinicians. Nutr Clin Care 1999; 2(4): 250-7.
[http://dx.doi.org/10.1046/j.1523-5408.1999.00114.x]

[175] Wan D, Wu Q, Kuča K. Spirulina. In Nutraceuticals 2021 Jan 1 (pp. 959-974). Academic Press.

[176] Belay A, Ota Y, Miyakawa K, Shimamatsu H. Current knowledge on potential health benefits of Spirulina. J Appl Phycol 1993; 5(2): 235-41. [http://dx.doi.org/10.1007/BF00004024]

[177] Ciferri O. Spirulina, the edible microorganism. Microbiol Rev 1983; 47(4): 551-78. [http://dx.doi.org/10.1128/mr.47.4.551-578.1983] [PMID: 6420655]

[178] Usharani G, Saranraj P, Kanchana D. Spirulina cultivation: a review. Int J Pharm Biol Arch 2012; 3(6): 1327-41.

[179] Bchir B, Felfoul I, Bouaziz MA, *et al.* Investigation of physicochemical, nutritional, textural, and sensory properties of yoghurt fortified with fresh and dried spirulina (Arthrospira platensis). Int Food Res J 2019; 26(5).

[180] Priyanka S , Varsha R , Riya Verma , Ayenampudi SB. Spirulina: A spotlight on its nutraceutical properties and food processing applications. J Microbiol Biotechnol Food Sci 2023; 12(6): e4785. [http://dx.doi.org/10.55251/jmbfs.4785]

[181] Baicus C, Baicus A. Spirulina did not ameliorate idiopathic chronic fatigue in four N-of-1 randomized controlled trials. Phytother Res 2007; 21(6): 570-3. [http://dx.doi.org/10.1002/ptr.2114] [PMID: 17335116]

[182] Kim HM, Lee EH, Cho HH, Moon YH. Inhibitory effect of mast cell-mediated immediate-type allergic reactions in rats by spirulina. Biochem Pharmacol 1998; 55(7): 1071-6. [http://dx.doi.org/10.1016/S0006-2952(97)00678-3] [PMID: 9605430]

[183] Hayashi T, Hayashi K, Maeda M, Kojima I. Calcium spirulan, an inhibitor of enveloped virus replication, from a blue-green alga Spirulina platensis. J Nat Prod 1996; 59(1): 83-7. [http://dx.doi.org/10.1021/np960017o] [PMID: 8984158]

[184] Ramamoorthy A, Premakumari S. Effect of supplementation of Spirulina on hypercholesterolemic patients. Journal of Food Science and Technology-Mysore 1996; 33: 124-7.

[185] Patel P, Jethani H, Radha C, *et al.* Development of a carotenoid enriched probiotic yogurt from fresh biomass of *Spirulina* and its characterization. J Food Sci Technol 2019; 56(8): 3721-31. [http://dx.doi.org/10.1007/s13197-019-03844-0] [PMID: 31413399]

[186] Ashok SA. Phytochemical and pharmacological screening of wheatgrass juice (Triticum aestivum L.). Int J Pharm Sci Rev Res 2011; 9(1): 159-64.

[187] Smith BH. Generalization of spatially variant apodization to noninteger Nyquist sampling rates. IEEE Trans Image Process 2000; 9(6): 1088-93. [http://dx.doi.org/10.1109/83.846250] [PMID: 18255478]

[188] Ben-Arye E, Goldin E, Wengrower D, Stamper A, Kohn R, Berry E. Wheat grass juice in the treatment of active distal ulcerative colitis: a randomized double-blind placebo-controlled trial. Scand J Gastroenterol 2002; 37(4): 444-9. [http://dx.doi.org/10.1080/003655202317316088] [PMID: 11989836]

[189] de Vogel J, Jonker-Termont DSML, Katan MB, van der Meer R. Natural chlorophyll but not chlorophyllin prevents heme-induced cytotoxic and hyperproliferative effects in rat colon. J Nutr 2005; 135(8): 1995-2000. [http://dx.doi.org/10.1093/jn/135.8.1995] [PMID: 16046728]

[190] Ferruzzi MG, Blakeslee J. Digestion, absorption, and cancer preventative activity of dietary chlorophyll derivatives. Nutr Res 2007; 27(1): 1-12. [http://dx.doi.org/10.1016/j.nutres.2006.12.003]

[191] Meyerowitz S. Wheatgrass, Natures Finest Medicine. Book Publishing Company. 2006.

[192] Marawaha RK, Bansal D, Kaur S, Trehan A. Wheat grass juice reduces transfusion requirement in

patients with thalassemia major: a pilot study. Indian Pediatr 2004; 41(7): 716-20. [PMID: 15297687]

[193] Sareen M, Baghla P, Dhaka P, Mathur E, Sobti P, Khajuria S. Wheat grass-a wonder herb. Systematic Reviews in Pharmacy 2016; 5(1): 4-5. [http://dx.doi.org/10.5530/srp.2014.1.2]

[194] Rana S, Kamboj JK, Gandhi V. Living life the natural way – Wheatgrass and Health. Funct Food Health Dis 2011; 1(11): 444-56. [http://dx.doi.org/10.31989/ffhd.v1i11.112]

[195] Bar-Sela G, Cohen M, Ben-Arye E, Epelbaum R. The medical use of wheatgrass: Review of the gap between basic and clinical applications. Mini Rev Med Chem 2015; 15(12): 1002-10. [http://dx.doi.org/10.2174/138955751512150731112836] [PMID: 26156538]

[196] Tandon S, Arora A, Singh S, Monga J, Arora S. Antioxidant profiling of Triticum aestivum (wheatgrass) and its antiproliferative activity in MCF-7 breast cancer cell line.

[197] Rani K, Sandal N, Sahoo PK. A comprehensive review on chlorella-its composition, health benefits, market and regulatory scenario. Pharma Innovation Journal 2018; 7(7): 584-9.

[198] Saad A, Atia A. Review on freshwater blue-green algae (Cyanobacteria): occurrence, classification and toxicology. Biosci Biotechnol Res Asia 2014; 11(3): 1319-25. [http://dx.doi.org/10.13005/bbra/1522]

[199] Northcote DH, Goulding KJ, Horne RW. The chemical composition and structure of the cell wall of *Chlorella pyrenoidosa*. Biochem J 1958; 70(3): 391-7. [http://dx.doi.org/10.1042/bj0700391] [PMID: 13596355]

[200] Safi C, Zebib B, Merah O, Pontalier PY, Vaca-Garcia C. Morphology, composition, production, processing and applications of Chlorella vulgaris: A review. Renew Sustain Energy Rev 2014; 35: 265-78. [http://dx.doi.org/10.1016/j.rser.2014.04.007]

[201] Merchant RE, Andre CA. A review of recent clinical trials of the nutritional supplement Chlorella pyrenoidosa in the treatment of fibromyalgia, hypertension, and ulcerative colitis. Altern Ther Health Med 2001; 7(3): 79-91. [PMID: 11347287]

[202] Samac DA, Austin-Phillips S. Alfalfa (Medicago sativa L.). Agrobacterium protocols. 2006; 301: 12.

[203] Shi S, Nan L, Smith K. The current status, problems, and prospects of alfalfa (Medicago sativa L.) breeding in China. Agronomy (Basel) 2017; 7(1): 1. [http://dx.doi.org/10.3390/agronomy7010001]

[204] Hong YH, Chao WW, Chen ML, Lin BF. Ethyl acetate extracts of alfalfa (Medicago sativa L.) sprouts inhibit lipopolysaccharide-induced inflammation *in vitro* and *in vivo*. J Biomed Sci 2009; 16(1): 64. [http://dx.doi.org/10.1186/1423-0127-16-64] [PMID: 19594948]

[205] Karimi E, Oskoueian E, Oskoueian A, Omidvar V, Hendra R, Nazeran H. Insight into the functional and medicinal properties of Medicago sativa (Alfalfa) leaves extract. J Med Plants Res 2013; 7(7): 290-7.

[206] Doss A, Parivuguna V, Vijayasanthi M, Surendran S. Antibacterial evaluation and phytochemical analysis of Medicago sativa L. against some microbial pathogens. Indian J Sci Technol 2011; 4(5): 550-2. [http://dx.doi.org/10.17485/ijst/2011/v4i5.23]

[207] Rana MG, Katbamna RV, Padhya AA, Dudhrejiya AD, Jivani NP, Sheth NR. *In vitro* antioxidant and free radical scavenging studies of alcoholic extract of Medicago sativa L. Romanian Journal of Biology-Plant Biology 2010; 55(1): 15-22.

[208] Massiot G, Lavaud C, Guillaume D, Le Men-Olivier L. Reinvestigation of the sapogenins and

prosapogenins from alfalfa (Medicago sativa). J Agric Food Chem 1988; 36(5): 902-9. [http://dx.doi.org/10.1021/jf00083a005]

[209] Oleszek W. Alfalfa saponins: structure, biological activity, and chemotaxonomy 1996. [http://dx.doi.org/10.1007/978-1-4613-0413-5_13]

[210] Caunii A, Pribac G, Grozea I, Gaitin D, Samfira I. Design of optimal solvent for extraction of bio–active ingredients from six varieties of Medicago sativa. Chem Cent J 2012; 6(1): 123. [http://dx.doi.org/10.1186/1752-153X-6-123] [PMID: 23098128]

[211] Al-Snafi Ali Esmail, Khadem Hanaa Salman, Al-Saedy Hussein Ali, Alqahtani Ali M, Batiha Gaber El-Saber, Abolfazl Jafari-Sales. A review on Medicago sativa: A potential medicinal plant 2021. [http://dx.doi.org/10.30574/ijbpsa.2021.1.2.0302]

[212] Mehranjani MS, Shariatzadeh MA, Desfulian AR, Noori M, Abnosi MH, Moghadam ZH. Effects of *Medicago sativa* on nephropathy in diabetic rats. Indian J Pharm Sci 2007; 69(6): 768. [http://dx.doi.org/10.4103/0250-474X.39431]

[213] Adaay MH, Al-Dujaily SS, Khazzal FK. Effect of aqueous extract of Medicago sativa and Salvia officinalis mixture on hormonal, ovarian and uterine parameters in mature female mice. J Mater Environ Sci 2013; 4(4): 424-33.

[214] Choi KC, Hwang JM, Bang SJ, *et al.* Chloroform extract of alfalfa (Medicago sativa) inhibits lipopolysaccharide-induced inflammation by downregulating ERK/NF-κB signaling and cytokine production. J Med Food 2013; 16(5): 410-20. [http://dx.doi.org/10.1089/jmf.2012.2679] [PMID: 23631491]

[215] Zadeh MZ, Mirzaei A, Mohammad F. Effects of hydro-alcoholic extract of Medicago sativa on the chemical burn injuries in rats, 2014.

[216] Liu XueGui LX, Lv MengChao LM, Huang MingYuan HM, Sun YuQiu SY, Gao PinYi GP, Li DanQi LD. A network pharmacology study on the triterpene saponins from Medicago sativa L. for the treatment of neurodegenerative diseases. J Food Biochem. 2019 Aug; 43(8): e12955. [http://dx.doi.org/10.1111/jfbc.12955] [PMID: 31368545]

[217] Gomathi R, Vijipriya M, Usha K. Cardioprotective effect of ethanolic extract of Medicago sativa stem on isoproterenol-induced myocardial infarction in Wistar albino rats. Int J Pharm Pharm Sci 2014; 6(2): 839-42.

[218] Al-Dosari MS. *In vitro* and *in vivo* antioxidant activity of alfalfa (Medicago sativa L.) on carbon tetrachloride intoxicated rats. Am J Chin Med 2012; 40(4): 779-93. [http://dx.doi.org/10.1142/S0192415X12500589] [PMID: 22809031]

[219] Vyas S, Collin SM, Bertin E, Davys GJ, Mathur B. Leaf concentrate as an alternative to iron and folic acid supplements for anaemic adolescent girls: a randomised controlled trial in India. Public Health Nutr 2010; 13(3): 418-23. [http://dx.doi.org/10.1017/S1368980009991224] [PMID: 19706212]

[220] Servatyari K, Ahmadi A, Kashefi H, Manbari MN, Rostami A, Moulodi MR. The effect of hydroalcoholic extract of Medicago sativa on liver function tests, blood biochemical factors and coagulation system in male rats. Scientific Journal of Kurdistan University of Medical Sciences, 2017, Vol. 21, No. 6, Pe16-Pe26, En2 ref. 40.

[221] Beauchemin KA, Rode LM. Compressed baled alfalfa hay for primiparous and multiparous dairy cows. J Dairy Sci 1994; 77(4): 1003-12. [http://dx.doi.org/10.3168/jds.S0022-0302(94)77036-3] [PMID: 8201037]

[222] Haque T, Muhsin MDA, Akhter T, Haq ME, Begum R, Chowdhury SFUA. Antimicrobial and analgesic activity of leaf extracts of Phyllanthus reticulatus Poir. (Family- Euphorbiaceae). Jahangirnagar University Journal of Biological Sciences 2016; 5(1): 81-5. [http://dx.doi.org/10.3329/jujbs.v5i1.29746]

[223] Devi S, Kumar D, Kumar M. *In-Vitro* antioxidant activities of methanolic extract of whole plant of

Phyllanthus amarus (Euphorbiaceae). *In-Vitro* 2016; 1(3).

[224] Devi S, Kumar M. *In vitro* Antioxidant potential of methanolic extract of whole plant of Phyllanthus amarus Schum (Euphorbiaceae). Int J Bot Stud 2017; 2: 100-2.

[225] Kaur B, Kaur N, Gautam V. Evaluation of anti-helicobacter pylori (DSMZ 10242) activity and qualitative analysis of quercetin by HPLC in Phyllanthus niruri Linn. World J Pharm Pharm Sci 2016; 5: 1691-706.

[226] Cabieses Molina F. Apuntes de medicina tradicional. La racionalización de lo irracional. Tomo I. InApuntes de medicina tradicional. La racionalización de lo irracional. Tomo 1993; I: 414-4.

[227] Chevallier A. Encyclopedia of herbal medicine: natural health. USA: Dorling Kindersley Book 2000; p. 336.

[228] Patel JR, Tripathi P, Sharma V, Chauhan NS, Dixit VK. Phyllanthus amarus: Ethnomedicinal uses, phytochemistry and pharmacology: A review. J Ethnopharmacol 2011; 138(2): 286-313. [http://dx.doi.org/10.1016/j.jep.2011.09.040] [PMID: 21982793]

[229] Mao X, Wu LF, Guo HL, *et al.* The genus Phyllanthus: an ethnopharmacological, phytochemical, and pharmacological review. Evid Based Complement Alternat Med 2016; 2016(1): 7584952. [http://dx.doi.org/10.1155/2016/7584952] [PMID: 27200104]

[230] Lee NYS, Khoo WKS, Adnan MA, Mahalingam TP, Fernandez AR, Jeevaratnam K. The pharmacological potential of *Phyllanthus niruri*. J Pharm Pharmacol 2016; 68(8): 953-69. [http://dx.doi.org/10.1111/jphp.12565] [PMID: 27283048]

[231] Yang B, Kortesniemi M, Liu P, Karonen M, Salminen JP. Analysis of hydrolyzable tannins and other phenolic compounds in emblic leafflower (Phyllanthus emblica L.) fruits by high performance liquid chromatography-electrospray ionization mass spectrometry. J Agric Food Chem 2012; 60(35): 8672-83.
[http://dx.doi.org/10.1021/jf302925v] [PMID: 22889097]

[232] Hasan HH, Habib IH, Gonaid MH, Islam M. Comparative phytochemical and antimicrobial investigation of some plants growing in Al Jabal Al-Akhdar. J Nat Prod Plant Resour 2011; 1(1): 15-23.

[233] Judd PA. The oxford book of health foods: a comprehensive guide to natural remedies. Oxford University Press 2003.

[234] Oyewo EB, Akanji MA, Adekunle AS. Immunomodulation capabilities of aqueous leaf extract of Phyllanthus amarus in male Wistar rats. Rep Opinion 2012; 4(1): 22-37.

[235] Peter S, Dey S, Veerakyathappa B, Kumar SR, Paulad C. Therapeutic activity of partially purified fractions of Emblica officinalis (Syn. Phyllanthus emblica) dried fruits against Trypanosoma evansi. J Pharm Pharmacol 2016; 4: 546-58.

[236] Putakala M, Gujjala S, Nukala S, Bongu SBR, Chintakunta N, Desireddy S. Cardioprotective effect of Phyllanthus amarus against high fructose diet induced myocardial and aortic stress in rat model. Biomed Pharmacother 2017; 95: 1359-68.
[http://dx.doi.org/10.1016/j.biopha.2017.09.054] [PMID: 28946183]

[237] Guo JR, Chen QQ, Lam C, *et al.* Effect of Phyllanthus amarus extract on 5-fluorouracil-induced perturbations in ribonucleotide and deoxyribonucleotide pools in HepG2 cell line. Molecules 2016; 21(9): 1254.
[http://dx.doi.org/10.3390/molecules21091254] [PMID: 27657029]

[238] Tamayo MV, Schuch AP, Yagura T, Gil LB, Menck CFM, Sánchez-Lamar A. Genoprotective effect of Phyllanthus orbicularis extract against UVA, UVB, and solar radiation. Photochem Photobiol 2018; 94(5): 1026-31.
[http://dx.doi.org/10.1111/php.12939] [PMID: 29768722]

[239] Thyagarajan SP, Thirunalasundari T, Subramanian S, Venkateswaran PS, Blumberg BS. Effect of

Phyllanthus amarus on chronic carriers of hepatitis B virus. Lancet 1988; 332(8614): 764-6. [http://dx.doi.org/10.1016/S0140-6736(88)92416-6] [PMID: 2901611]

[240] Papp V. The Lingzhi naming dilemma: Overlooked and long-forgotten names threaten nomenclatural stability. Fungal Biol Rev 2024; 47: 100338. [http://dx.doi.org/10.1016/j.fbr.2023.100338]

[241] Wachtel-Galor S, Yuen J, Buswell JA, Benzie IF. Ganoderma lucidum (*Lingzhi or Reishi*): a medicinal mushroom. In: Benzie IFF, Wachtel-Galor S, editors. Herbal Medicine: Biomolecular and Clinical Aspects. 2nd ed. Boca Raton (FL): CRC Press/Taylor & Francis; 2011. [PMID: 22593926]

[242] Mushroom AM. 9 Ganoderma lucidum (Lingzhi or Reishi). Lester Packer, Ph.D. 2011; p. 175.

[243] Shazia F, Siddiqui MA, Ahmed K, *et al.* Clinical efficacy and safety of Bhui Amla (Phyllanthous niruri) in liver disease: A case series. The Pharma Innovation Journal 2019; 8: 565-6.

[244] Wasser SP. Reishi or ling zhi (*Ganoderma lucidum*). Encyclopedia of dietary supplements 2005; 1: 603-22.

[245] Borchers AT, Krishnamurthy A, Keen CL, Meyers FJ, Gershwin ME. The immunobiology of mushrooms. Exp Biol Med (Maywood) 2008; 233(3): 259-76. [http://dx.doi.org/10.3181/0708-MR-227] [PMID: 18296732]

[246] Boh B, Berovic M, Zhang J, Zhi-Bin L. *Ganoderma lucidum* and its pharmaceutically active compounds. Biotechnol Annu Rev (Amst) 2007; 13: 265-301. [http://dx.doi.org/10.1016/S1387-2656(07)13010-6] [PMID: 17875480]

[247] Zhou X, Lin J, Yin Y, Zhao J, Sun X, Tang K. Ganodermataceae: natural products and their related pharmacological functions. Am J Chin Med 2007; 35(4): 559-74. [http://dx.doi.org/10.1142/S0192415X07005065] [PMID: 17708623]

[248] Chang ST, Buswell JA. Mushroom nutriceuticals. World J Microbiol Biotechnol 1996; 12(5): 473-6. [http://dx.doi.org/10.1007/BF00419460] [PMID: 24415377]

[249] Borchers AT, Stern JS, Hackman RM, Keen CL, Gershwin ME. Mushrooms, tumors, and immunity. Proc Soc Exp Biol Med 1999; 221(4): 281-93. [http://dx.doi.org/10.1046/j.1525-1373.1999.d01-86.x] [PMID: 10460691]

[250] Zhang Y, Lin Z, Hu Y, Wang F. Effect of *Ganoderma lucidum* capsules on T lymphocyte subsets in football players on "living high–training low". Br J Sports Med 2008; 42(10): 819-22. [http://dx.doi.org/10.1136/bjsm.2007.038620] [PMID: 18048435]

[251] Sohretoglu D, Huang S. *Ganoderma lucidum* polysaccharides as an anti-cancer agent. Anti-Cancer Agents in Medicinal Chemistry (Formerly Current Medicinal Chemistry-Anti-Cancer Agents). 2018; 18(5): 667-74.

[252] Tang W, Gao Y, Chen G, *et al.* A randomized, double-blind and placebo-controlled study of a *Ganoderma lucidum* polysaccharide extract in neurasthenia. J Med Food 2005; 8(1): 53-8. [http://dx.doi.org/10.1089/jmf.2005.8.53] [PMID: 15857210]

[253] Rajasekaran M, Kalaimagal C. Cardioprotective effect of a medicinal mushroom, *Ganoderma lucidum* against Adriamycin-induced toxicity. Int. J. Pharmacol. 2012, 8(4), 252–258.

[254] Zhang HN, He JH, Yuan L, Lin ZB. *In vitro* and *in vivo* protective effect of *Ganoderma lucidum* polysaccharides on alloxan-induced pancreatic islets damage. Life Sci 2003; 73(18): 2307-19. [http://dx.doi.org/10.1016/S0024-3205(03)00594-0] [PMID: 12941433]

[255] Wachtel-Galor S, Tomlinson B, Benzie IFF. *Ganoderma lucidum* ('Lingzhi'), a Chinese medicinal mushroom: biomarker responses in a controlled human supplementation study. Br J Nutr 2004; 91(2): 263-9. [http://dx.doi.org/10.1079/BJN20041039] [PMID: 14756912]

[256] Cardi T, D'Ambrosio E, Consoli D, Puite KJ, Ramulu KS. Production of somatic hybrids between

frost-tolerant Solanum commersonii and S. tuberosum: characterization of hybrid plants. Theor Appl Genet 1993; 87(1-2): 193-200.
[http://dx.doi.org/10.1007/BF00223764] [PMID: 24190212]

[257] Bent S, Kane C, Shinohara K, *et al.* Saw palmetto for benign prostatic hyperplasia. N Engl J Med 2006; 354(6): 557-66.
[http://dx.doi.org/10.1056/NEJMoa053085] [PMID: 16467543]

[258] Gordon AE, Shaughnessy AF. Saw palmetto for prostate disorders. Am Fam Physician 2003; 67(6): 1281-3.
[PMID: 12674456]

[259] Ham B, Jolly S, Triche G, Williams PR, Wallace F. A study of the physical and chemical properties of saw palmetto berry extract. 2002.

[260] Farnsworth MB. Evidence-Based Health Care: Using Saw Palmetto in the Treatment of Symptoms Associated with Benign Prostatic Hyperplasia/Hypertrophy (Doctoral dissertation, Chatham University).

[261] Sudeep HV, Thomas JV, Shyamprasad K. A double blind, placebo-controlled randomized comparative study on the efficacy of phytosterol-enriched and conventional saw palmetto oil in mitigating benign prostate hyperplasia and androgen deficiency. BMC Urol 2020; 20(1): 86.
[http://dx.doi.org/10.1186/s12894-020-00648-9] [PMID: 32620155]

[262] Ulbricht C. What every clinician should know about herb–supplement–drug interactions. Altern Complement Ther 2012; 18(2): 67-70.
[http://dx.doi.org/10.1089/act.2012.18202]

[263] Avins AL, Lee JY, Meyers CM, Barry MJ. Safety and toxicity of saw palmetto in the CAMUS trial. J Urol 2013; 189(4): 1415-20.
[http://dx.doi.org/10.1016/j.juro.2012.10.002] [PMID: 23063633]

CHAPTER 10

Synergistic Effects of Dietary Supplements and Nutraceuticals

Mukesh Singh Sikarwar[1,*]

[1] *Amity Institute of Pharmacy, Amity University, Gwalior, Madhya Pradesh, India*

Abstract: Synergism means the interaction of two or more elements that produce a combined effect greater than the sum of their individual effects. In traditional medicine, the concept of holistic medicine utilizes the synergy of phytochemicals in treating mild to complex health conditions. The polyherbal nature of traditional medicine is also deeply rooted in the key concept of synergism. Nutraceuticals are mostly natural products that exhibit medicinal values along with nutritional values, for example, isolated nutrients, herbal products, and processed foods, whereas dietary supplements are specific dietary ingredients such as vitamins, minerals, herbs, amino acids, and enzymes with the goal of providing essential nutrients like vitamins and minerals to support general health. Synergism in nutraceuticals is the interaction of multiple bioactive compounds, ingredients, or nutrients that work together to produce enhanced health benefits compared to their individual effects. The benefits of synergism in nutraceuticals include enhanced therapeutic efficacy, targeted health support, and a broader spectrum of health benefits. The present chapter includes the description of the synergistic effects of fatty acids and antioxidants, vitamin D and vitamin K, vitamin C and zinc, the synergistic effects of piperine, and the synergistic effects of probiotics. Synergistic nutraceuticals pave the way for personalized nutrition *via* advances in nutrigenomics, innovative delivery systems due to nanoencapsulation and liposomal technologies, and holistic approaches due to integrating traditional medicine knowledge with modern research to design synergistic nutraceuticals.

Keywords: Dietary supplements, Holistic medicine, Polyherbal, Synergism.

INTRODUCTION

Synergism is a phenomenon where multiple agents interact to produce a combined effect greater than their individual effects, a concept widely used in fields like medicine, pharmacology, biology, ecology, and technology. In Herbal drugs, the

* **Corresponding author Mukesh Singh Sikarwar:** Amity Institute of Pharmacy, Amity University, Gwalior, Madhya Pradesh, India; E-mail: mukeshsikarwar@gmail.com

polyherbal therapy involves combining multiple compounds to improve therapeutic effects on the same physiological target, like piperine in black pepper, which enhances the bioavailability of curcumin in turmeric. Compounds, like valerian root and hops, work together to enhance the sedative effects *via* additive synergism. Synergistic effects may allow lower dosages of each herb, reducing side effects. Herb synergy emphasizes the significance of holistic approaches in herbal medicine, where the whole is often greater than its parts.

SYNERGISTIC NUTRACEUTICALS

Synergistic nutraceuticals are natural bioactive compounds that work together through pharmacokinetic or pharmacodynamic synergy to enhance their health benefits by acting on similar or complementary biological targets (Fig. **1**).

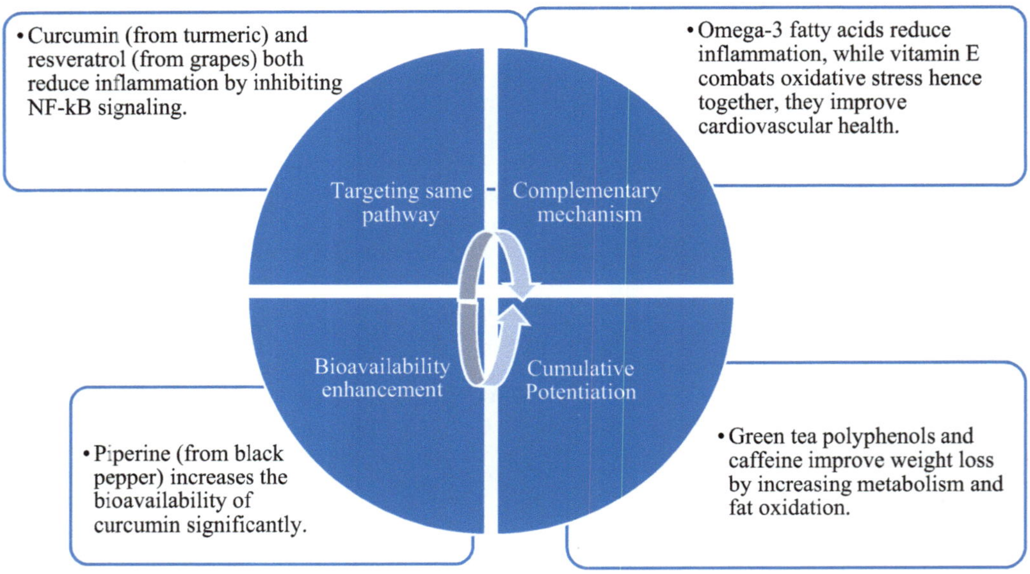

Fig. (1). A general diagram showing different principles of pharmacodynamic synergism in nutraceuticals.

Fatty Acids and Antioxidants

ω-6 Polyunsaturated fatty acids (PUFAs) are essential fatty acids involved in various cellular metabolism. Studies show their antistress activity, including reducing oxidative stress, regulating cyclooxygenase activity, and altering membrane phospholipid composition and receptor function [1]. One of the most important problems with unsaturated lipids is lipid oxidation, which causes radical-initiated oxidative degradation in unsaturated lipids. Off-flavors, harmful aldehydes, and the co-oxidation of proteins and colourants are formed during lipid oxidation. The food industry faces a significant challenge in controlling lipid oxidation due to the complexity of food products and the influence of multiple elements. This process produces volatile chemicals like aldehydes, ketones, and alcohols, leading to rancidity [2]. Antioxidants are molecules that prevent food product deterioration by minimizing lipid oxidation, scavenging free radicals, chelating metal ions, and quenching singlet oxygen [2]. A study reported that combining Astaxanthin and omega-3 fatty acids individually and in combination protects against oxidative stress *via* the Nrf2-ARE pathway. It is shown that lower concentrations of Astaxanthin show synergistic effects when combined with Docosahexaenoic Acid (DHA) or Eicosapentaenoic Acid (EPA) [3].

Research on synergism was carried out on fatty acid, carotenoid, and tocopherol compositions of 20 Canadian lentil cultivars. Results showed that Carotenoids and tocopherols showed weak correlation with DPPH activity; however, their combination showed good correlation, suggesting they may act synergistically [4]. There have been reports of both synergistic and non-synergistic effects of omega-3 fatty acids and salmon calcitonin on haematological, anti-inflammatory, and antioxidant indices in diabetic rats. The combination of salmon calcitonin and omega-3 fatty acids showed synergistic effects on total bilirubin and antioxidant capacity, but non-synergistic effects on malondialdehyde, uric acid, interleukin-6, lactate dehydrogenase, superoxide dismutase, catalase, glutathione peroxidase, and haematological parameters, comparable to metformin's therapeutic action, which was more or less than that of omega-3 fatty acids [5]. Edible oils lose their qualities and nutritional value as a result of oxidation during production and storage. In order to prevent this oxidation and preserve the nutritional value and biological activity of edible oils, lipophilic antioxidants are essential [6]. A study showed that the oxidative stability of blended oils high in unsaturated fatty acids is improved by combining the natural antioxidants β-carotene, sesamol, and caffeic acid. The primary antioxidant in the early phases of oxidation is β-carotene. The primary antioxidants in the middle and late phases of oxidation are sesamol and caffeic acid [7].

Vitamin D and Vitamin K

Vitamin D, also known as calciferol, is a fat-soluble vitamin found in some foods and supplements. It is produced endogenously when sunlight hits the skin, triggering vitamin D synthesis [8]. Vitamin D, obtained from sun exposure, foods, and supplements, undergoes two hydroxylations in the body for activation. The first hydroxylation occurs in the liver, converting vitamin D to 25-hydroxyvitamin D, or calcidiol, and the second hydroxylation occurs primarily in the kidney, forming the physiologically active 1,25-dihydroxyvitamin D, or calcitriol [9]. Vitamin K is a lipid-soluble vitamin found in two forms: K1 (phylloquinone) and K2 (menaquinones). The derivative without the side chain, called menadione or K3, lacks vitamin K activity. K1, the main form in the liver, is crucial for the synthesis and carboxylation of vitamin K-dependent coagulation factors, while K2 plays a more significant role in peripheral tissues and skeletal diseases [10].

To find out if vitamin K1 and 25(OH)D were linked to a higher risk of hip fractures and whether bone turnover markers mediated the potential synergistic effect of these two micronutrients, a study was conducted. The study indicates that Vitamin K1 and 25(OH) D are linked to hip fracture risk, suggesting that intervention studies should incorporate both vitamins [11]. Vitamin K and D combination enhances bone mineral density and reduces undercarboxylated osteocalcin, with a more favorable effect expected when vitamin K2 is used [12]. A review of the data supporting the synergistic effect of vitamin K and vitamin D3 indicates that maintaining bone health appears to be enhanced by both an adequate supply of vitamin K and an optimal level of vitamin D [13]. Vitamin K and Vitamin D work together to maintain bone health and blood clotting. Vitamin D aids in calcium absorption, while Vitamin K directs calcium into bones, promoting bone density and cardiovascular health [14].

The study suggests that continuous therapy with vitamin K(2) and D(3) can increase vertebral bone mass in postmenopausal women. For 24 months, this therapy significantly increased bone mineral density, indicating stimulation of both bone formation and resorption activity [15]. Evidence supports the notion that joint supplementation of vitamins D and K might be more effective than the consumption of either alone for bone and cardiovascular health [16]. Glycoxidation in human osteoblast cell cultures can hinder osteoblast maturation, potentially affecting bone markers. However, the addition of vitamins D and K can reverse this negative effect, causing beneficial biochemical changes in bone. This could potentially help treat bone metabolic diseases like osteoporosis, highlighting the potential of vitamins D and K as therapeutic interventions [17].

Vitamin C and Zinc

According to Pauling, ascorbic acid is a necessary dietary component for humans. People who don't get enough ascorbic acid, or vitamin C, get sick. Vitamin C is primarily found in fruits and vegetables, with citrus fruits like orange, lemon, amla, watermelon, berries, pineapple, strawberries, cherries, kiwi fruits, mangoes, and tomatoes being particularly rich sources. Although l-ascorbic acid is generically known as vitamin C, it also goes by several other chemical names, such as ascorbate and antiscorbutic vitamin. The structurally similar l-ascorbic acid molecule is composed of asymmetrical six-carbon atoms ($C_6H_8O_6$) [18]. Ascorbic acid, a vitamin C antioxidant, donates a single reducing equivalent, forming a radical called monodehydroascorbate. This radical reacts preferentially with radicals, unlike non-radical compounds. This is because the removal of an electron from monodehydroascorbate would create an unfavored tricarbonyl structure. Instead, ascorbic acid oxidizes monodehydroascorbate, which reacts with other radicals, potentially circumventing the formation of this unfavored structure [19].

Zinc is a metallic element with atomic number 30 and stable isotopes of mass 66, 67, 68, and 70, averaging 65.38 a.m.u. Zinc sites in proteins are zinc polyhedra with apical S, N, or O, linked to cysteine, histidine, glutamic acid, aspartic acid, and water [20]. Zinc biology is based on the complexation and solution chemistry of zinc ions. The only valence state of zinc in living things is Zn (II), and it is redox-inert. Zinc, found in 10% of human proteins, has catalytic or structural functions and remains bound throughout the protein's lifetime. In other proteins, zinc ions bind reversibly with dissociation and association rates suited to regulation, transport, transfer, sensing, signaling, and storage [21]. Supplementation of zinc and vitamin C is crucial for the functioning of the central nervous system, as zinc ions are involved in neurotransmission and protein degradation. Vitamin C, a zinc synergist, aids brain antioxidants, synaptic activity, and detoxification, and daily doses of 130-500 mg are recommended to prevent dementia and neurodegenerative pathology [22].

Vitamin C, D, and zinc are essential for the immune system to fight infections, supporting both innate and adaptive immunity. Through their complementary and synergistic effects, they help maintain epithelial barriers, cellular defense, and antibodies, which are the three main lines of immune defense [23]. A study found that vitamin C and zinc supplementation significantly improve the management of *Plasmodium berghei*-infected individuals by improving packed cell volume and haemoglobin concentration levels, lowering mortality rates, and complementing the therapeutic effect of artemether [24]. Research shows that adequate intakes of vitamin C and zinc can improve symptoms and shorten the duration of respiratory tract infections, including the common cold. Natural defenses only provide full protection when the body has sufficient zinc and high levels of vitamin C. Zinc complements vitamin C's actions, providing double protection and potentially synergizing with it. Recent research has demonstrated that zinc is essential for effective immune defense at various levels [25].

Vitamin C and zinc are crucial for nutrition, immune defense, and health maintenance. Two preliminary trials showed that a combination of 1000 mg vitamin C plus 10 mg zinc was more effective than a placebo in reducing rhinorrhoea duration over five days. Symptom relief was quicker, and the product was well-tolerated. This suggests that vitamin C plus zinc may be an effective and safe measure against the common cold, given its significant burden [26]. Vitamin C and zinc are essential nutrients for immune function and reducing the risk of infectious diseases. Vitamin C improves immune system components like antimicrobial and natural killer cell activities, while zinc impairs cellular mediators of innate immunity. Insufficient intake of these nutrients is prevalent in populations like the developing world and the elderly. Research shows adequate intakes of vitamin C and zinc can ameliorate symptoms and shorten the duration of respiratory tract infections, pneumonia, malaria, and diarrhea, especially in children [27].

Synergistic Effects of Piperine

Piperine, an alkaloid from black pepper, has been found to have numerous pharmacological activities, including antioxidant, anti-asthma, anti-carcinogenic, anti-inflammatory, anti-ulcer, and anti-amoeba properties. It also has the ability to alter gastrointestinal disorders, drug-metabolizing enzymes, and drug bioavailability [28]. Curcumin, given alone at a dose of 2 g/kg to rats, achieved moderate serum concentrations over 4 hours. When piperine was administered 20 mg/kg, the serum concentration of curcumin increased for 1-2 hours post-drug, leading to a significant increase in time to maximum, decreased elimination half-life and clearance, and a 154% increase in bioavailability. Concomitant administration of piperine at 20 mg significantly increased the concentration of curcumin from 0.25 to 1 hour post-drug, with a 2000% increase in bioavailability. This indicates that piperine enhances the absorption and bioavailability of curcumin in rats and humans without any adverse effects [29].

The interaction analysis indicated a synergistic effect between low doses of Ferulic acid and piperine, enhancing monoaminergic function. Neurochemical evidence, including monoamine levels in the frontal cortex, hippocampus, and hypothalamus, also supported this as a synergistic effect in the enhancement of monoaminergic function [30]. Study reported the combination of Ciprofloxacin and Piperine, extracted from *Piper nigrum*, demonstrated synergistic activity against *Bacillus subtilis* and *E. coli*, even at a low concentration (20 μg/mL) [31]. Ursolic acid and piperine work synergistically to protect against carbon tetrachloride-induced liver damage in rats. Piperine enhances ursolic acid's pharmacokinetic properties and oral bioavailability by tenfold when combined [32]. A combination of Rutin and Piperine exhibits synergistic antioxidant and cytotoxic effects, and the study thus provides more insight into the mechanism of the hepatoprotective action of the combinational sample for the management of hepatotoxicity [33]. The study found that the combination of curcumin, piperine, and resveratrol in diets is more effective than isolated forms, suggesting potential use in future clinical trials for breast cancer treatment, especially in MCF-7 and MDA-MB-231 cells [34]. The combination of paclitaxel with piperine produces synergistic effects in human ovarian adenocarcinoma SKOV3 cells *via* the modulation of pro- and anti-apoptotic genes and may compensate for the toxicity and side effects of paclitaxel [35]. Piperine in combination with cisplatin could trigger p53-mediated apoptosis more effectively than cisplatin alone in MCF-7 breast cancer cells, reducing the toxic dose of cisplatin used in cancer chemotherapy [36].

Synergistic Effects of Probiotics

The term "probiotic" originates from the Greek, meaning "for life." Ferdinand Vergin likely invented it in 1954 in his article "Anti-und Probiotika," comparing the harmful effects of antibiotics on intestinal microbiota with the beneficial effects of beneficial bacteria. "Probiotics are live strains of strictly selected microorganisms which, when administered in adequate amounts, confer a health benefit on the host. "Prebiotics as a nonviable food component that confers a health benefit on the host associated with modulation of the microbiota". Prebiotics can be used as an alternative to probiotics or as a supplement, but they stimulate the growth of different gut bacteria. Prebiotics have the potential to modify gut microbiota, but these changes occur at individual strains and species levels and are not easily predicted. Synbiotics, which possess both probiotic and prebiotic properties, were developed to address potential issues with probiotic survival in the gastrointestinal tract. Combining these components in a single product can provide superior effects compared to the activity of either probiotic or prebiotic alone [37]. The study investigated the synergistic antibacterial activities of probiotic lactic acid bacteria and *Curcuma longa* rhizome extract against *Cutibacterium acnes*. Results indicated that these synbiotics showed antibacterial effects, suggesting potential therapeutic potential for cosmetics or medicine development against *Cutibacterium acnes* [38]. The study found that combining probiotic (*Lactobacillus fermentum*) and cinnamon powder can improve growth performance, intestinal microbiota, immunity, antioxidant defense, and resistance to *Yersinia ruckeri* infection in rainbow trout. This suggests that a combination of these ingredients can be more effective in improving digestive enzyme performance and resistance to *Y. ruckeri* infection in rainbow trout, suggesting a synergistic effect for them [39]. Probiotic strains like Bifidobacterium, Lactobacilli, S. boulardii, and B. coagulans are commonly used. Prebiotics like FOS, GOS, XOS, and Inulin, particularly fructans, are used in synbiotics to enhance probiotic viability. Proper symbiotic selection requires the use of prebiotics to maintain good synergy and maximize beneficial effects [40].

The etiopathogenesis of Inflammatory Bowel Disease (IBD) is linked to changes in bowel microflora due to environmental or dietary factors. Researchers are exploring the effectiveness of prebiotics, probiotics, and synbiotics in treating IBD by restoring the balance between microflora and host defense mechanisms.

Probiotics, such as Lactobacillus species and Bifidobacterium species, suppress pathogen growth, immunomodulate immune responses, enhance barrier activity, and suppress human T-cell proliferation. Prebiotics, like lactulose, lactosucrose, oligofructose, and inulin, induce host microflora growth and exert anti-inflammatory effects [41]. The study examined the synergistic effect of n-3 Polyunsaturated Fatty Acids (PUFA) and probiotics on depression-induced bone loss in rats. Results showed that n-3 PUFA and probiotics enhanced bone mass, calcium, and osteoprotegerin, while decreasing cytokines and enhancing brain serotonin, thereby demonstrating the synergistic bone-protective effects of these substances [42].

The study explores the development of next-generation probiotics, specifically *Faecalibacterium prausnitzii*, which is associated with human health. The researchers co-isolated *Faecalibacterium prausnitzii* and *Desulfovibrio piger*, a sulfate-reducing bacterium, to tolerate oxygen exposure. The resulting symbiotic product is tolerated by mice and humans and detected in the human gut [43]. The study found that the bacterial consortium MPRO, including *Lactiplantibacillus plantarum, Bifidobacterium animalis ssp. lactis, and Lacticaseibacillus casei,* showed enhanced therapeutic efficacy in experimental models of atopic dermatitis and inflammatory colitis, suggesting a preference for bacterial consortia over single strains [44]. The study explores the synergistic effects of prebiotic chitooligosaccharide and commercial prebiotics on probiotic growth. Combinations of chitooligosaccharide with inulin, fructooligosaccharide, and lactulose were evaluated. The results showed that chitooligosaccharide and fructooligosaccharide showed higher synergism than lactulose or inulin. The synergistic effect increased with prebiotic concentration and strain, with higher synergism observed with *Bifidobacterium lactis* [45].

This study examined the microbial interactions between Lactobacillus plantarum AKK30 and yeast S. cerevisiae B18 and their potential as probiotics for animal feed additives. The results showed a synergistic effect between the two microorganisms, with good viability on low pH, gastric juice, and bile salt, suggesting their potential use as probiotics [46]. This study investigates the effectiveness of combination therapy for Multidrug-Resistant Acinetobacter Baumannii (MRAB) infections. It identifies the synergistic effect of four probiotic culture extracts and Lactobacillus preparations against 33 strains of A. baumannii. Results show that 79% of the strains were MRAB, with ST191 being the predominant type. Combination therapy with meropenem and colistin had the highest synergistic effect, with Lactobacillus paracasei showing the fastest antimicrobial reactivity and longest sustained activity. The findings provide valuable data for treating MRAB infections in clinical settings [47]. The study evaluated the modulation of cytokine production by probiotics Bifidobacterium animalis and Lactobacillus casei in human intestinal Caco-2 cells exposed to different EAEC strains. Results showed that probiotics increased cytokine production, but not IL-8 production. This reinforces the synergistic immunomodulatory activity of probiotics [48].

The gut microbiota, a community of bacterial species, plays a crucial role in health. Dysbiosis, caused by factors like diet, antibiotic use, age, and stress, can lead to diseases like diabetes, obesity, colon cancer, inflammatory bowel disease, and neurodegeneration. A probiotic regime with prebiotics can reverse dysbiosis, promoting health and wellness in older individuals. A study developed a new probiotic and synbiotic formulation, including three active probiotics and a polyphenol-rich prebiotic called Triphala. The study found that Triphala supported beneficial bacteria growth while inhibiting pathogenic species. The combination of probiotics and synbiotics was found to be more effective in modulating the gut microbiota [49].

Miscellaneous

Vitamin C with Vitamin E, β-Carotene

A combination of vitamin C with other antioxidants (vitamin E, β-carotene) provides synergic antihypertensive effects. Vascular biology, nutrient-gene interactions, nutrition, antioxidants, and whole foods are key factors in preventing and treating hypertension and CVD. Lifestyle modifications like exercise, weight reduction, smoking cessation, and alcohol and caffeine restriction can also help manage hypertension [50].

Rutin and Cisplatin

The study found that rutin, a prophylactic oral treatment of cisplatin, effectively prevented nephrotoxicity in Wistar rats. Rutin reduced oxidative stress, caspase-3, TNF-α, and NFκB protein expression levels, and restored histopathological changes. This protective mechanism was partially mediated by its inhibitory effect on NFκB and TNF-α pathway-mediated inflammation [51].

Dietary Flavonoids with Antibiotics Gentamicin and Ceftriaxone

Antimicrobial resistance is a global health concern, affecting drug regimens. A study investigates the synergistic effects of dietary flavonoids rutin and quercetin with antibiotics gentamicin and ceftriaxone against drug-resistant superbugs. Results show rutin and quercetin restore antibiotic activity against multidrug-resistant and extensively drug-resistant strains, promising a potential therapeutic strategy [52].

Rutin Hydrate, Quercetin Dihydrate, Hydroquinone, Kaempferol, and Resveratrol

This study tested dual combinations of five phenolic compounds, including rutin hydrate, quercetin dihydrate, hydroquinone, kaempferol, and resveratrol, for their antioxidant activities. The results showed synergistic antioxidant interactions among these compounds, with quercetin dihydrate showing the highest activity. Antagonistic interactions were also identified. The findings could help industries develop more potent nutraceutical supplements or guide researchers for further bioactivity validation using *in vivo* assays [53].

Rutin and Vitamin C

Supplementing with vitamin C alone for 16 weeks may have affected the antioxidant GPx activity. Furthermore, the lower MDA levels were reported to indicate a protective function for both vitamin C alone and the rutin/vitamin C combination (Ruta C) against lipid peroxidation. Lastly, rutin and vitamin C reduced TG and TNF-α levels and raised HDL-C levels in a positive synergistic impact [54].

Naringin and Sericin

A possible clinical application for psoriasis and other inflammation-related disorders was indicated by the combination of naringin and sericin's ability to down-regulate these pro-inflammatory cytokines. The combination may be used to enhance clinical efficacy and tolerability in psoriasis as a supplemental therapy to traditional treatment [55].

Quercetin with Sitagliptin and Soybean Fiber

Research indicates quercetin, when combined with sitagliptin and soybean fiber, has better antidiabetic effects than either substance alone. However, scientists face challenges with the low bioavailability of quercetin. Using nano-emulsions or nano-hydrogels, quercetin improves bioavailability and release. These findings suggest quercetin's anti-diabetic activity, suggesting it could be an alternative for managing diabetes without side effects [56].

Curcumin with Boswellic Acids

Boswellia serrata and *Curcuma longa*, natural ingredients used in Ayurvedic medicine for thousands of years, have been found to reduce inflammation and pain in various illnesses. *In vitro* data suggest that these ingredients influence gene expression through NF-κB, reducing inflammation pathways and matrix degradation. Studies have shown that these extracts, which contain curcumin and boswellic acids, relieve pain from osteoarthritis (OA) and other inflammatory conditions, offering alternatives to nonsteroidal anti-inflammatory agents. Further research is needed to understand the effects of curcumin on the microbiome and intestinal metabolism [57].

SUMMARY

Synergistic nutraceuticals are gaining momentum in clinical practice due to their multifactorial role in the prevention and treatment of diseases. Vitamin D with K2, curcumin with boswellic acids, Vitamin C with Zinc, curcumin with piperine, and many other such combinations are already sold as synergistic nutraceuticals. This chapter summarizes the various combinations of nutraceuticals with herbal drugs and synthetic drugs, covering the synergistic effects on biological activities, including antioxidants, cancer treatment, antimicrobial, immune boosting, antidepressant, apoptosis, osteoarthritis, osteoporosis, anti-inflammatory, antihepatotoxic, synbiotic, probiotic, *etc*. Synergistic Nutraceuticals are transforming the nutraceutical industry and paving the way for personalized nutrition, creating a shift toward more effective and tailored health solutions.

EXERCISE

1. Differentiate between saturated, monounsaturated, and polyunsaturated fatty acids, providing examples of each and their general dietary sources. Discuss their respective impacts on cardiovascular health.
2. Explain the concept of essential fatty acids. Name two essential fatty acids and describe their critical roles in human physiology. What are the consequences of their deficiency?
3. Describe the mechanism by which free radicals cause cellular damage. How do antioxidants counteract this damage, and what are the main classifications of antioxidants found in the human body and diet?
4. Discuss the relationship between lipid peroxidation and oxidative stress. How do dietary antioxidants, particularly those found in fruits and vegetables, contribute to mitigating this process?
5. Compare and contrast water-soluble and fat-soluble antioxidants, providing an example of each. Explain where they primarily function in the body to exert their protective effects.
6. Explain the process of Vitamin D synthesis in the skin and its subsequent activation in the liver and kidneys. What is the active form of Vitamin D, and what are its primary physiological roles?
7. Discuss the role of Vitamin K in blood coagulation. Name at least three Vitamin K-dependent clotting factors and describe how Vitamin K contributes to their activation.

8. Beyond bone health, what are some emerging roles of Vitamin D in immune modulation and chronic disease prevention? Provide specific examples.
9. Describe the different forms of Vitamin K (K1 and K2) and their respective dietary sources. How does the body acquire and utilize each form?
10. Explain the potential for synergistic interaction between Vitamin D and Vitamin K in bone metabolism. How do they complement each other in maintaining bone health?
11. Describe the key biochemical functions of Vitamin C in the human body, focusing on its role as an antioxidant and its involvement in collagen synthesis.
12. Explain how Zinc contributes to immune system function. Discuss at least two specific mechanisms by which Zinc supports immunity.
13. What are the clinical manifestations of severe Vitamin C deficiency (scurvy)? How does understanding its biochemical roles explain these symptoms?
14. Discuss the importance of Zinc in enzyme catalysis. Provide an example of a Zinc-dependent enzyme and describe its function.
15. Explain how Vitamin C can enhance the absorption of non-heme iron. Why is this interaction clinically significant, especially for individuals with iron deficiency?
16. Describe the primary mechanism by which Piperine enhances the bioavailability of various compounds. Illustrate this with an example.
17. Beyond bioavailability, discuss any other reported synergistic effects of Piperine that contribute to its therapeutic potential.
18. Explain how Piperine's interaction with drug-metabolizing enzymes can impact the efficacy and safety of co-administered drugs.
19. Discuss the potential applications of Piperine in improving the absorption of nutraceuticals. Provide a theoretical example of a supplement that could benefit from co-administration with Piperine.
20. What are the considerations and potential challenges in utilizing Piperine for synergistic effects in pharmaceutical or nutraceutical formulations?
21. Define probiotics and prebiotics, and explain the concept of synbiotics. Provide examples of each.
22. Discuss how probiotics can exert synergistic effects with other compounds or therapies, particularly in the context of gut health.
23. Explain the mechanism by which certain probiotic strains might improve nutrient absorption or metabolism.
24. Describe how probiotics can modulate the immune system through their interactions with the gut microbiota.
25. Discuss the potential benefits and challenges of using probiotic interventions in conjunction with conventional medical treatments.
26. Explain the antioxidant cascade involving Vitamin C, Vitamin E, and Beta-

carotene. How do these three antioxidants work together to provide enhanced protection against oxidative damage?

27. Discuss the potential synergistic effects of Rutin and Cisplatin in cancer therapy. What mechanisms might underlie this interaction?
28. Describe how dietary flavonoids (*e.g.*, in combination with Gentamicin and Ceftriaxone) can influence the efficacy of antibiotics.[1] What are the implications for combating antibiotic resistance?
29. Compare and contrast the individual and potential combined antioxidant or anti-inflammatory properties of Rutin hydrate, Quercetin dihydrate, Hydroquinone, Kaempferol, and Resveratrol.
30. Explain the synergistic relationship between Rutin and Vitamin C. How do they enhance each other's stability and bioavailability, and what are the implications for their physiological roles?
31. Describe the potential synergistic interaction between Naringin and Sericin, outlining possible mechanisms and applications.
32. Discuss the synergistic effects observed when Quercetin is combined with Sitagliptin and soybean fiber, particularly in the context of metabolic health.
33. Explain the reported synergistic anti-inflammatory effects of Curcumin when combined with Boswellic acids. What are the biochemical pathways involved?

Case Studies

Case 1: *Chronic Fatigue and Bone Health: A 45-year-old female presents with persistent fatigue, muscle weakness, and recurrent bone pain. Her blood tests reveal low serum 25-hydroxyvitamin D levels and slightly elevated Parathyroid Hormone (PTH). She also has a history of mild bleeding gums.*

Questions: Propose a dietary and/or supplementation strategy that addresses her symptoms, specifically considering the synergistic roles of Vitamin D and Vitamin K, and another relevant vitamin mentioned in the topics. Justify your choices with a brief explanation of the mechanism of action for each nutrient.

Case 2: *Post-Antibiotic Gut Dysbiosis: A 30-year-old male recently completed a 7-day course of broad-spectrum antibiotics for a bacterial infection. He is now experiencing significant gastrointestinal discomfort, including bloating, diarrhea, and indigestion. He is concerned about restoring his gut health.*

Questions: How would you advise this patient regarding the use of probiotics and prebiotics to mitigate the effects of antibiotic-induced gut dysbiosis? Explain the synergistic benefits of a synbiotic approach in this scenario.

Case 3: *Enhanced Bioavailability for Chronic Inflammation: A patient with a chronic inflammatory condition is considering a supplement regimen that* *includes Curcumin for its anti-inflammatory properties. However, they are aware of Curcumin's low bioavailability. They inquire about ways to enhance its effectiveness.*

Questions: Based on the provided topics, recommend a specific natural compound that could be co-administered with Curcumin to enhance its anti-inflammatory effects and bioavailability. Explain the mechanism of this synergistic interaction and why it's beneficial in managing inflammation.

Case 4: *Oxidative Stress and Cardiovascular Risk: A 55-year-old male with a family history of cardiovascular disease is advised to reduce oxidative stress. He is considering increasing his intake of antioxidants through diet and supplements.*

Questions: Design a strategy incorporating at least three key antioxidants discussed (two vitamins and one carotenoid) that work synergistically to protect against oxidative damage. Describe how each chosen antioxidant contributes to the overall protective effect and how their combined action offers enhanced benefits.

Case 5: *Dietary Flavonoids and Antibiotic Efficacy: A research team is investigating ways to improve the efficacy of existing antibiotics, specifically Gentamicin and Ceftriaxone, against increasingly resistant bacterial strains. They are exploring natural compounds that could act as adjuvants.*

Questions: Based on the provided topics, suggest a class of dietary compounds that could potentially exert synergistic effects with these antibiotics. Explain the theoretical mechanisms by which these compounds might enhance antibiotic effectiveness or overcome resistance, and discuss the implications for future antimicrobial strategies.

REFERENCES

[1] Yang B, Zhou Y, Wu M, Li X, Mai K, Ai Q. ω-6 Polyunsaturated fatty acids (linoleic acid) activate both autophagy and antioxidation in a synergistic feedback loop *via* TOR-dependent and TOR-independent signaling pathways. Cell Death & Disease 2020 11:7 [Internet]. 2020 Jul 30 [cited 2024 Dec 30]; 11(7): 1–19. Available from: https://www.nature.com/articles/s41419-020-02750-0

[2] Bayram I, Decker EA. Underlying mechanisms of synergistic antioxidant interactions during lipid oxidation. Trends Food Sci Technol 2023; 133: 219-30. [http://dx.doi.org/10.1016/j.tifs.2023.02.003]

[3] Saw CLL, Yang AY, Guo Y, Kong ANT. Astaxanthin and omega-3 fatty acids individually and in combination protect against oxidative stress *via* the Nrf2–ARE pathway. Food Chem Toxicol 2013; 62: 869-75. Available from: https://pubmed.ncbi.nlm.nih.gov/24157545/ [http://dx.doi.org/10.1016/j.fct.2013.10.023] [PMID: 24157545]

[4] Zhang B, Deng Z, Tang Y, *et al.* Fatty acid, carotenoid and tocopherol compositions of 20 Canadian lentil cultivars and synergistic contribution to antioxidant activities. Food Chem 2014; 161: 296-304. [http://dx.doi.org/10.1016/j.foodchem.2014.04.014] [PMID: 24837953]

[5] Adeyemi WJ, Olayaki LA. Synergistic and non-synergistic effects of salmon calcitonin and omega - 3 fatty acids on antioxidant, anti-inflammatory, and haematological indices in diabetic rats. Biomed Pharmacother 2018; 99: 867-75. Available from: https://pubmed.ncbi.nlm.nih.gov/29710486/ [http://dx.doi.org/10.1016/j.biopha.2018.01.085] [PMID: 29710486]

[6] Liu X, Zheng Z, Liu Y. Lipophilic antioxidants in edible oils: Mechanisms, applications and interactions. Food Res Int 2025; 200: 115423. [http://dx.doi.org/10.1016/j.foodres.2024.115423] [PMID: 39779163]

[7] Wang G, Liu L, Peng F, Ma Y, Deng Z, Li H. Natural antioxidants enhance the oxidation stability of blended oils enriched in unsaturated fatty acids. J Sci Food Agric 2024; 104(5): 2907-16. Available from: https://onlinelibrary.wiley.com/doi/full/10.1002/jsfa.13183 [http://dx.doi.org/10.1002/jsfa.13183] [PMID: 38029376]

[8] Rockwell M, Kraak V, Hulver M, Epling J. Clinical management of low vitamin D: A scoping review of physicians' practices. Nutrients 2018; 10(4): 493. [http://dx.doi.org/10.3390/nu10040493] [PMID: 29659534]

[9] Chalcraft JR, Cardinal LM, Wechsler PJ, *et al.* Vitamin D synthesis following a single bout of sun exposure in older and younger men and women. Nutrients 2020; 12(8): 2237. [http://dx.doi.org/10.3390/nu12082237] [PMID: 32727044]

[10] Aaseth JO, Finnes TE, Askim M, Alexander J. The importance of vitamin k and the combination of vitamins k and d for calcium metabolism and bone health: a review. nutrients 2024, vol 16, page 2420 [Internet]. 2024 Jul 25 [cited 2024 Dec 30]; 16(15): 2420. Available from: https://www.mdpi.com/2072-6643/16/15/2420/htm

[11] Torbergsen AC, Watne LO, Wyller TB, *et al.* Vitamin K1 and 25(OH)D are independently and synergistically associated with a risk for hip fracture in an elderly population: A case control study. Clin Nutr 2015; 34(1): 101-6. Available from: https://pubmed.ncbi.nlm.nih.gov/24559841/ [http://dx.doi.org/10.1016/j.clnu.2014.01.016] [PMID: 24559841]

[12] Kuang X, Liu C, Guo X, Li K, Deng Q, Li D. The combination effect of vitamin K and vitamin D on human bone quality: a meta-analysis of randomized controlled trials. Food Funct 2020; 11(4): 3280-97. Available from: https://pubmed.ncbi.nlm.nih.gov/32219282/ [http://dx.doi.org/10.1039/C9FO03063H] [PMID: 32219282]

[13] Aaseth JO, Finnes TE, Askim M, Alexander J. The importance of vitamin k and the combination of vitamins k and d for calcium metabolism and bone health: a review. nutrients 2024, vol 16, page 2420 [internet]. 2024 Jul 25 [cited 2024 Dec 30]; 16(15): 2420. Available from: https://www.mdpi.com/2072-6643/16/15/2420/htm

[14] Maresz K. Proper calcium use: vitamin k2 as a promoter of bone and cardiovascular health. Integr Med (Encinitas) 2015; 14(1): 34-9. Available from: https://pmc.ncbi.nlm.nih.gov/articles/PMC4566462/ [Internet]. [PMID: 26770129]

[15] Ushiroyama T, Ikeda A, Ueki M. Effect of continuous combined therapy with vitamin K2 and vitamin D3 on bone mineral density and coagulofibrinolysis function in postmenopausal women. Maturitas 2002; 41(3): 211-21. Available from: https://pubmed.ncbi.nlm.nih.gov/11886767/ [http://dx.doi.org/10.1016/S0378-5122(01)00275-4] [PMID: 11886767]

[16] Van Ballegooijen AJ, Pilz S, Tomaschitz A, Grübler MR, Verheyen N. The synergistic interplay between vitamins d and k for bone and cardiovascular health: a narrative review. Int J Endocrinol [Internet]. 2017 [cited 2024 Dec 30]; 2017: 7454376. Available from: https://pmc.ncbi.nlm.nih.gov/articles/PMC5613455/

[17] Gigante A, Torcianti M, Boldrini E, *et al.* Vitamin K and D association stimulates *in vitro* osteoblast differentiation of fracture site derived human mesenchymal stem cells. J Biol Regul Homeost Agents 2008; 22(1): 35-44. [PMID: 18394316]

[18] Yussif NM, Yussif NM. Vitamin C. Vitamin C - an update on current uses and functions [Internet]. 2018 Dec 5 [cited 2024 Dec 30]; Available from: https://www.intechopen.com/chapters/64659

[19] Njus D, Kelley PM, Tu YJ, Schlegel HB. Ascorbic acid: The chemistry underlying its antioxidant properties. Free Radic Biol Med 2020; 159: 37-43. [http://dx.doi.org/10.1016/j.freeradbiomed.2020.07.013] [PMID: 32738399]

[20] Barak P, Helmke PA. The chemistry of zinc. zinc in soils and plants [Internet]. 1993 [cited 2024 Dec 30]; 1–13. Available from: https://link.springer.com/chapter/10.1007/978-94-011-0878-2_1 [http://dx.doi.org/10.1007/978-94-011-0878-2_1]

[21] Krężel A, Maret W. The biological inorganic chemistry of zinc ions. Arch Biochem Biophys 2016; 611: 3-19. [http://dx.doi.org/10.1016/j.abb.2016.04.010] [PMID: 27117234]

[22] Gromova OA, Torshin IY, Pronin AV, Kilchevsky MA. Synergistic application of zinc and vitamin C to support memory, attention and the reduction of the risk of the neurological diseases. Zh Nevrol Psikhiatr Im S S Korsakova 2017; 117(7): 112-9. Available from: https://pubmed.ncbi.nlm.nih.gov/28805771/ [http://dx.doi.org/10.17116/jnevro201711771112-119] [PMID: 28805771]

[23] Maggini S, Maldonado P, Cardim P, Fernandez Newball C, Sota Latino ER. Vitamins C, D and Zinc: Synergistic roles in immune function and infections. 2017.

[24] Ekeh FN, Ekechukwu NE, Chukwuma CF, *et al.* Mixed vitamin C and zinc diet supplements co-administered with artemether drug improved haematological profile and survival of mice infected with Plasmodium berghei. Food Sci Hum Wellness 2019; 8(3): 275-82. [http://dx.doi.org/10.1016/j.fshw.2019.05.003]

[25] Beveridge S, Wintergerst ES, Maggini S, Hornig D. Immune-enhancing role of vitamin C and zinc and effect on clinical conditions. Ann Nutr Met [Internet]. [cited 2024 Dec 30]; 50:83. [http://dx.doi.org/10.1017/S0029665108006927]

[26] Maggini S, Beveridge S, Suter M. A combination of high-dose vitamin C plus zinc for the common cold. J Int Med Res 2012; 40(1): 28-42. Available from: https://pubmed.ncbi.nlm.nih.gov/22429343/ [http://dx.doi.org/10.1177/147323001204000104] [PMID: 22429343]

[27] Wintergerst ES, Maggini S, Hornig DH. Immune-enhancing role of vitamin C and zinc and effect on clinical conditions. Ann Nutr Metab 2006; 50(2): 85-94. Available from: https://pubmed.ncbi.nlm.nih.gov/16373990/ [http://dx.doi.org/10.1159/000090495] [PMID: 16373990]

[28] Tripathi AK, Ray AK, Mishra SK. Molecular and pharmacological aspects of piperine as a potential molecule for disease prevention and management: evidence from clinical trials 2022. Available from: https://bjbas.springeropen.com/articles/10.1186/s43088-022-00196-1 [http://dx.doi.org/10.1186/s43088-022-00196-1]

[29] Shoba G, Joy D, Joseph T, Majeed M, Rajendran R, Srinivas P. Influence of piperine on the pharmacokinetics of curcumin in animals and human volunteers. Planta Med 1998; 64(4): 353-6. Available from: https://pubmed.ncbi.nlm.nih.gov/9619120/ [http://dx.doi.org/10.1055/s-2006-957450] [PMID: 9619120]

[30] Li G, Ruan L, Chen R, *et al.* Synergistic antidepressant-like effect of ferulic acid in combination with piperine: involvement of monoaminergic system. Metab Brain Dis 2015; 30(6): 1505-14. Available from: https://link.springer.com/article/10.1007/s11011-015-9704-y [http://dx.doi.org/10.1007/s11011-015-9704-y] [PMID: 26220010]

[31] Maitra J. Shilpi. Synergistic Effect of Piperine, Extracted from Piper nigrum, with Ciprofloxacin on *Escherichia coli, Bacillus subtilis*. Pharm Sin 2017; 8(3). Available from: https://www.imedpub.com/articles/ synergistic-effect-of-piperine-extracted-from-piper-nigrum-withciprofloxacin-on-escherichia-coli-bacillus-subtilis.php?aid=21392 [Internet].

[32] Biswas S, Kar A, Sharma N, Haldar PK, Mukherjee PK. Synergistic effect of ursolic acid and piperine in CCl_4 induced hepatotoxicity. Ann Med 2021; 53(1): 2009-17. Available from: https://www.tandfonline. com/doi/abs/10.1080/07853890.2021.1995625 [http://dx.doi.org/10.1080/07853890.2021.1995625] [PMID: 34751064]

[33] Prapurnachandra Yadala A. Viswanathswamy, *In vitro* antioxidant and cytotoxic activity of rutin and piperine and their synergistic effect | International Journal of Pharmacy and Pharmaceutical Sciences [Internet]. [cited 2024 Dec 31]. Available from: Available from: https://journals.innovareacademics.in/index. php/ijpps/article/view/10426/5011.

[34] Schmidt B, Luan C, Passos A, Ferreira C, Lima Da Silva J, Fialho E. Synergistic effect of curcumin, piperine and resveratrol in MCF-7 and MDA MB-231 breast cancer cells. Biomed Res 2020; 31(5): 113-7. Available from: https://www.alliedacademies.org/articles/synergistic-effect-of-curcu-in-piperine-and-resvera trol-in-mcf7-and-mda-mb231-breast-cancer-cells-14432.html [Internet].

[35] Pal MK, Jaiswar SP, Srivastav AK, *et al.* Synergistic effect of piperine and paclitaxel on cell fate *via* cyt-c, Bax/Bcl-2-caspase-3 pathway in ovarian adenocarcinomas SKOV-3 cells. Eur J Pharmacol 2016; 791: 751-62. Available from: https://cris.bgu.ac.il/en/publications/synergistic-effect--f-piperine-and-paclitaxel-on-cell-fate-via-cy-2 [http://dx.doi.org/10.1016/j.ejphar.2016.10.019] [PMID: 27756602]

[36] Fattah A, Morovati A, Niknam Z, *et al.* The synergistic combination of cisplatin and piperine induces apoptosis in mcf-7 cell line. Iran J Public Health 2021; 50(5): 1037-47. Available from: https://publish.kne-publishing.com/index.php/ijph/article/view/6121 [http://dx.doi.org/10.18502/ijph.v50i5.6121] [PMID: 34183962]

[37] Markowiak P, Śliżewska K. Effects of probiotics, prebiotics, and synbiotics on human health. Nutrients 2017; 9(9): 1021. Available from: https://pmc.ncbi.nlm.nih.gov/articles/PMC5622781/ [http://dx.doi.org/10.3390/nu9091021] [PMID: 28914794]

[38] Kim J, Kim H, Jeon S, Jo J, Kim Y, Kim H. Synergistic antibacterial effects of probiotic lactic acid bacteria with curcuma longa rhizome extract as synbiotic against cutibacterium acnes 2020. Available from: https://www.mdpi.com/2076-3417/10/24/8955/htm [http://dx.doi.org/10.3390/app10248955]

[39] Jasim SA, Hafsan H, Saleem HD, Kandeel M, Khudhair F, Yasin G, *et al.* The synergistic effects of the probiotic (Lactobacillus fermentum) and cinnamon, Cinnamomum sp. powder on growth performance, intestinal microbiota, immunity, antioxidant defence and resistance to Yersinia ruckeri infection in the rainbow trout (Oncorhynchus mykiss) under high rearing density. Aquac Res [Internet]. 2022 Dec 1 [cited 2024 Dec 31]; 53(17): 5957–70. Available from: https://onlinelibrary.wiley.com/doi/full/10.1111/are.16064

[40] Pandey KR, Naik SR, Vakil BV. Probiotics, prebiotics and synbiotics- a review. J Food Sci Technol 2015; 52(12): 7577-87. Available from: https://pmc.ncbi.nlm.nih.gov/articles/PMC4648921/ [http://dx.doi.org/10.1007/s13197-015-1921-1] [PMID: 26604335]

[41] Roy S, Dhaneshwar S. Role of prebiotics, probiotics, and synbiotics in management of inflammatory bowel disease: Current perspectives. World J Gastroenterol 2023; 29(14): 2078-100. Available from: https://pmc.ncbi.nlm.nih.gov/articles/PMC10130969/ [http://dx.doi.org/10.3748/wjg.v29.i14.2078] [PMID: 37122604]

[42] Lee Y, Oh H, Jo M, *et al.* Synergistic effect of n-3 PUFA and probiotic supplementation on bone loss induced by chronic mild stress through the brain–gut–bone axis. J Funct Foods 2023; 100: 105363. [http://dx.doi.org/10.1016/j.jff.2022.105363]

[43] Khan MT, Dwibedi C, Sundh D, *et al.* Synergy and oxygen adaptation for development of next-generation probiotics. Nature 2023 620:7973 [Internet]. 2023 Aug 2 [cited 2024 Dec 31]; 620(7973): 381–5. Available from: https://www.nature.com/articles/s41586-023-06378-w [http://dx.doi.org/10.1038/s41586-023-06378-w]

[44] Lee C, Kim SW, Verma R, *et al.* Probiotic consortium confers synergistic anti-inflammatory effects in

inflammatory disorders. nutrients [Internet]. 2024 Mar 1 [cited 2024 Dec 31]; 16(6). Available from: https://quillbot.com/flow
[http://dx.doi.org/10.3390/nu16060790] [PMID: 38542701]

[45] Fayed B, El-Sayed H, Ismail S. Novel assessment of synergistic stimulatory effect of prebiotic chitooligosaccharide and some commercial prebiotics on the probiotic growth: A preliminary study. J Microbiol Biotechnol Food Sci 2021; 11(1): e3341-1. Available from: https://office2.jmbfs.org/index.php/JMBFS/article/view/3341 [Internet].
[http://dx.doi.org/10.15414/jmbfs.3341]

[46] Istiqomah L, Damayanti E, Suryani AE, Karimy MF, Maknuna D, Lutfiani . Synergistic effect between *Lactobacillus plantarum* AKK30 and *Saccharomyces cerevisiae* B18 and the probiotic properties of microencapsulated cultures. IOP Conf Ser Earth Environ Sci 2019; 251(1): 012062. Available from: https://iopscience.iop.org/article/10.1088/1755-1315/251/1/012062 [Internet].
[http://dx.doi.org/10.1088/1755-1315/251/1/012062]

[47] Lee JH, Kim J, Kim GY. Synergistic effects of a probiotic culture extract and antimicrobial combinations against multidrug-resistant *Acinetobacter baumannii.* Medicina (Kaunas) 2023; 59(5): 947. Available from: https://pmc.ncbi.nlm.nih.gov/articles/PMC10222653/
[http://dx.doi.org/10.3390/medicina59050947] [PMID: 37241179]

[48] Ferreira AF, Braga RLL, Andrade MF, Rosa ACP, Pereira-Manfro WF. Synergistic immunomodulatory activity of probiotics Bifidobacterium animalis and *Lactobacillus casei* in enteroaggregative *Escherichia coli* (EAEC)-infected CACO-2 cells. Arq Gastroenterol 2021; 58(4): 433-8. Available from: https://www.scielo.br/j/ag/a/cJM44PcHJR7GG66ZmmFsC9m/?lang=en
[http://dx.doi.org/10.1590/s0004-2803.202100000-79] [PMID: 34909846]

[49] Westfall S, Lomis N, Prakash S. A novel polyphenolic prebiotic and probiotic formulation have synergistic effects on the gut microbiota influencing Drosophila melanogaster physiology 2018. Available from: https://www.tandfonline.com/doi/abs/10.1080/21691401.2018.1458731
[http://dx.doi.org/10.1080/21691401.2018.1458731]

[50] Houston M. Nutraceuticals, vitamins, antioxidants, and minerals in the prevention and treatment of hypertension. Prog Cardiovasc Dis 2005; 47(6): 396-449.
[http://dx.doi.org/10.1016/j.pcad.2005.01.004] [PMID: 16115519]

[51] Arjumand W, Seth A, Sultana S. Rutin attenuates cisplatin induced renal inflammation and apoptosis by reducing NFκB, TNF-α and caspase-3 expression in wistar rats. Food Chem Toxicol 2011; 49(9): 2013-21. Available from: https://pubmed.ncbi.nlm.nih.gov/21605616/
[http://dx.doi.org/10.1016/j.fct.2011.05.012] [PMID: 21605616]

[52] Alnour TMS, Ahmed-Abakur EH, Elssaig EH, Abuduhier FM, Ullah MF. Antimicrobial synergistic effects of dietary flavonoids rutin and quercetin in combination with antibiotics gentamicin and ceftriaxone against *E. coli* (MDR) and P. mirabilis (XDR) strains isolated from human infections: Implications for food–medicine interactions. Ital J Food Sci 2022; 34(2): 34-42. Available from: https://www.itjfs.com/index.php/ijfs/article/view/2196/813
[http://dx.doi.org/10.15586/ijfs.v34i2.2196]

[53] Joshi T, Deepa PR, Sharma PK. Effect of different proportions of phenolics on antioxidant potential: pointers for bioactive synergy/antagonism in foods and nutraceuticals. Proc Natl Acad Sci, India, Sect B Biol Sci 2022; 92(4): 939-46. Available from: https://pubmed.ncbi.nlm.nih.gov/35935740/
[http://dx.doi.org/10.1007/s40011-022-01396-6] [PMID: 35935740]

[54] Omar S, El Borolossy RM, Elsaid T, Sabri NA. Evaluation of the combination effect of rutin and vitamin C supplementation on the oxidative stress and inflammation in hemodialysis patients. Front Pharmacol 2022; 13: 961590. Available from: https://pubmed.ncbi.nlm.nih.gov/36160426/
[http://dx.doi.org/10.3389/fphar.2022.961590] [PMID: 36160426]

[55] Deenonpoe R, Prayong P, Thippamom N, Meephansan J, Na-Bangchang K. Anti-inflammatory effect of naringin and sericin combination on human peripheral blood mononuclear cells (hPBMCs) from patient with psoriasis. BMC Complement Altern Med 2019; 19(1): 168. Available from:

https://bmccomplementmedtherapies.biomedcentral.com/articles/10.1186/s12906-019-2535-3 [http://dx.doi.org/10.1186/s12906-019-2535-3] [PMID: 31291937]

[56] Michala AS, Pritsa A. Quercetin: A Molecule of Great Biochemical and Clinical Value and Its Beneficial Effect on Diabetes and Cancer. Diseases 2022; 10(3): 37. Available from: https://pmc.ncbi.nlm.nih.gov/articles/PMC9326669/ [http://dx.doi.org/10.3390/diseases10030037] [PMID: 35892731]

[57] Sethi V, Garg M, Herve M, Mobasheri A. Potential complementary and/or synergistic effects of curcumin and boswellic acids for management of osteoarthritis. Ther Adv Musculoskelet Dis 2022; 14: 1759720X221124545. Available from: https://pubmed.ncbi.nlm.nih.gov/36171802/ [http://dx.doi.org/10.1177/1759720X221124545] [PMID: 36171802]

CHAPTER 11

Standardization and Quality Control of Nutraceuticals

Mukesh Singh Sikarwar[1,*] and **Vaibhav Kumar Rathi**[2]

[1] *Amity Institute of Pharmacy, Amity University, Gwalior, Madhya Pradesh, India*

[2] *Department of Pharmacy, Quantum University, Roorkee (Haridwar), Uttarakhand, India*

Abstract: Standardization in nutraceuticals is essential due to biochemical variation in crude drugs influenced by environmental factors, adulteration, substitution, and other factors affecting the quality of crude drugs used in the preparation of nutraceuticals. Standardization is crucial for the safety, efficacy, quality, and consistency of nutraceuticals, which are derived from natural sources and can vary significantly depending on source, processing, and storage. Standardization of nutraceuticals is a regulatory requirement in different countries covered under different guidelines. The European Food Safety Authority (EFSA) controls the nutraceutical sector in Europe; the Dietary Supplement Health and Education Act (DSHEA) 1994 governs it in the United States; the Food for Specified Health Uses (FOSHU) governs it in Japan; and the Food Safety and Standards Authority of India (FSSAI) oversees it in India. This chapter includes the profiles of a few chosen nutraceuticals, including their names and chemical contents. Therapeutic uses, dosages, and forms. The topic also includes WHO recommendations for standardisation and quality control of plant preparations, completed products, and crude pharmaceuticals for their efficacy, safety, and quality.

Keywords: FSSAI, Functional food, Quality control, Standardization, Specified health uses.

INTRODUCTION

Nutraceuticals are naturally derived, bioactive compounds with health benefits. To ensure quality, a systems approach is needed from farm gate to plate, starting with optimizing the agricultural crop and ensuring the quality of functional food products containing nutraceuticals. Phytochemical fingerprinting, employing botanical, farm-site, biodata, and agronomic approaches to identify crops, is the key to standardisation. For ascertaining real-time compliance, standardisation,

* **Corresponding author Mukesh Singh Sikarwar:** Amity Institute of Pharmacy, Amity University, Gwalior, Madhya Pradesh, India; E-mail: mukeshsikarwar@gmail.com

Mukesh Singh Sikarwar, Arunachalam Muthuraman & Sohrab A. Shaikh (Eds.)

documentation, and change monitoring in handling, harvesting, processing, and manufacturing, such knowledge requires the establishment of rapid assay methods. Quick tests can also ensure chemical and microbiological safety throughout the shelf life of the product.

Bigger vitamin/mineral companies scaled up their herb business during and after the passage of the 1994 Dietary Supplement Health and Education Act (DSHEA). Due to this, the business from health food stores shifted towards the pharmacies and dollar stores through partnering and buying acquisitions. People in the USA purchased natural medication with the structuring-function assurance, causing dietary supplement consumption in the US to rise from $8 billion in 1993 to $14 billion in 1999. Standardized biomarker products lack pre-market safety testing and FDA approval, causing consumer value issues. Consumers are becoming more educated about these products' differences in market forms [1].

Nutraceuticals' efficacy and safety assessment depend on their raw materials, with traditional foods requiring a toxicity study, while non-traditional ones require a genotoxicity, carcinogenicity, teratogenicity, and 90-day toxicity study [2]. Nutraceutical regulations worldwide are diverse and often unclear, leading to potential danger. Manufacturers and consumers should be aware of their country's regulations to make informed decisions, as information and expectations can be misleading and potentially dangerous [3]. The European Food Safety Authority (EFSA) defines nutraceuticals as food supplements containing vitamins, minerals, and amino acids. They must adhere to Good Manufacturing Practices for quality assurance. In the USA, nutraceuticals are regulated by the Dietary Supplement Health and Education Act (DSHEA), which includes specific regulations for finished supplements and dietary ingredients.

FOOD FOR SPECIFIED HEALTH USES (FOSHU)

By FOSHU, foods are ingredients with health-giving attributes that are officially recognized to have physiological effects in individuals.

Types of FOSHU

Qualified FOSHU: Foods with health benefits but which have not been demonstrated at the FOSHU level, or for which there is some efficacy but no action mechanism for the beneficial ingredient, will be permitted to qualify as qualified FOSHU. Standardised FOSHU: Foods having sufficient FOSHU certification and accumulated evidence are subject to standards and specs. Standardised FOSHU that meets standards and requirements is authorized.

The reducing the risk of disease FOSHU: If there is clinical and nutritional evidence to support an ingredient's disease risk-reducing claim, then it is granted approval [4]. In India, the Food Safety and Standards Authority of India regulates the nutraceutical industry, with proposed 2022 regulations aiming to enhance safety, labelling, and quality control. To comply with FSSAI regulations, manufacturers must obtain approval before marketing their products. Consumer confidence can be strengthened by requesting independent testing in third-party laboratories. Transparency is also crucial, with easy-to-understand labelling about nutraceuticals' composition and effects [3].

Indian food business operators are allowed to declare flavour additions on the label of a product in accordance with the Food Safety and Standards (Labelling and Packaging) Regulations, 2011, by virtue of the Food Safety and Standards (Health Supplements, Nutraceuticals, Food for Special Dietary Use, Food for Special Medical Purpose, Functional Food, and Novel Food) Regulations, 2016. Tablets, capsules, and syrups should comply with the general quality requirements and regulations as provided in the Indian Pharmacopoeia, British Pharmacopoeia, or United States Pharmacopoeia. As per the Indian Council of Medical Research, the level of nutrients added to foods cannot exceed the daily recommended intake. International food standard bodies like the Codex Alimentarius Commission use it if no standards are available. The highest nutritional value for any health supplement category is 15% of a day's intake. Food business operators are authorized to use food colouring, but with some restrictions. Articles intended for the correct age groups, sexes, and physiological phases must supply the necessary number of calories, protein, vitamins, minerals, and other essential elements for standard nutrient or nutritionally complete formulations for the correct age groups, sexes, and physiological phases. Purity standards for food ingredients to be used in food articles should be established and notified by the Food Authority. The permissible limit of variation in food articles covered under these regulations is not more than 10% from the value declared on the label of nutrients or nutritional ingredients. Production of ingredients and products should be in accordance with good manufacturing practices established [5].

Nutraceuticals' yearly growth rate in India was determined to be 25%, comparable to that of the developed nation of Japan. According to this perspective, a large number of new businesses have started producing nutraceuticals in India. The growing demand for nutraceuticals in India suggests their potential for disease prevention and treatment. Therefore, regulatory authorities must ensure product quality and safety to minimize adverse events like toxicity, adulteration, misuse, and overdose. As food products are transported across borders, maintaining safety and quality standards is crucial. New and existing companies should follow FSSAI's regulatory guidance to ensure the best use of nutraceuticals [6]. Quality

Assurance (QA) is a crucial component in maintaining quality standards, and systems like Good Manufacturing Practices (GMP) help measure product quality benchmarks. Adhering to guidelines and meeting requirements of regulatory bodies like the FDA and FSSAI can lead to significant resource savings and performance improvements. However, global regulatory frameworks for nutraceuticals remain unclear, creating an imbalance between claims and new product arrivals. Policies and agencies for approval, registration, and marketing vary globally and are regulated by various factors. Innovations with QA and compliance with standard requirements are the major market differentiators for scientific credibility, success, and sustainability [7].

TOP KEY REGULATION THAT GOVERNS THE NUTRACEUTICAL EXPORT COMPANIES IN INDIA

ISO: The most industry-relevant standard, ISO is a globally recognised standard that assists exporters in maintaining a generally recognised food safety procedure for their company. The purpose of these ISO certificates is to ensure the safety, efficacy, and quality testing of the exported nutraceutical products.

GMP: If your supplement bears the GMP (Good Manufacturing Procedures) label, it complies with the Natural Products Association's (NPA) certifications and the FDA's most recent good manufacturing procedures. The initial stand-alone testing standard and product certification scheme, NSF, has to be complied with by nutritional supplement exporters. The scheme serves to safeguard customers through contaminant level testing for harmful contaminants and ensuring that supplements include only labelled ingredients.

The Food Safety and Standards Authority of India (FSSAI) is responsible for ensuring that nutraceutical goods are manufactured, labelled, consumed, and exported in accordance with the Food Safety and Standards Act, 2006 (FSS Act) and its regulations. Regulations for Nutraceutical Export-Import Law: The "law and regulations" established by the Directorate General of Foreign Trade (DGFT) to guarantee seamless export operations are one of the Top 10 Things to Take into Account for Quality Assurance in Nutraceuticals Exports. These guidelines include following international commerce laws and operating within customer processes [8].

PROFILE OF SELECTED NUTRACEUTICALS

Garlic (*Allium sativum*) (Standardized Active Principles: Allicin, S-allylcysteine)

Medicinal Uses: Lower blood pressure in people with hypertension, lowers fasting blood glucose in Type 2 diabetics, promotes the immune system, and also helps in regulating elevated cholesterol levels.

Available Dosage Forms: Tablets, powder, capsules filled with oil, tablets of extract, and liquid dosage forms. Bulbs are shown in Fig. (**1**).

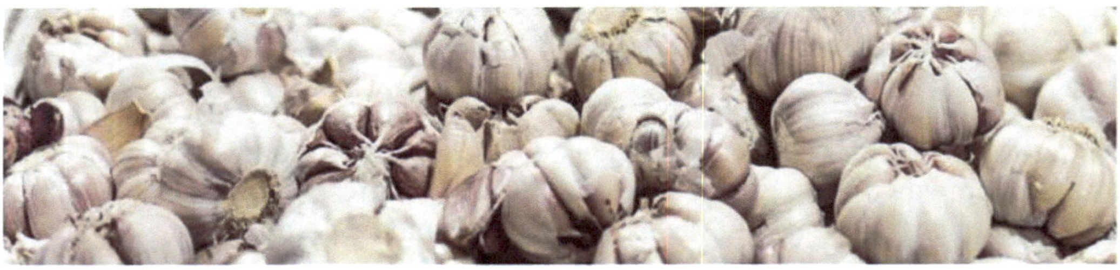

Fig. (1). Garlic.

Dose: In hypertension: 900 mg garlic powder daily, in hyperlipidaemia: 600 - 5600 mg garlic powder; 4 - 10 grams of raw garlic, In Hyperglycaemia: 1200 - 1500 mg/day, and for Immunity: Equivalent to 180 mg allicin/day.

Caution: With Metformin, garlic may have an additive hypoglycaemic effect, may cause bloating, reflux, flatulence, garlic breath, not recommended in pregnancy, not recommended for people with bleeding disorders [9 - 12].

Turmeric (Curcuma longa)

Medicinal Uses: Anti-inflammatory, hepatoprotective, and antioxidant.

Available Dosage Forms: Powder, tablets, and capsules.

Dose: Curcumin, 500 – 1200 mg for Rheumatoid arthritis, 360 mg three to four times a day for inflammatory bowel disease, for at least 3 months is recommended. Fig. (**2**) shows the turmeric being mixed with water.

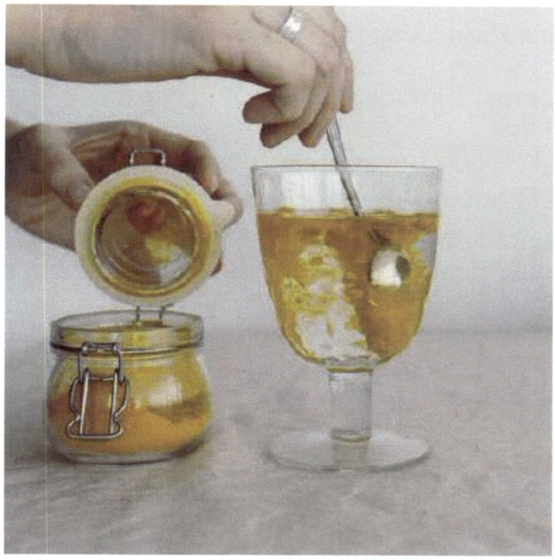

Fig. (2). Turmeric.

Caution: People with bile duct obstruction should avoid high doses, as they may cause irritation [13 - 15].

Milk Thistle (*Silybum marianum*)

The flowers of Milk thistle are shown in Fig. (**3**). The Active component of silymarin is silibinin, also known as silybin (mixture of silybin A and B).

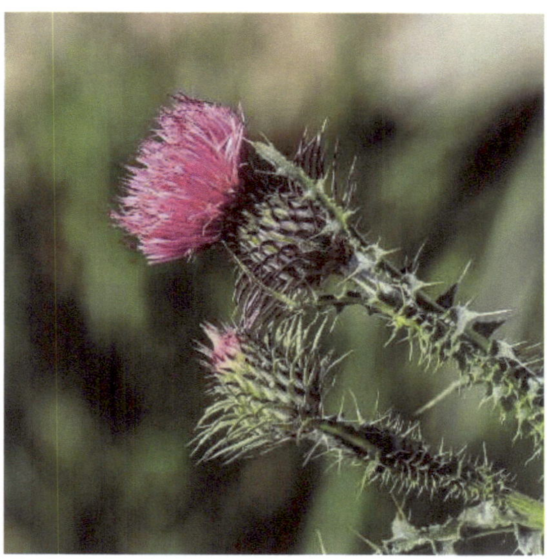

Fig. (3). Milk Thistle.

Medicinal Uses: Hepatoprotective, anti-inflammatory, and antioxidant.

Available Dosage Forms: Extracts, tablets, and capsules.

Dose: Liver support 420-600 mg silymarin/daily, which is equivalent to raw herb ~35-50 g/day. Extract contains 65-80% silymarin (100 mg is equivalent to 65-80 mg silymarin), and Silymarin contains 50-70% silibinin/ silybin (100 mg silibinin/silybin is equivalent to 143-200 mg of silymarin).

Caution: Milk thistle is contraindicated in pregnancy and lactation; it may cause allergic reactions in people who have an allergy to *Asteraceae* family plants [16, 17].

St John's Wort (Hypericum perforatum)

Bioactive Components: hypericin and hyperforin.

Medicinal Uses: Antidepressant, anxiolytic, and neuroprotective.

Available Dosage Forms: Extracts, tablets, and capsules.

Dosage Range: Depression: 500 to 1200 mg daily, Benefits for Menopause symptoms: 900 mg three times daily.

Caution: Light-skinned persons taking a high hypericin content should be advised to take extra precautions in the sun to avoid photosensitisation, not recommended in pregnancy and lactation, check for Interactions with some medicines (Fig. **4**) [18, 19].

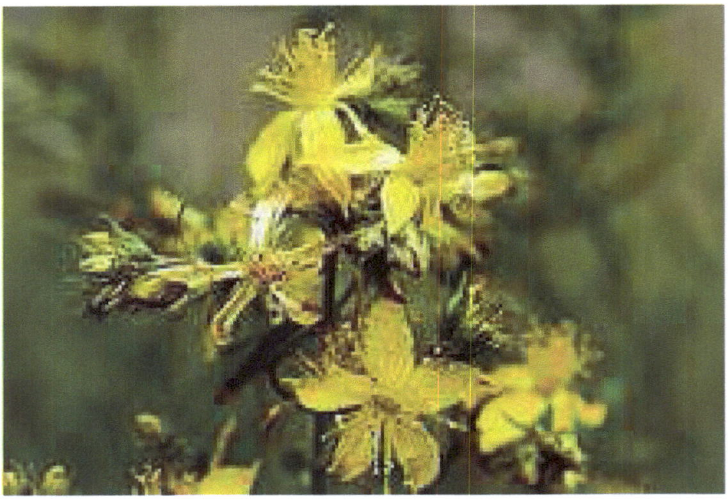

Fig. (4). St John's Wort.

Ginkgo (*Ginkgo biloba*) Ginkgoaceae Family

Standardized extract contains ginkgo flavone glycosides 24% and terpenoids 6% (Fig. **5**).

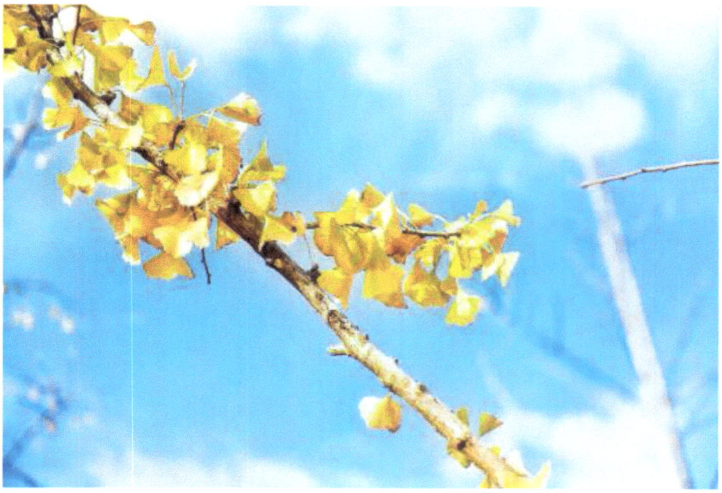

Fig. (5). Ginkgo.

Medicinal Uses: Protection against damage done by cerebral ischaemia, Working memory.

Available Dosage Forms: Extracts, tablets, and capsules.

Dosage Range: 120-240 mg/day in divided doses for 22-26 weeks in treatment of Dementia/ Cognitive Impairment, 120 mg/day standardised extract used for six seeks for Working memory (6 weeks).

Caution: Stop using if unusual bleeding occurs in any part of the body, interaction is possible with food and medicines [20 - 22].

Ginger, *Zingiber Officinale* Roscoe, Zingiberaceae Family

Rhizome of Ginger, which contains Gingerol, the main bioactive component in ginger, is responsible for its unique taste as well as therapeutic properties (Fig. **6**). It has proven anti-inflammatory and antioxidant properties. Zingerone, another compound, also has antioxidant activity [23]. Ginger is identified for its anti-inflammatory properties, as it decreases prostaglandin production by blocking enzymes cyclooxygenase-1 and cyclooxygenase-2. It also has digestive benefits, alleviating nausea and indigestion. Ginger is also found to have antioxidant and antidiabetic activities, being particularly effective against Type-2-diabetes [24].

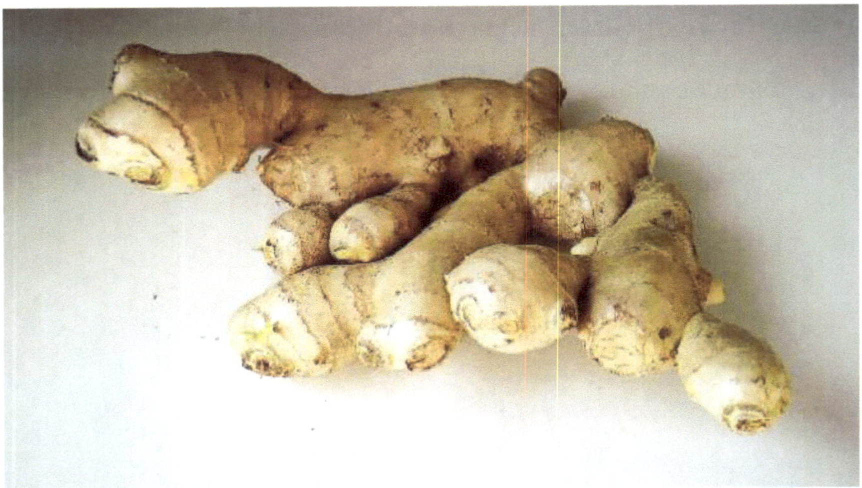

Fig. (6). Ginger.

Black Pepper, *Piper nigrum*, Piperaceae Family

Pepper contains a pungent taste and heat due to its main chemical constituent, piperine, which has antioxidant and anti-inflammatory activities. It contains essential oils like β-caryophyllene, pinene, limonene, and sabinene, and minerals like iron, manganese, and magnesium. Pepper also contains peptidase, which may aid digestion, and piperidine alkaloids [25]. Black pepper, known for its spice and flavor enhancement, has medicinal uses as a spice. Piperine, the active constituent, enhances the bioavailability of nutrients like curcumin, has anti-inflammatory and antioxidant activities, and stimulates digestive enzyme production. Pepper also relieves respiratory symptoms like congestion [26].

Green Tea Powder Camellia sinensis (Theaceae)

Green tea (Fig. 7) is rich in flavonoid-like catechins like epicatechin gallate, epigallocatechin, and epicatechin, which have antioxidant properties. It contains lower caffeine levels than black tea and coffee, but still carries a minor stimulant effect. The flavor of green tea is calming, and it contains vitamins B and C, as well as minerals such as magnesium, calcium, and potassium. Green tea, rich in phenolics, has antioxidant properties, preventing diseases like malignancy and diabetes, enhancing metabolic rate, and promoting fat oxidation for weight management. It also enhances cognitive functions by combining theanine and caffeine. Regular consumption reduces cholesterol levels and improves cardiac functions [27 - 29].

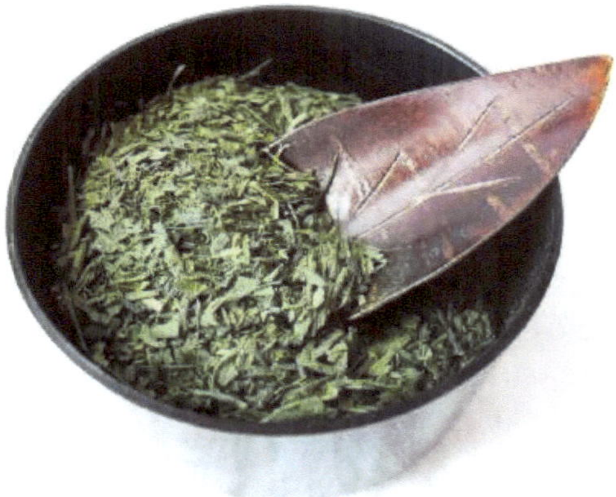

Fig. (7). Green tea.

Soy Isoflavones *Glycine max* of Family Fabaceae

Soybeans (Fig. **8**) contain genistein, a highly researched soy isoflavone that has been associated with improved heart health, decreased menopausal symptoms, and even a decreased risk of cancer. Microbes in the intestines convert the soy isoflavone daizein, well known for being present in most soy products, into an equal. The third prominent isoflavone in soy, glycitein, is often present in lower concentrations. Genistein isoflavones, found in soy, have estrogen-like effects that alleviate menopausal symptoms. They also have bone protective effects, reduced osteoporosis risk, improved cardiac health, cancer prevention, cognitive function improvement, and skin benefits. Soy is a good nutraceutical due to its high protein and various elements content [29, 30].

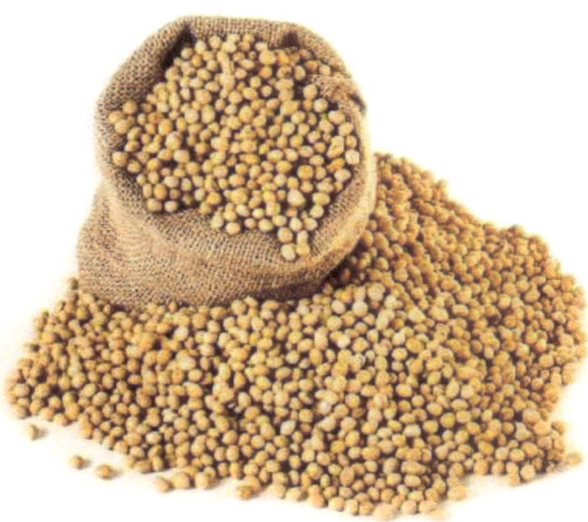

Fig. (8). Soy.

Vitamin D (Cholecalciferol)

Vitamin D is a fat-soluble vitamin that plays a crucial role in bone metabolism, the immune system, and calcium homeostasis. It is endogenously synthesized primarily from sun exposure, from UVB radiation and cholesterol, and thus sun exposure is the primary source, and diet accounts for only 5–10%. Fatty fish, egg yolks, and fortified foods provide small amounts and are frequently inadequate. Sun deprivation, the use of sunscreen, and low-sunlight lifestyles are risk factors for deficiency. Therefore, safe sun exposure and supplementation are frequently necessary for sufficient levels.

Key Functions and Indications

- Immunomodulation, regulation of calcium and phosphorus homeostasis, inhibits bone resorption, maintains heart and skeletal muscle function, brain function, insulin secretion, cell growth, differentiation, and proliferation.
- Vitamin D usually co-exists with calcium and exists in the blood as 25-hydroxyvitamin D (25(OH)D).
- Certain animal foods and certain fish oils contain cholecalciferol (D3), which the body synthesizes in sunlight. Certain plants contain ergocalciferol (D2), which is used in certain supplements. D3 is better than D2 at increasing serum levels.

Dosage Range

- Treatment for moderate to severe deficit (≤29 nmol/L): 3000-5000 IU daily for 6-13 weeks, followed by continuous maintenance at 1000-2000 IU daily.

Caution: Excessive vitamin D intake can be harmful. Toxicity manifestations such as headache, nausea, vomiting, loss of appetite, muscle ache, and lethargy are provoked by consuming high doses for months [31, 32].

Vitamin B12 (Cobalamin)

B12 is transformed to active forms in the body, including methylcobalamin and 5-deoxyadenosylcobalamin. Serum B12 is not an accurate guide to B12 status. Elevated serum or plasma homocysteine in association with methylmalonic acid (MMA) testing is a more reliable measure.

Key Functions and Indications

Red blood cell production, Nervous system function, Cognitive health, and Homocysteine metabolism.

Dosage Range: Adults (13 + years): 2.4 mcg/day, Pregnancy/lactation: 2.4-2.8 mcg/day, 1000-2000 mcg/day taken 30 mins before breakfast, Sublingually. Vitamin B12 contains many compounds with the same structures to one another, such as aquacobalamin, nitrocobalamin, and cyanocobalamin. It is easier for the body to utilize methylcobalamin, an active compound.

Interaction: Proton pump inhibitors led to a reduction in stomach acid, which may reduce B12 absorption [33].

WHO GUIDELINES FOR STANDARDIZATION AND QUALITY CONTROL

Ready-to-administer drug formulations comprise active plant principles, aerial or subterranean, crude or processed, present in juices, gums, fixed oils, essential oils, or other plant materials. Other ingredients, such as excipients, are added to herbal medicine along with the active component.

Assessment of Quality

This should include all aspects relevant to the assessment of the quality of herbal medicines. One can be content with the mention of a pharmacopoeial monograph in the event that such is available. Where such is not available, one must submit one prepared in accordance with an official pharmacopoeia. All processes must be in accordance with Good Manufacturing Practices.

The standardization of crude drug materials includes the following steps:

1. Identity and Authentication
   - Botanical/Taxonomic Identity: Phytomorphology, taxonomical verification.
   - Diagnostic Microscopy/Histology: Microscopical and histological analysis; tissues of diagnostic importance in the drug powder.
   - Chromatographic/Spectroscopic Evaluation:
   - Qualitative and semi-quantitative analysis *via* TLC, HPTLC, and HPLC.
   - Chemical marker identification (*e.g.*, fingerprint evaluation).

2. Physical and Sensory Evaluation
   - Organoleptic Evaluation: Sensory attributes (taste, odor, appearance, texture).
   - Foreign Matter: Absence of soil, insect parts, animal excreta, *etc.*
   - Moisture Content: Determination of water content.
   - Volatile Matter: Assessment of volatile components.

3. Chemical and Analytical Parameters
   - Ash Values: Total ash, acid-insoluble ash, *etc.*

- Extractive Values: Soluble extractives (water, alcohol, *etc.*).
- Heavy Metals: Limits for cadmium, lead, arsenic, *etc.*
- Pesticide Residues: Compliance with WHO/FAO limits (*e.g.*, DDT, BHC, aldrin).

4. Safety and Contaminant Testing
   - Microbial Contamination:
   - Limits for *E. coli*, moulds, and aflatoxins.
   - Assessment of harvesting/production practices.

5. Radioactive Contamination:
   - Screening per IAEA (International Atomic Energy Agency) and WHO guidelines.
   - Risk evaluation from sterilization *via* irradiation.

Plant Preparations

Plant preparations include crushed or powdered plant materials, extracts, tinctures, fatty or essential oils, expressed juices, and preparations made by concentration, fractionation, or purification. A thorough explanation of the production process is necessary. Any additional chemicals used during the production process to raise the plant preparation to a specific level of active or distinctive components, or for any other reason, should be disclosed in the manufacturing procedure. A way to identify the plant preparation and, if feasible, test it must exist. If an active component cannot be identified, it should be enough to identify a distinguishing ingredient or combination of compounds (such as a "chromatographic fingerprint") to guarantee constant quality of the mixture.

Finished Product: The formula, quantity of additives, and production procedure must all be thoroughly explained. How the plant material found in the final product is recognised and, if feasible, quantified must be described. If an active principle cannot be identified, identifying a distinctive substance or combination of components (such as a "chromatographic fingerprint") should be adequate to guarantee consistent product quality. For certain dosage forms, the final product must meet the general standards. For imported completed goods, verification of the regulatory status in the nation of origin is necessary.

Assessment of Safety

An overarching principle should be that, unless new information requires an updated risk-benefit assessment, no specific, limited regulatory intervention is undertaken if the product has historically been used without resulting in harm. Original references or references to the original references must be included along with an evaluation of the relevant literature. Official review or monograph outcomes may be referred to if available. Long-term use of a drug without any evidence of hazards, however, can imply that the drug is safe. Documentation of spontaneously reported adverse events should be in accordance with standard pharmacovigilance practice. Toxicological studies should be included if available.

Documentation of Safety Based on Experience

Generally, during safety evaluation, reports of widespread use should be considered. The length of use, the dose-response conditions treated, the number of individuals exposed, and the countries with experience should be specified. If a risk is known, toxicological information should be supplied. Risk assessment should be documented, whether or not it is related to dose. In the latter case, a substantial part of the risk assessment should involve the dose specification. Wherever possible, a description of the hazards should be given. Documentation of any abuse potential, dependency, or misuse is required. Toxicological information should be given if long-term traditional use cannot be established or if safety is in doubt.

Assessment of Efficacy

All major aspects of effectiveness evaluation must be covered in this section. The original papers or proper citations to them must be provided, along with a discussion of the relevant literature. If there are studies, they should be taken into account. Activity: Specification or characterization of the pharmacological and clinical actions of the active ingredients, as well as of any compounds with therapeutic activity, if any are recognized, is crucial.

Evidence Required to Support Indications

There is a need to give the indication or indications for the use of the drug. The type of indication should decide the criteria for demonstrating the efficacy of traditional medicines. With the commonality of traditional use, some loosening of the standards for demonstration of efficacy may be tolerated for the treatment of mild illness and for non-specific indications. Even when used prophylactically, the same considerations may be applicable. Personal experience recorded in accounts from medical practitioners, traditional healers, or their patients must be taken into account. Sufficient clinical evidence must be required in instances where traditional use has not been demonstrated.

Combination Products

Since most herbal remedies contain numerous active ingredients, and because traditional medicines are often comprised of combination products, analyses must separate new and old combination products. Historical records of traditional use (*e.g.*, traditional Chinese medicine, Ayurvedic classics, Unani, Siddha, *etc.*) and practice may be used as evidence of effectiveness in the instance of long-used combination products. The documentation of traditional knowledge for each individual constituent must be complemented with the explanation of a novel combination of known chemicals, such as compatibility and therapeutic ranges of the effective dose. In order to illustrate the effectiveness of a new ingredient and its therapeutic effect on the whole combination, clinical studies can be required [34].

SUMMARY

There are several processes involved in standardising nutraceuticals, starting with the agricultural process of growing the raw medications required to make them. Among the crucial processes in standardising nutraceuticals are authentication, harvesting, collecting, storage, HPTLC fingerprinting, marker compound identification, and extract standardisation with % of active ingredients. The profiles of several nutraceuticals demonstrate that various health issues are managed with varying dosages of these products. The WHO provided recommendations for evaluating herbal medicine's effectiveness, safety, and quality. Students and readers will benefit from this chapter's coverage of the many facets of herbal medication quality management.

EXERCISE

Short Answer Questions

1. What are the two primary active compounds in Garlic for which it is standardized, and what is the key chemical transformation that links them?
2. Explain the primary challenge in maintaining the stability of allicin in commercial garlic supplements.
3. Name the three main curcuminoids found in Turmeric and identify which one is most abundant.
4. Why is piperine from Black Pepper often formulated with curcumin in nutraceutical products?
5. What are the key bioactive compounds in St. John's Wort responsible for its neurological effects, and why is their standardization critical for safety?
6. Describe the primary quality control issue related to hyperforin content in St. John's Wort extracts.

7. List two distinct groups of active compounds found in Ginkgo biloba extracts that are subject to standardization.
8. What is a common adulterant found in Ginkgo supplements, and what analytical method is used to detect it?
9. Identify the main pungent compounds in Ginger and describe how their profile can vary based on the rhizome's drying process.
10. What specific role does the Food Safety and Standards Authority of India (FSSAI) play in governing the domestic sale and production of nutraceuticals?
11. Name the primary catechins in Green Tea powder, with a focus on the most biologically active one.
12. How does the processing of green tea differ from black tea, and how does this impact its final chemical profile?
13. What are the two major Soy Isoflavones, and in what form (aglycone or glycoside) are they typically found in soybeans?
14. Explain the significance of standardizing nutraceuticals based on S-allyl cysteine for Garlic products.
15. What is the chemical name for Vitamin D3, and why is it preferred over Vitamin D2 in fortifications?
16. Describe the core chemical structure of Vitamin B12 (cobalamin) that features a metal ion.
17. According to WHO guidelines, what is the fundamental difference between 'quality' and 'efficacy' in the context of a nutraceutical product?
18. In the WHO's framework for safety assessment, what does the term 'margin of safety' refer to?
19. Which regulatory body, besides FSSAI, is critical for an Indian company aiming to export its nutraceutical products to the European Union or the USA?
20. For Black Pepper, what quality parameter other than piperine content is crucial for ensuring its commercial grade and stability?

Long Answer Questions

1. Discuss the comprehensive regulatory framework an Indian nutraceutical company must navigate for exporting its products. Elaborate on the roles of at least two key governmental/regulatory bodies.
2. Compare and contrast the challenges of standardizing a whole-herb extract like Turmeric (Curcuma longa) with a pure compound like Vitamin D (cholecalciferol). Address aspects of sourcing, extraction, and analytical validation.
3. Elaborate on the WHO guidelines for assessing the *quality* of a finished herbal nutraceutical product. What specific physical, chemical, and microbiological parameters must be evaluated?
4. "The assessment of efficacy for a nutraceutical is more complex than for a

pharmaceutical drug." Critically evaluate this statement, using Ginkgo biloba or St. John's Wort as an example.

5. Design a quality control protocol for a batch of Green Tea Powder (Camellia sinensis) intended for use in a high-potency antioxidant supplement. Your protocol should cover raw material identification, extraction, standardization of the final product, and stability testing.
6. Explain the chemistry of Soy Isoflavones (Glycine max) and their mechanism of action in the human body. Discuss the controversies and regulatory considerations surrounding their use in supplements for hormonal health.
7. Describe the process of assessing the *safety* of a novel nutraceutical ingredient according to WHO guidelines. What types of toxicological studies are essential before the product can be marketed?
8. A company wants to launch a high-potency Ginger (Zingiber officinale) extract standardized for its gingerol content. Explain the entire process from raw material sourcing to finished product, focusing on the critical quality control checkpoints at each stage.
9. Discuss the stability issues associated with Vitamin B12 (cobalamin) and Vitamin D (cholecalciferol) in fortified foods and supplements. What formulation strategies can be employed to protect them from degradation?
10. Compare the regulatory status and scientific evidence for St. John's Wort in the European Union *versus* the United States. Why do these differences exist, and what are the implications for global nutraceutical companies?
11. Explain the concept of 'chemoprofiling' or 'fingerprinting' in the context of herbal nutraceuticals. Why is this approach often superior to standardization based on a single active marker? Use Garlic or Ginkgo as an example.
12. What are the key differences in the quality control requirements for a nutraceutical sold as a food supplement *versus* one making a specific health claim under FSSAI regulations?
13. Discuss the potential for adulteration in the Black Pepper supply chain. What analytical techniques are most effective for detecting common adulterants and ensuring the authenticity of the product?
14. Explain the physiological importance of both Vitamin D and Vitamin B12. Why has their role in preventative health led to their widespread use as nutraceuticals?
15. Analyze the challenges in establishing a scientifically valid 'Recommended Daily Allowance' (RDA) for a complex nutraceutical like Green Tea extract compared to a single nutrient like Vitamin D.

Case Studies

Case 1: *A nutraceutical company in India sources Ginkgo biloba extract from a new supplier in China at a significantly lower cost. The supplier's Certificate of*

Analysis (CoA) shows that the extract meets the standard of 24% flavone glycosides and 6% terpene lactones. However, after launching a new memory support product, the company receives consumer complaints of inefficacy. As the Head of Quality Control, you are tasked with investigating. Outline your investigation plan. What specific advanced analytical tests would you conduct to confirm the identity and quality of the extract, and what potential adulterants would you be looking for?

Case 2: *A start-up has developed a novel enteric-coated tablet of Garlic powder designed to maximize allicin delivery to the intestines. Initial lab tests show high allicin yield. However, stability testing reveals that the allicin content drops by 60% within 3 months of storage at room temperature. The product launch is in six months. Analyze the potential biochemical and formulation-based reasons for this instability. Propose a multi-pronged strategy to reformulate the product to ensure allicin stability and meet the quality claims at the time of expiry.*

Case 3: *An established Indian herbal company wants to export its St. John's Wort (Hypericum perforatum) extract to Germany. Their current extract is standardized to 0.3% hypericin. However, German regulatory authorities (BfArM) have strict limits on hyperforin content due to its potential for drug interactions. The company's current extract has a high and variable hyperforin level. As the Regulatory Affairs Manager, what steps must you take to make this product compliant for the German market? Discuss the necessary changes in sourcing, extraction technology, and the quality control documentation required for the export dossier.*

Case 4: *A company plans to market a Soy Isoflavone supplement with a specific health claim related to menopausal symptom relief. The FSSAI requires them to submit data supporting this claim. You are hired to design a study to assess the product's efficacy. Describe the key elements of the clinical trial protocol you would design. Include details on participant selection criteria, study duration, dosage, primary and secondary outcome measures, and the type of control group you would use to ensure the results are scientifically valid and unbiased.*

Case 5: *An exporter of Turmeric (Curcuma longa) powder to the USA has had a large shipment rejected by the FDA due to "filth and microbiological contamination" and levels of lead that exceed safety limits. This is a major financial and reputational blow. You are brought in as a consultant to overhaul their quality management system. Develop a comprehensive corrective and preventive action (CAPA) plan. Your plan should address the entire supply chain, from the farm level (sourcing of rhizomes) through processing, drying, grinding, packaging, and final pre-shipment testing.*

REFERENCES

[1] Lachance PA, Saba RG. Quality management of nutraceuticals: intelligent product-delivery systems and safety through traceability. 2002. Available from: https://pubs.acs.org/sharingguidelines

[2] van Breemen RB, Fong HHS, Farnsworth NR. The role of quality assurance and standardization in the safety of botanical dietary supplements. Chem Res Toxicol 2007; 20(4): 577-82. Available from: https://pmc.ncbi.nlm.nih.gov/articles/PMC2570109/ [http://dx.doi.org/10.1021/tx7000493] [PMID: 17362032]

[3] Das L, Bhaumik E, Raychaudhuri U, Chakraborty R. Role of nutraceuticals in human health. J Food Sci Technol 2012; 49(2): 173-83. [http://dx.doi.org/10.1007/s13197-011-0269-4] [PMID: 23572839]

[4] Food with Health Claims, Food for Special Dietary Uses, and Nutrition Labeling. Available from: https://www.mhlw.go.jp/english/topics/foodsafety/fhc/02.html

[5] Food Safety and Standards Authority of India. Food safety and standards (Health supplements, nutraceuticals, food for special dietary use, food for special medical purpose, functional food and novel food) regulations, 2016. The Gazette of India 2016.

[6] FSSAI guidance and notification on nutraceuticals – An insight. Available from: https://fssai.gov.in/upload/media/FSSAI_News_Guidance_FNB_09_06_2020.pdf

[7] Inbathamizh L, Prabavathy D, Sudha S. Quality assurance of nutraceuticals and their approval, registration, marketing. Handbook of Nutraceuticals and Natural Products 2022; 337-60. Available from: https://onlinelibrary.wiley.com/doi/full/10.1002/9781119746843.ch27

[8] United Laboratories Top Points to Consider for Quality Assurance in Nutraceuticals Exports. Available from: https://www.unitedlabs.in/top-points-to-consider-for-quality-assur-nce-in-nutraceuticals-exports/

[9] Ried K, Toben C, Fakler P. Effect of garlic on serum lipids: an updated meta-analysis. Nutr Rev 2013; 71(5): 282-99. Available from: https://pubmed.ncbi.nlm.nih.gov/23590705/ [http://dx.doi.org/10.1111/nure.12012] [PMID: 23590705]

[10] Sobenin IA, Andrianova IV, Fomchenkov IV, Gorchakova TV, Orekhov AN. Time-released garlic powder tablets lower systolic and diastolic blood pressure in men with mild and moderate arterial hypertension. Hypertens Res 2009; 32(6): 433-7. Available from: https://pubmed.ncbi.nlm.nih.gov/19390538/ [http://dx.doi.org/10.1038/hr.2009.36] [PMID: 19390538]

[11] Lissiman E, Bhasale AL, Cohen M. Garlic for the common cold. Cochrane Database Syst Rev 2014; 2014(11)CD006206 Available from: https://pubmed.ncbi.nlm.nih.gov/25386977/ [Internet]. [PMID: 25386977]

[12] Ashraf Phil RM, Alam Khan R, Ashraf I. Effects of garlic on blood glucose levels and HbA1c in patients with type 2 diabetes mellitus. J Med Plants Res 2011; 5(13): 2922-8. Available from: http://www.academicjournals.org/JMPR [Internet].

[13] Kedia S, Bhatia V, Thareja S, *et al.* Low dose oral curcumin is not effective in induction of remission in mild to moderate ulcerative colitis: Results from a randomized double blind placebo controlled trial. World J Gastrointest Pharmacol Ther 2017; 8(2): 147-54. Available from: https://pmc.ncbi.nlm.nih.gov/articles/PMC5421114/ [http://dx.doi.org/10.4292/wjgpt.v8.i2.147] [PMID: 28533925]

[14] Preliminary study on antirheumatic activity of curcumin (diferuloyl methane). Available from: https://pubmed.ncbi.nlm.nih.gov/7390600/

[15] Chandran B, Goel A. A randomized, pilot study to assess the efficacy and safety of curcumin in patients with active rheumatoid arthritis. Phytother Res 2012; 26(11): 1719-25. Available from: https://pubmed.ncbi.nlm.nih.gov/22407780/ [http://dx.doi.org/10.1002/ptr.4639] [PMID: 22407780]

[16] Freedman ND, Curto TM, Morishima C, *et al.* Silymarin use and liver disease progression in the Hepatitis C Antiviral Long-Term Treatment against Cirrhosis trial. Aliment Pharmacol Ther 2011; 33(1): 127-37. Available from: https://pubmed.ncbi.nlm.nih.gov/21083592/ [http://dx.doi.org/10.1111/j.1365-2036.2010.04503.x] [PMID: 21083592]

[17] Freedman ND, Curto TM, Morishima C, *et al.* Silymarin use and liver disease progression in the Hepatitis C Antiviral Long-Term Treatment against Cirrhosis trial. Aliment Pharmacol Ther 2011; 33(1): 127-37. Available from: https://pubmed.ncbi.nlm.nih.gov/21083592/ [http://dx.doi.org/10.1111/j.1365-2036.2010.04503.x] [PMID: 21083592]

[18] Liu YR, Jiang YL, Huang RQ, Yang JY, Xiao BK, Dong JX. *Hypericum perforatum L.* preparations for menopause: a meta-analysis of efficacy and safety. Climacteric 2014; 17(4): 325-35. Available from: https://pubmed.ncbi.nlm.nih.gov/24188229/ [http://dx.doi.org/10.3109/13697137.2013.861814] [PMID: 24188229]

[19] Linde K, Berner MM, Kriston L. St John's wort for major depression. Cochrane Database Syst Rev 2008; 2008(4)CD000448 Available from: https://pubmed.ncbi.nlm.nih.gov/18843608/ [Internet]. [PMID: 18843608]

[20] Sakatani K, Tanida M, Hirao N, Takemura N. Ginkobiloba extract improves working memory performance in middle-aged women: role of asymmetry of prefrontal cortex activity during a working memory task. Adv Exp Med Biol 2014; 812: 295-301. Available from: https://pubmed.ncbi.nlm.nih.gov/24729246/ [http://dx.doi.org/10.1007/978-1-4939-0620-8_39] [PMID: 24729246]

[21] Gauthier S, Schlaefke S. Efficacy and tolerability of Ginkgo biloba extract EGb 761® in dementia: a systematic review and meta-analysis of randomized placebo-controlled trials. Clin Interv Aging 2014; 9: 2065-77. Available from: https://pubmed.ncbi.nlm.nih.gov/25506211/ [http://dx.doi.org/10.2147/CIA.S72728] [PMID: 25506211]

[22] von Gunten A, Schlaefke S, Überla K. Efficacy of *Ginkgo biloba* extract EGb 761 ® in dementia with behavioural and psychological symptoms: A systematic review. World J Biol Psychiatry 2016; 17(8): 622-33. Available from: https://pubmed.ncbi.nlm.nih.gov/26223956/ [http://dx.doi.org/10.3109/15622975.2015.1066513] [PMID: 26223956]

[23] Semwal RB, Semwal DK, Combrinck S, Viljoen AM. Gingerols and shogaols: Important nutraceutical principles from ginger. Phytochemistry 2015; 117: 554-68. Available from: https://pubmed.ncbi.nlm.nih.gov/26228533/ [http://dx.doi.org/10.1016/j.phytochem.2015.07.012] [PMID: 26228533]

[24] Mahluji S, Attari VE, Mobasseri M, Payahoo L, Ostadrahimi A, Golzari SEJ. Effects of ginger (*Zingiber officinale*) on plasma glucose level, HbA1c and insulin sensitivity in type 2 diabetic patients. Int J Food Sci Nutr 2013; 64(6): 682-6. Available from: https://pubmed.ncbi.nlm.nih.gov/23496212/ [http://dx.doi.org/10.3109/09637486.2013.775223] [PMID: 23496212]

[25] Butt MS, Pasha I, Sultan MT, Randhawa MA, Saeed F, Ahmed W. Black pepper and health claims: a comprehensive treatise. Crit Rev Food Sci Nutr 2013; 53(9): 875-86. Available from: https://pubmed.ncbi.nlm.nih.gov/23768180/ [http://dx.doi.org/10.1080/10408398.2011.571799] [PMID: 23768180]

[26] Meghwal M, Goswami TK. Piper nigrum and piperine: an update. Phytother Res 2013; 27(8): 1121-30. Available from: https://pubmed.ncbi.nlm.nih.gov/23625885/ [http://dx.doi.org/10.1002/ptr.4972] [PMID: 23625885]

[27] Cabrera C, Artacho R, Giménez R. Beneficial effects of green tea--a review. J Am Coll Nutr 2006; 25(2): 79-99. Available from: https://pubmed.ncbi.nlm.nih.gov/16582024/ [http://dx.doi.org/10.1080/07315724.2006.10719518] [PMID: 16582024]

[28] Hursel R, Viechtbauer W, Westerterp-Plantenga MS. The effects of green tea on weight loss and weight maintenance: a meta-analysis. Int J Obes 2009; 33(9): 956-61. Available from: https://pubmed.ncbi.nlm.nih.gov/19597519/

[http://dx.doi.org/10.1038/ijo.2009.135] [PMID: 19597519]

[29] Tang GY, Meng X, Gan RY, Zhao CN, Liu Q, Feng Y. Health functions and related molecular mechanisms of tea components: an update review. Int J Mol Sci 2019; 20(24) Available from: https://pubmed.ncbi.nlm.nih.gov/31817990/

[30] Taku K, Melby MK, Kronenberg F, Kurzer MS, Messina M. Extracted or synthesized soybean isoflavones reduce menopausal hot flash frequency and severity. Menopause 2012; 19(7): 776-90. Available from: https://pubmed.ncbi.nlm.nih.gov/22433977/ [http://dx.doi.org/10.1097/gme.0b013e3182410159] [PMID: 22433977]

[31] Dietary Supplement Fact Sheets National Institutes of Health, Office of Dietary Supplements 2025. Available from: https://ods.od.nih.gov/factsheets/list-all/

[32] Vitamin D. Vitamin D | Eat For Health National Health and Medical Research Council 2025. Available from: https://www.eatforhealth.gov.au/nutrient-reference-values/nutrients/vitamin-d

[33] NatMed Pro - Food, Herbs and Supplements Therapeutic Research Faculty 2025. Available from: https://naturalmedicines.therapeuticresearch.com/databases/food,-herbs-supplements.aspx

[34] World Health Organization. Guideline for Assessing Quality of Herbal Medicines with Reference to Contaminants and Residues. 3rd ed.. Geneva: World Health Organization 2007; pp. 130-43.

CHAPTER 12

Current Regulations and Clinical Applications of Nutraceuticals

Khian Giap Lim[1], **Nazmun Nahar Alam**[2] and **Arunachalam Muthuraman**[3,*]

[1] *Clinical Pharmacy and Pharmacy Practice Unit, Faculty of Pharmacy, AIMST University, Bedong 08100, Kedah, Malaysia*

[2] *Faculty of Medicine, AIMST University, Bedong 08100, Kedah, Malaysia*

[3] *Pharmacology, Toxicology, and Basic Health Sciences Unit, Faculty of Pharmacy, AIMST University, Bedong 08100, Kedah, Malaysia*

Abstract: The global nutraceutical market has a higher impact, and in the coming decades, it will become a multibillion-dollar business. Nutraceuticals are comprised of multiple diverse food product categories, including vitamins (water and fat-soluble); micro and macronutrients, essential fatty acids, prebiotics and probiotics, phytochemicals, and herbs. Pharmacological aspects, nutraceuticals, and dietary supplements possess synergistic effects. However, standardization and quality control checking of nutraceuticals can be useful for the safe and effective management of illness in clinical settings. The key driving forces of nutraceutical usage in clinical applications are wider due to its possible usage over a longer period, ease of administration to aged populations, compatibility with consumer lifestyle, and a higher rate of cost-benefits. However, the major challenges regarding safety and efficacy concern the scientific evidence and rationality-based therapy in clinical trials. This kind of study may reach out to the patient with consistent and well-defined regulatory clearance, and it provides greater opportunities for growth and expansion, and encourages nutraceutical applications in a clinical setup. Hence, this book chapter focused on expressing the possibilities and current perspectives of nutraceuticals for clinical applications.

Keywords: Chelation, Fenton reactions, Mammalian target of rapamycin, Mitochondrial protection, Natural health products, Nuclear factor kappa B.

INTRODUCTION

Nutraceuticals like dietary supplements and their isolated products are commercialized for medicinal use, and it is claimed that they produce physio-

* **Corresponding author Arunachalam Muthuraman:** Pharmacology, Toxicology, and Basic Health Sciences Unit, Faculty of Pharmacy, AIMST University, Bedong 08100, Kedah, Malaysia; E-mail: muthuraman.a@aimst.edu.my

Mukesh Singh Sikarwar, Arunachalam Muthuraman & Sohrab A. Shaikh (Eds.)

logical benefits and also support chronic disorders [1]. However, the major questions raised by the scientific community are about the evidence of the molecular mechanism and chemical structure of the responsible compounds. Sometimes, nutraceuticals fail to address the scientific evidence for the management of chronic disorders due to their multi-functional (pleiotropic) physiological/pharmacological actions, mechanisms of action, and safety and efficacy in clinical conditions [2]. Hence, numerous studies are required to establish the use of nutraceuticals in various chronic disorders in clinical conditions. Therefore, the challenges and therapeutic action of nutraceuticals in chronic disorders and the use of nutraceuticals with evidence-based clinical applications in various disorders can be warranted [3]. The basic approaches of clinical applications of nutraceuticals are categorized into nutrition, pharmaceuticals, and nutraceutical products [4]. Nutrition products provide support for essential physiological functions, and they are required daily. Pharmaceutical products provide the mitigation/treatment of abnormal physiological functions, and they are required in pathological conditions. Nutraceutical products play both functions and also produce the enhancement of physiological function and fight against the progression of the disease [5]. Hence, the net effects are producing the maximal benefits and more safety and efficacious action in clinical conditions.

The classification of nutraceuticals is wider, *i.e.*, vitamins (water and lipid-soluble vitamins); micro/macronutrients; essential fatty acids; pre- and probiotics; and phytochemicals (herbs). The broader definition of nutraceuticals is known as optimized food products with health benefits and treats chronic disorders [6, 7]. More precisely nutraceuticals are also considered non-nutrient secondary metabolites type of nutraceuticals *i.e.*, such as terpenoids, polyphenols, and glucosinolates, illustrated in Fig. (**1**). It has synergistic, agonistic, and antagonist actions. The standardization, quality control, and clinical benefits of nutraceuticals are well established [8]. However, the approval and recognition of the use of nutraceuticals in clinical conditions remains to be established with more scientific evidence. However, the regulatory process to approve the nutraceuticals in clinical conditions remains delayed and questionable. Certain regulatory bodies have started to approve nutraceuticals in various clinical conditions for the management of various disorders [9].

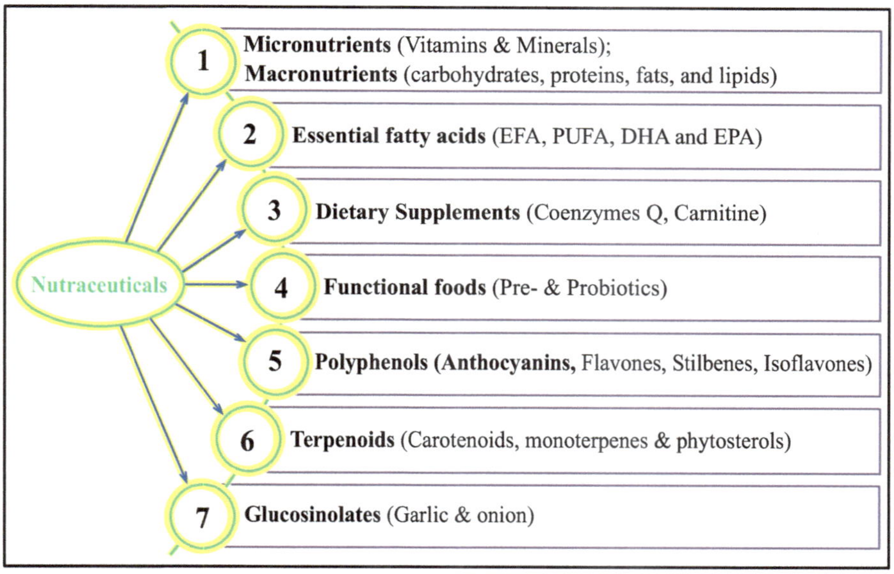

Fig. (1). Classification of nutraceuticals (Nutrient and non-nutrient types). *Abbreviations:* DHA, Docosahexaenoic Acid; EFA, Essential Fatty Acids; EPA, Eicosapentaenoic Acid; and PUFA, Polyunsaturated Fatty Acids.

Nutraceuticals have organ-protective roles in various disorders like cardiovascular diseases (hypertension, atherosclerosis), metabolic disorders (diabetes mellitus), arthritis, obesity, and cancer. Hence, it is also known as preventive medicine [10, 11]. Nevertheless, the legislation for the sales, marketing, safety, and efficacy of nutraceuticals in various regions around the world with cultural influence is a challenge [12]. This chapter discussed and summarized the use of nutraceuticals with regulatory requirements in various regions of the world. From the regulatory perspective, nutraceuticals are classified according to the regulatory framework and nutraceutical policy of the specific country [13]. Canada considers Natural Health Products (NHPs) and supplemented foods to be nutraceuticals. However, the European Food Safety Authority, the USA Food and Drug Administration (FDA), and Health Canada agencies allow use in clinical conditions based on the strength of scientific evidence and evaluation reports [9, 14]. Evidence-based medicines are integrated based on the available evidence for the decision-making process with Randomized Clinical Trials (RCTs). RCT permits a strong correlation between the interventions and outcomes [15].

Furthermore, RCT plays a central role in the regulatory process for the approval of drugs and health claims of nutraceuticals. However, the limitation of this RCT method of drug evaluation model is either sensitive or not relevant to nutraceuticals due to i) the inability of true placebos applications; ii) the effect size of healthy populations are often modest conditions; iii) the analysis with statistical methods always refocused; iv) endpoints should be multifunctional or global aspects; v) the proof of efficacy must be better than the probability of harmful actions which is always lacking in the RCT intervention; and vi) challenge to recruit the healthy participants [16, 17]. Furthermore, the major challenges and systems-based approaches of nutraceuticals in RCT trials are 1) weak interaction with diverse proteins (non-specific protein interactions); 2) adopting the rapid metabolic process and oxidized leads to generate the abundant quantity of reactive oxygen species (ROS); 3) the comprehensive omics (proteomics, metabolomics and genomics) approaches causes the protein enrichment, dysregulation of net physiological actions and difficult to differentiate the specific targets based actions leads to causalities with complex physiological actions [18, 19]. Crucially, the comparison of nutraceuticals and pharmaceuticals has a wide variety of actions, *i.e.*, nutraceuticals are consumed as normal food ingredients [1]. It has low potency, weak interaction with target proteins, can correlate with pleiotropic actions with physiological mechanisms, and inhibits the disease progression in chronic disorders and has very low levels of casualties [20]. However, pharmaceuticals are highly potent, have strong and specific interactions with targets for minimal physiological mechanisms, and treat the disease in short time intervals, unfortunately causing frequent casualties [21].

Current Landscape and Evaluation of Nutraceuticals

Currently, the market for nutraceuticals is high-impact in healthcare sectors, and it is a multi-billion-dollar industry. It is rapidly growing every decade. It comprises myriad food-derived products and is widely spread over the globe due to the rise in consumer education and awareness of the health benefits of nutraceuticals [22]. Nutraceutical markets cover products for aging populations, consumer health awareness, and consumer lifestyle changes. However, some nutraceuticals also hold promising preventive and therapeutic benefits. The major challenge to the legalization of nutraceutical products in the global market is the lack of an international definition, awareness, and framework of regulatory guidelines internationally and among countries. Furthermore, there is a lack of scientific evidence of nutraceutical efficacy, safety, and effectiveness [9, 23]. Moreover, food items also claim to have additional health benefits; hence, there needs to be proper regulation for nutraceutical products to be used in the healthcare system and launched in the global market [24].

The global market for nutraceutical products is influenced by the Food and Drug Administration (FDA). The FDA looks into the labeling of nutritional foods *via* "The Nutrition Labelling and Education Act, 1990". Besides, the FDA also controls the secure environment of food safety and innovation to prevent the misconduct of nutraceutical product manufacturing on an international level [25].

The USA adopted its own regulatory principles for nutraceutical products *via* the Dietary Supplement and Health Education Act (DSHEA) – 1994 [26]. Poland adopted the Food and Nutrition Safety Act (FNSA) in 2006 [27]. India also adopted the Food Safety and Standards Act (FSSA) in 2006 [28]. Furthermore, the Brazilian Health Regulatory Agency, *i.e.*, Anvisa, also connected with the Ministry of Health (part of the Brazilian National Health System and Brazilian Health Regulatory System, SNVS) regulates the multiple nutraceutical products that are used in our daily life [29]. The summary of the landscape and evaluation of nutraceutical products and the set of international regulations is depicted in Fig. (**2**).

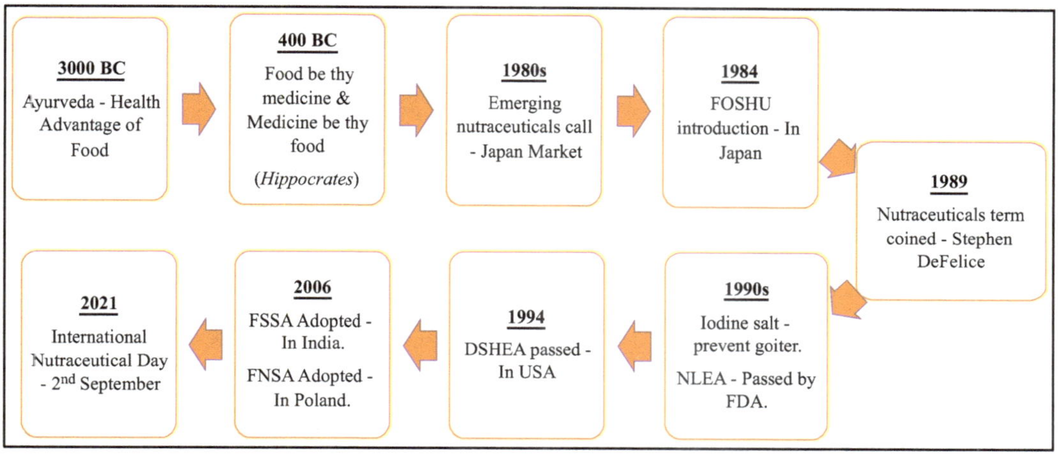

Fig. (2). Landscape and evaluation of nutraceuticals regulations. *Abbreviations:* DSHEA, Dietary Supplement Health and Education Act; FDA, Food and Drug Administration; FNSA, Food, Nutrition Safety Act; FOSHU, food for specific health uses; FSSA, Food Safety and Standard Act; NLEA, Nutrition Labelling and Education Act; and USA, United States of America.

Benefits of Nutraceuticals

Nutraceutical products are promising to improve health conditions. However, the evidence of pre-clinical data shows that the beneficial effects of nutraceuticals, phytochemical-enriched products, and food extracts are reducing the inflammatory reactions and free radical-associated injury [30]. According to the expert of the International Lipid Expert Panel (ILEP), nutraceutical approval applications claim that it reduces the risk factors for inflammation, lipid-associated disorders, statin intolerance, and heart failure [31]. Current literature data also revealed that it possesses the potential prophylactic actions or adjunct molecules for the treatment of various chronic disorders like aging, Alzheimer's disease, mental health, cancers, and metabolic disorders like diabetes mellitus [5]. However, multi-targeted and pleiotropic actions with safety concern in clinical trials needs to be investigated. Hence, consumers want to be safe and effective nutraceuticals to enhance their health, life, and well-being [29]. The primary molecular mechanism of nutraceuticals is proven to have free radical scavenging actions. Beyond that, it has inhibitory actions on the activation of Nuclear Factor kappa B (NF-κB); Phosphoinositide 3-kinases (PI3Ks)-Protein Kinase B (PKB)-mammalian target of rapamycin (mTOR) pathway; prevents the protein-DNA damage; reduce the Fenton reactions; chelate the metals; regulates the apoptotic and immunological proteins; mitochondrial protections; and enhance the cell proliferation [32, 33]. The mechanism of nutraceuticals for their clinical benefit is summarized in Fig. (**3**).

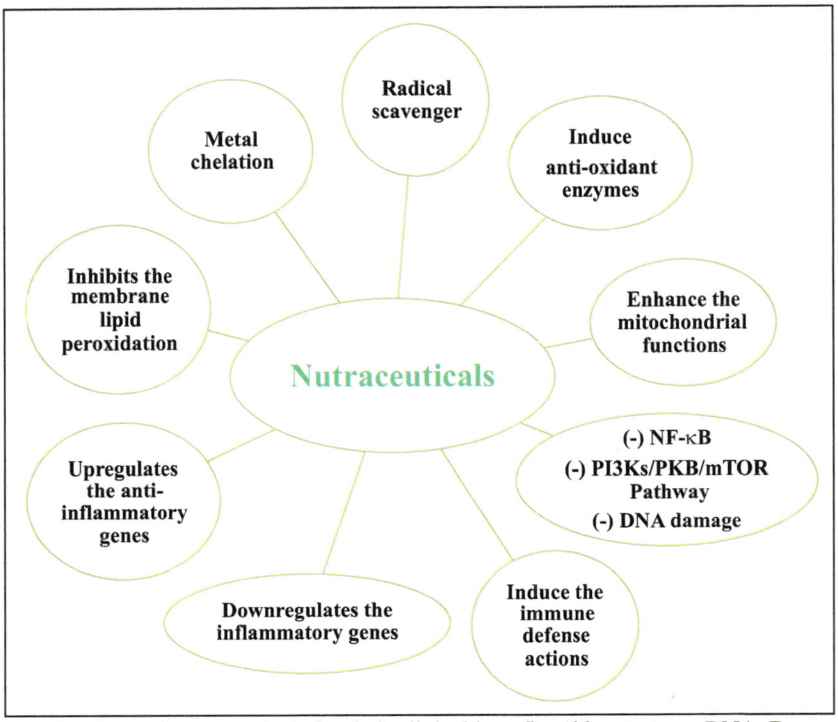

Fig. (3). The mechanisms of nutraceuticals for their clinical benefit. *Abbreviations:* DNA, Deoxyribonucleic Acid; mTOR, Mammalian Target of Rapamycin; NF-κB, Nuclear Factor Kappa B; PI3Ks, Phosphoinositide 3-kinases; and PKB, Protein Kinase B.

Insights into the Global Market of Nutraceutical Products

Over the last few decades, the healthcare sector has emerged to emphasize nutraceutical products, including diet and nutrition. Even health-conscious consumers have raised and shifted the trends to purchase dietary supplement products, functional foods, and nutraceuticals. It promises optimal health benefits and lacks negative health consequences [34]. It is an innovative concept to achieve the nutritive supplements with therapeutic benefits over the basic nutritional value. Moreover, multiple bioactive molecules and extracts of food and/or herbal and phytochemicals-enriched extracts are launched in the market, similar to pharmaceutical formulations like solutions, powders, gels, and capsules [35, 36]. The global nutraceutical product market was appraised at around 383 billion USD in 2016; around 561 billion USD in 2022; and reached 712.97 billion USD in 2023. Hence, the nutraceutical industry is flourishing and diversifying rapidly every year [37]. The current scenario of the nutraceutical product market is geared towards preventive health care management of disease rather than the treatment of disease. Due to the rising healthcare costs, the global market is turning towards the management of chronic disease with nutraceutical products in both developing and developed countries [38, 39]. According to the report of Klynveld Peat Marwick Goerdeler (KPMG), the nutraceuticals market was expected to be worth around 250 billion USD in 2018. However, the growth of the nutraceutical industry reached about 7.3% of the Compound Annual Growth Rate (CAGR) between 2018 and 2021 [40, 41].

The USA is the largest consumer of nutraceuticals and has the largest nutraceutical market. The USA nutraceuticals market has raised CAGR value from 5.5 to 6.0% between 2016 and 2022. It covers the supplementary products of dietary and immune-boosting products; energy drinks; protein supplements, and pre- and probiotics [42]. In Canada, 750 Canadian nutraceutical companies gained more than 11 billion USD in revenue in 2011 based on specializing in Functional Foods and Natural Health Products (FFNHP). The Canadian nutraceuticals market has experienced a 5.62% growth rate between 2019 and 2024 due to rising concerns about the potential health benefits [43]. Now, the Natural Health Products Directorate (NHPD) is known as the Natural and Non-prescription Health Products Directorate (NNHPD). NNHPD granted 27,900 nutraceutical product licenses over 43,000 natural health products. It indicates that nutraceutical products have a greater demand in the global market [9, 44]. The nutraceutical products market in the Asia-Pacific is also experiencing rapid growth. The market value of nutraceuticals was 31% in 2019, and it rose to more than 89.6 billion USD in 2021 with a CAGR of 8.52% between 2016 and 2021. Furthermore, the functional food ingredients market is expected to reach a CAGR of 5.9% between 2016 and 2026 and 5.04 billion USD by the end of 2026 [45, 46]. The Chinese nutraceutical market is the second-largest market in the world. According to a 2017 report, China created 39.5% of the growth and 80.9 billion USD value of nutraceutical products [45]. Japan's nutraceuticals market is in fifth position in the Asia-Pacific nutraceutical market share value. In the year 1991, the Japanese government introduced the Foods for Specified Health Use (FOSHU) regulatory bodies. It covers the functional foods market and its use in off-label health claims. The total retail value of FOSHU-approved nutraceutical products was 6.2 billion USD in 2007 [9].

The nutraceutical products industry in India has shown rapid flourishing markets in the Asia-Pacific region. It reached 2.2-2.8 213 billion USD values in 2015. The growth rate reached around 20% with 6.1 billion USD between the years 2019 and 2020, and rose to 8.5 billion USD in the year 2022 [26]. Indian nutraceutical products were claimed to treat sedentary lifestyles associated with disorders like hyperlipidemia, obesity, hypertension, cardiovascular diseases, and diabetes mellitus [47]. The United Kingdom (UK) and European Union (EU) markets for nutraceutical products are the third-largest market value in the world [48]. Germany, France, and Italy are key areas for nutraceutical product markets. Moreover, the UK and Spain are employed in the sales markets for nutraceutical products [49, 50]. The European market value reached 79.7 billion USD in the year 2016. The CAGR percentage reached 6.39% between 2018 and 2023. Germany covers 23.02% of the nutraceutical products' share of Europe, followed by the UK and France. Furthermore, the value is raised 11.0 billion USD in the year 2016 with a 6.37% CAGR value [45, 51]. Central and Latin America (Brazil and Argentina) are the fourth-largest nutraceutical product market in the world. Hence, the rapid expansion of the nutraceutical market is due to the trend of interest and awareness of healthy living. Brazil's market reached 13 billion USD value in 2005 and rose to around 13.25 billion USD in 2021 with a CAGR percentage of 7.96%. It is expected to raise 19.4 billion USD in 2026. Brazil is gaining 5.3% of shares of global revenues *via* the nutraceutical products market [46, 52].

Key Factors to Drive the Nutraceutical Market

The nutraceutical product industry is mainly driven by consumer interest in developing a healthy lifestyle and therapy for chronic disease in both developing and developed countries. The understanding of primary factors and other key factors about the nutraceutical market driving force will support the capture of the opportunities for growth, expansion, and segmentation of the global market [12]. The key factors of the nutraceutical market are 1) the *aging population*; 2) *Consumer awareness*; 3) the *Increasing cost of healthcare*; and 4) the *increasing number of distribution channels* [34]. The aging process is a natural biological event that leads to certain apparent chronic diseases like dementia, Alzheimer's disease, cardiovascular disorders, respiratory problems, osteoporosis, and cataracts [53]. Healthy aging is one of the best ways to live a healthy, happy life. Nutraceuticals with a nutritious diet promise to support the living of an active and healthy life. Furthermore, nutraceuticals are proven to protect the organs from rapid aging and stress. Some of the nutraceuticals are also evidenced to raise concern for promoting cellular longevity and well-being for the elderly population [54].

The awareness of consumer health is raising the benefits to their healthy life. The intake of improved lifestyles, nutritional diets, nutraceutical products, education programs, and active health awareness information (social media) is driving the growth of the nutraceuticals market [55]. This market growth is steadily rising with consumers' awareness and interest in the USA and Canada. In the Asia-Pacific region, the growth of the nutraceuticals market has risen based on middle-class consumers due to urbanization and the incidence of lifestyle-associated disorders like diabetes mellitus, hypertension, and other cardiovascular diseases [56]. The management of chronic disorders with pharmaceuticals is rising every year. Nutraceuticals are an alternative option to manage chronic disorders. The low-cost factors make the raising of nutraceuticals consumers and the nutraceuticals market than the pharmaceuticals market [57]. Moreover, nutraceuticals not only support the improvement of health but also reduce healthcare expenses. This is one of the reasons to raise the substantial nutraceutical market in the USA, Canada, the Asia-Pacific region, and Mexico. However, raising the number of distribution channels of nutraceutical products helps to reach the products to consumers and expand the nutraceuticals market [58]. The distribution channels, like online ordering and selling, direct telemarketing, business-to-business channels, and business-to-consumer channels, are promising to capture the nutraceutical market value [59]. Euromonitor International Research report evidenced that the vitamin and supplement market is worth 60.2 billion EUR by internet sales. Globally, 44% of nutraceuticals were purchased through online methods. India was well established in the online market for nutraceuticals with the largest online population [39, 60].

CURRENT REGULATIONS SPECIFIC TO NUTRACEUTICALS

The concept of nutraceutical products and related terms and definitions remains a grey area between food, food supplements, and pharmaceuticals. The definition of nutraceutical products and assessment of their potential therapeutic actions is subject to debate for global acceptance by regulatory bodies [61]. For instance, in Japan, functional foods are considered based on their use of natural ingredients; whereas in the USA, they are considered as ingredients that are produced with biotechnological methods [9]. This kind of divergence in the definitions of nutraceuticals across different countries and regulatory bodies has critical implications. Moreover, the global arrangement of harmonized legislation and regulations for nutraceutical product growth and distribution is also an additional complication [34]. However, the existence of different regulations in various countries can result in avoiding ambiguity and inconsistency when defining nutraceutical products in the presence of multiple countries [62]. In the year 1992, the major millstone was set by the United Nations Food and Agriculture Organization (FAO) and the World Health Organization (WHO) in the Codex

Alimentarius for the evaluation of the efficacy and safety of food [63]. However, this internationally recognized guideline helps to find the general rules for producing and marketing foodstuffs and their derivatives in many countries. It also helps to define the health claims, terms of nutrient function, enhanced function, and risk reduction to market nutraceutical products among the nations and regions.

European Regulations

The European Food Safety Authority (EFSA) covers the guidelines for defining and marketing food supplements. However, officially, it does not mention or recognize nutraceutical products. Furthermore, it does not describe the divergence between food supplements and nutraceuticals in the application of the healthcare process [14]. The claim of nutraceuticals' medicinal value is required to conform to regulatory bodies with evidence of efficacy, safety, and quality testing reports. Hence, European regulations recommended that nutraceuticals must be monitored as a food component under Directive 2002/46/EC or a medicinal product under Directive 2004/27/EC sections [64]. Besides, the safety of nutraceutical supplements is monitored under Directive 2002/46/EC by EFSA and the European Commission. It is synchronized with various legislations, *i.e.*, Regulation EC 1924/2006 for claiming nutritional health [61]. The primary aim of this European regulation is to instill confidence among nutraceutical consumers by making the availability of understandable product information and ensuring the safety and efficacy of nutraceutical products [40]. According to EFSA guidelines, the claim of nutraceuticals must be labeled on the packaging of products. Since 2005, Europe has also been the home of the European Nutraceutical Association (ENA) to evaluate nutraceuticals [65].

USA Regulations

The Food and Drug Administration (FDA) partially plays a role in the regulation of nutraceuticals *via* the Dietary Supplement Health and Education Act and the Food and Drug Administration Modernization Act (FDAMA) of 1997. Furthermore, botanical preparation doesn't require any clinical testing for marketing [13]. Anyway, botanical preparation is labeled as a drug substance for diagnosis, prevention, and curative purposes; the manufacturer needs to provide the data on clinical efficacy and safety for the review of Over-The-Counter (OTC) drugs [66]. According to the DSHEA, the manufacturer is responsible for the evidence of nutraceutical safety. Furthermore, the marketing of nutraceuticals must meet certain criteria *i.e.*, i) it should be intended for ingestion in the form of capsule, tablet, pill, powder, or liquid; ii) It is not used as a conventional food or sole item of meal/diet; and iii) It should be labeled as a "*dietary supplement*" [67].

The FDA also established the Office of Dietary Supplement Programs (ODSP) to ensure the safety and efficacy of nutraceutical products for production and marketing. This also raises the concern and responsibility to take manufacturers to task for adequate protection of consumers [68]. Truly, manufacturers are not required to get approval or registration for their nutraceutical products from the FDA for marketing [13]. Sometimes, it engages the consumer at risky, unsafe, and inefficient conditions due to a lack of preclinical and clinical evidence.

Canadian Regulations

The regulation of nutraceutical products in Canada is governed by the Food and Drugs Authority of Health Canada (FDAHC). Most of the drugs are regulated than food products [69]. It covers homeopathic medicines, herbal remedies, traditional Chinese medicines, vitamins and minerals, probiotics, and other products like amino acids and fatty acids [70, 71].

Russian Regulations

The Russian Federation Food Security Doctrine regulates nutraceutical products with the Biologically Active Dietary Supplements (BADS) process scheme [62, 72]. According to Russian regulations, nutraceuticals are considered foodstuffs with clinically proven data evidence for their effectiveness for the actions of prophylaxis for the prevention of pharmaceutical products associated side effects and the accomplishment of complete remission [73]. Furthermore, the definition of nutraceutical products includes amino acids, dietary fibers, minerals, vitamins, and para-pharmaceutical products like alkaloids, bioflavonoids, essential oils, and polysaccharides [74].

Indian Regulations

Indian regulations don't provide the legal status for the marketing of nutraceuticals. The Food Safety and Standards Act (FSSA) was established in 2006. However, it does not differentiate dietary supplements, nutraceuticals, and functional foods [75]. In the market, it is indicated as food for a specialized dietary application. In India, for more than 1000 years, Ayurvedic medicines have been practiced with natural medicinal products [76]. It is also made a well-practiced and tested medicine with supervised administration of natural products [60].

Asia-Pacific Region and Other Countries Regulations

Japan is the first country to regulate food supplements and foodstuff-related issues by its regulatory authority, *i.e.*, Foods for Specified Health Use (FOSHU) [9]. However, other countries like Australia and China regulate nutraceuticals marketing with consideration of the food category [72, 77]. Some countries, like Argentina, Brazil, and Colombia, have the simplest registrations based on local authority approaches, *i.e.*, a notification-based approach [78]. It is valid in Mexico and Chile. China, Taiwan, and Brazil also have restricted stern requirements for nutraceutical registration without evidence of complete animal and/or human clinical data (Mandatory) [72].

Concerns of Nutraceutical Safety and Efficacy

Nutraceuticals are proven to show the potential for partial prevention and treatment of various ailments, including chronic disorders. In contrast, there is a lack of sufficient information on nutraceuticals to prove their safety and efficacy, possible mechanisms of action, and randomized clinical trials for their beneficial effects in the treatment of chronic disorders [65]. Moreover, single food constituents like micronutrients or secondary metabolites are reported *in vitro* studies and considered as safe, whereas still validated data with fastidious studies [79]. Therefore, it needs to conduct clinical trials for safety and efficacy assessments, and evaluation of bioavailability and mechanism of action of nutraceuticals [80]. Besides, the monitoring of nutraceutical production is also essential. Globally, this step is mostly overlooked in the consideration of nutraceutical regulations. Nutraceuticals may be toxic to consumers due to the presence of allergens, fertilizers, pesticides, heavy metals, mycotoxins, and residues of toxic plants during production [81]. Nutraceuticals as therapeutic agents must address the risk of adverse pharmacokinetic or pharmacodynamic interactions. On the other hand, patients opted for the consumption of supplements and pharmaceuticals, which causes complications to patient health [82]. For instance, peppermint oil readily interacts with isoforms of cytochrome P450, leading to modification of the various drugs' metabolism [83], and tyramine-containing nutraceuticals interact with monoamine oxidase inhibitors, leading to altered anti-depressive actions [84]. This kind of adverse reaction can cause life-threatening effects like hypertensive crisis, hyperthermia, cerebral hemorrhage, and cardiac arrhythmia. Herbal remedies like tonics, supplements, and nutraceuticals also have serious concerns due to the presence of natural botanical toxicants [85, 86]. *Aristolochia* herbs are used for the treatment of seizures in traditional Chinese medicine, whereas they are known to cause carcinogenic effects [87]. Therefore, Good Manufacturing Practices (GMP) and safety monitoring processes must be prosecuted by regulation bodies to ensure consumer's trust and safety in nutraceuticals.

Regulatory bodies have difficulty making a decree on the narcotics and cannabidiol industry. Phytocannabinoid, *i.e.*, cannabidiol, is extracted from *Cannabis* plants and mixed with sunflower oil, and it doesn't have a psychoactive isomer, *i.e.*, Δ9-tetrahydrocannabinol (THC) [88]. Moreover, the cannabidiol industry has a higher interest in manufacturing cannabidiol due to its medicinal value. This market value is 9.67 million USD and is expected to reach 5.3 billion USD in the year 2025 [43]. Clinical use of cannabidiol oil (Epidiolex®) was approved by the FDA for Dravet syndrome and Lennox-Gastaut syndrome (epileptic disorders) in children. Currently, it is used for neuropathic pain, anxiety, Parkinson's disease, and schizophrenia [89]. However, serious adverse reactions are also noted with cannabidiol in human trials. The 0.3% THC-containing *Cannabis* plant (industrial hemp) was removed by the USA Agriculture Improvement Act - Schedule I of the Controlled Substances Act in the year 2018. It means hemp was categorized as an agricultural raw material or a primary agricultural product, which raises the market value of hemp-derived cannabidiol [90]. Furthermore, cannabidiol is considered a "novel food" by EFSA in Europe. However, the safe consumption of cannabidiol is not demonstrated as per the amended Regulation (EU 2015/2283) of previous reiterations. Recent regulatory bodies of EFSA have not approved cannabidiol; however, numerous cannabidiol-derived products are available in European countries [91].

The approval of dietary supplements and nutraceuticals for treatment by the regulatory bodies is still challenging. Moreover, some of the nutraceuticals were approved with solid evidence of their safety and efficacy in clinical trials. The tomato-based nutraceutical product (Fruitflow®) of Provexis claims that it has anti-platelet actions and is granted permission by EFSA. This is the first nutraceutical product granted by EFSA [92]. The health claim of products is not only nutraceutical products, but also novel food and functional ingredients, which are also encouraged to get approval with evidence of clinical trial safety data. EFSA also approved a peptide obtained from *Pandalus borealis* in 2018 for the management of hypotensive conditions. This peptide was formulated by Medfiles for a Norwegian company [93]. Nevertheless, some of the products failed to get health claims MegaNatural®-BP grape seed extract was claimed to regulate normal blood pressure, but it was rejected by USA regulatory bodies due to a lack of clinical evidence [94]. It is evidenced that claiming nutraceutical product approval requires well-designed clinical trials with solid evidence of safety and efficacy to consumers. However, the requirement of clinical trial data may raise the burden on the manufacturers of nutraceutical products leading to engagement in the development of innovative nutraceutical products which can raise the cost of products for consumer usage.

FUTURE PERSPECTIVES OF NUTRACEUTICALS

Some of the nutraceuticals are proven to prevent and cure chronic disorders at a lower cost. Furthermore, the preparation and development of nutraceuticals are rapid in a short time, and they are administered as herbal compounds and as food ingredients [95]. The effect of nutraceuticals is mostly assessed by data obtained from epidemiological studies, safety profile information, and the cost involved in the clinical trials. Moreover, nutraceutical products minimize disease progression with low cost, minimal manufacturing time, lack of unpleasant side effects, and simpler clinical procedures than pharmaceutical products [96]. However, the approval and legal use of nutraceuticals as medicines need to address certain points in the clinical, regulatory, and research aspects [64]. In clinical aspects, nutraceuticals are considered for the management of certain diseases due to their multi-targeted pleiotropic actions [97]. For instance, curcumin is obtained from turmeric, and it is proven to reduce lipids, hypertension, free radical-associated injury, and inflammation, including the improvement of insulin sensitivity [30]. However, more interpretation is needed in the aspects of mechanisms, pharmacokinetics, and pharmacodynamics of nutraceutical compounds in clinical and preclinical research reports [98]. Besides, the evidence of safety and efficacy must also be addressed in clinical evaluations. It will help to change the nutraceutical products into drugs rather than as nutraceutical supplements [99]. Anyway, the fund allotment is mainly received for drug discovery and development, and testing at pre-clinical and clinical levels compared to fund allotment for nutraceuticals and supplements [100]. Therefore, more fund allotments for nutraceutical research for clinical trials will make the more interest in clinical research more interesting to scientists, increase the approval of more nutraceuticals as medicines, raise consumer trust in nutraceutical medicines, and raise the market value of nutraceutical products.

In regulatory aspects, the clear identification/classification of nutraceuticals as medicines is important, with evidence of safety and efficacy data in clinical trials similar to pharmaceuticals [95]. Furthermore, food supplement legislation must be focused on addressing the issues of nutraceutical safety and the labeling process [101]. The regulatory bodies must permit the identification/classification of nutraceutical products to prove their clinical benefits. It will help to give more clarity about the quality of nutraceuticals, the mechanism of action, efficacy, and safety awareness to consumers [61]. For instance, EFSA allowed exploring the novel food and its health benefits to consumers with evidence of clinical safety and efficacy of nutraceuticals. However, it will prevent small innovative nutraceutical companies from applying for novel food status and health claims due to the requirement of nutraceutical safety and efficacy data from clinical trials

[102]. The regulatory bodies and medical guidelines can offer the tools for bringing awareness about nutraceutical benefits and safety to consumers. The manufacturer of nutraceutical products needs to focus on the quality of products to obtain the identification and classification of nutraceuticals as medicine by providing a detailed description of the product specifications (on the label) [23, 96]. Moreover, it is used as an add-on therapy, not a first-line therapeutic agent; certain conditions prefer to use nutraceuticals over drugs like statins to avoid lower cholesterol, according to the recommendation of nutraceuticals [103]. In contrast, some physicians treat the patient with unproven effects of cannabidiol products instead of standard medical care [104]. Hence, well-structured guidelines need to be framed for the effective use of nutraceuticals in patients and support the growth of the nutraceuticals market.

The interest of regulatory bodies, consumers, public interest, and growing market value on nutraceuticals needs to be systematically identified with the benefits and safety of nutraceuticals [55]. More research needs to encourage the identification of the nutraceutical's health benefits to create opportunities and fill the gaps for nutraceutical product approval [105]. The data from a meta-analysis of clinical trials, epidemiological/observational, and pilot studies can be used to highlight the nutraceuticals and their (more nutraceutical) formulation's effectiveness and safety [106]. It makes the base for the rapid approval, clinical recommendation, and effective improvement of the nutraceutical market values.

SUMMARY

Current regulations about the use of nutraceuticals for chronic disorders emphasize consumer safety and efficacy. The regulation demands strong evidence about the nutraceutical products' safety based on pre-clinical and clinical data. However, the global recognition for the use of nutraceuticals as medicine is still debated due to their lack of a clear definition, classification, and category. Some regulations allow nutraceuticals to be used in practice to treat the disease. However, a few nutraceuticals/phytochemicals like cannabidiol are restricted from use as medicine in some countries. Hence, clear recommendations are needed to evaluate nutraceuticals in the aspects of clinical, regulatory, and research directions.

Therefore, globally acceptable and recognized nutraceutical products can be brought as medicine with clinical safety evidence, definitions, and classifications. This book chapter covers all aspects of the regulation of nutraceuticals, the regulatory requirements for nutraceuticals as medicine, and recommendations of nutraceutical-based medicine to bring to the market with consumer trust and health.

CASE STUDIES AND PRACTICE QUESTIONS

Case 1: *Malaysia's regulatory challenges highlight issues in using the pawpaw fruit, like the lack of specific legislation for nutraceuticals, leading to inconsistent regulation and unverified health claims on social media.*

Discussion Questions

a. Describe Malaysia's Control of Drugs and Cosmetics Regulation 1984.
b. What is the unsupervised production of nutraceutical products?
c. Briefly discuss the US-FDA description of nutraceutical products.
d. What are the "cure" claims of Pawpaw (*Asimina triloba*) fruit?
e. What are the major challenges in the efficacy and regulation of nutraceuticals?

Case 2: *According to Japanese regulations and innovation in dietary supplements, the foods with function claim (FFC) system facilitates the market entry of small and mid-size enterprises and promotes the creation of high-value products through innovative company efforts.*

Discussion Questions

a. Describe the food with function claims in Japan for dietary supplements.
b. Briefly discuss the "Food for Specified Health Uses" (FOSHU) and "Food with Nutrient Function Claims" (FNFC).
c. Does Japan have strict food regulations?
d. Discuss the arguments against the use of dietary supplements.
e. Are supplements regulated in Japan?

Case 3: *The United Nations Food and Agriculture Organization (FAO) and the World Health Organization (WHO) in the Codex Alimentarius (FAO/WHO 1992) describe assessing the safety and use of food.*

Discussion Questions

a. Describe how to safely use the food and dietary supplements.
b. Describe the terms of i) nutrient function, ii) enhanced function, and iii) reduction of risk according to the FAO/WHO 1992 guidelines of food and dietary supplements.
c. Briefly discuss the quality of nutraceutical formulation with physical and chemical stability, adequate safety, technological feasibility, and cost-effectiveness.

d. What are the major challenges for the various dosage formulations of dietary supplements?

MCQs Questions

1. Which one of the following properties supports the benefits of genetically modified food?
   A. Improved taste
   B. Low nutritional value
   C. Low crop productivity
   D. Higher production costs

2. What is a primary goal of applying evidence-based practice to deliver dietary supplements and complementary and alternative medicine (CAM)?
   A. To promote the use of all available supplements
   B. To discourage any use of supplements and CAM
   C. To rely solely on traditional use and anecdotal reports
   D. To critically evaluate and apply the best available evidence to guide patient care decisions

3. Which type of acts allows the manufacturers to make the dietary supplements without FDA pre-approval?
   A. Dietary Supplements Access Act
   B. Federal Food, Drug, and Cosmetic Act
   C. National Pharmaceutical Regulatory Agency (NPRA)
   D. Dietary supplements health and education act of 1994 (DSHEA)

4. Which type of claims allows the manufacturers under DSHEA?
   A. Drug claims
   B. Structure/function claims
   C. Disease-specific health claims
   D. Claims the product can diagnose, cure, mitigate, and treat

5. Which one of the clinical trial designs provides the highest level of evidence on dietary supplements?
   A. Case report
   B. Expert opinion
   C. Observational study
   D. Randomized controlled trial (RCT)

Answers: 1) A; 2) D; 3) D; 4) B; 5) D

REFERENCES

[1] Amanullah M, Nahid M, Hosen SMZ, Akther S, Kauser-Ul-Alam M. The nutraceutical value of foods and its health benefits: a review. Health Dynamics 2024; 1(8): 273-83. [http://dx.doi.org/10.33846/hd10802]

[2] Neha S. Chaudhary, P. Tiwari, S. Parvez, Amelioration of phytanic acid–induced neurotoxicity by nutraceuticals: mechanistic insights. Mol Neurobiol 2024; 1-16.

[3] Saxena S, Singh R, Dutta D, Gautam N, Setya S, Talegaonkar S. Nutraceuticals and their applications: recent trends and challenges. Anxiety, Gut Microbiome, and Nutraceuticals 2024; pp. 1-32.

[4] More BH, Bhat PS, Singh MR, Tasgaonkar RR. Nutraceuticals: an alternative to pharmaceuticals. World Journal of Biology Pharmacy and Health Sciences 2024; 19(1): 362-70. [http://dx.doi.org/10.30574/wjbphs.2024.19.1.0414]

[5] Ramesh V, Subbarayan K, Viswanathan S, Subramanian K. Role of nutraceuticals in the management of lifestyle diseases. Role of Herbal Medicines: Management of Lifestyle Diseases. Springer 2024; pp. 461-78.

[6] Gorain S. Functional Foods and Nutraceuticals. Micronutrients and Macronutrients as Nutraceuticals. Apple Academic Press 2024; pp. 1-45.

[7] Sharma DK. Immunity-boosting macronutrients and micronutrients. Micronutrients and Macronutrients as Nutraceuticals. Apple Academic Press 2024; pp. 131-66.

[8] Srivastav A, Shukla AK, Kumar M, Kumar S, Mishr RK. Nutraceutical bioactive compounds in fruits and vegetables. Plant Metabolites and Vegetables as Nutraceuticals. Apple Academic Press 2025; pp. 111-42.

[9] Thakur S, Gupta MM, Sharma D. Nutraceuticals regulation: an overview of the regulatory frameworks in USA. EU, and Japan, Nutraceutical Fruits and Foods for Neurodegenerative Disorders 2024; pp. 421-40.

[10] Singh AK, Mehta R, Singh A, Arya RKK. Nutraceutical herbs in obesity and diabetes. Herbals as Nutraceuticals. Apple Academic Press 2024; pp. 197-216. [http://dx.doi.org/10.1201/9781003488392-12]

[11] Bhuvaneshwari G, Ganiger VM, Narayanpur VB, Allolli TB. Nutraceuticals: classification, sources and relation with medicine. Frontiers in Food Biotechnology. Springer 2024; pp. 29-55. [http://dx.doi.org/10.1007/978-981-97-3261-6_3]

[12] Sen P, Khulbe P, Gupta M, Thapa R. Challenges for incorporation of nutraceuticals in food. Formulations, Regulations, and Challenges of Nutraceuticals. Apple Academic Press 2025; pp. 285-319.

[13] Bhardwaj M. Regulatory framework for the development of nutraceuticals. Formulations, Regulations, and Challenges of Nutraceuticals. Apple Academic Press 2025; pp. 213-24.

[14] Sharma G. Regulatory guidelines for the development of plant/phytochemical-based nutraceuticals. Formulations, Regulations, and Challenges of Nutraceuticals. Apple Academic Press 2025; pp. 171-91.

[15] Arnold R, Murphy-Smith J, Ng CH, *et al.* Predictors of the placebo response in a nutraceutical randomized controlled trial for depression. J Integr Med 2024; 22(1): 46-53. [http://dx.doi.org/10.1016/j.joim.2024.01.007] [PMID: 38331652]

[16] Bhattarai P, Rai S, Koirala P, Nirmal NP. Computational approach and its application in the nutraceutical industry. Bioactive Extraction and Application in Food and Nutraceutical Industries. Springer 2024; pp. 449-68. [http://dx.doi.org/10.1007/978-1-0716-3601-5_18]

[17] Gutiérrez-Romero SA, Torres-Narváez ES, Zamora-Gómez AC, *et al.* Effect of a nutraceutical combination on sleep quality among people with impaired sleep: a randomised, placebo-controlled

trial. Sci Rep 2024; 14(1): 8062.
[http://dx.doi.org/10.1038/s41598-024-58661-z] [PMID: 38580720]

[18] Mukherjee A, Maheshwari U, Sharma V, Sharma A, Kumar S. Functional insight into multi-omic--based interventions for climatic resilience in sorghum (Sorghum bicolor): a nutritionally rich cereal crop. Planta 2024; 259(4): 91.
[http://dx.doi.org/10.1007/s00425-024-04365-7] [PMID: 38480598]

[19] Missong H, Joshi R, Khullar N, *et al.* Nutrient-epigenome interactions: Implications for personalized nutrition against aging-associated diseases. J Nutr Biochem 2024; 127: 109592.
[http://dx.doi.org/10.1016/j.jnutbio.2024.109592] [PMID: 38325612]

[20] Li L, Wang L, Zhang L. Therapeutic potential of natural compounds from herbs and nutraceuticals in alleviating neurological disorders: targeting the wnt signaling pathway. J Agric Food Chem 2024; 72(5): 2411-33.
[http://dx.doi.org/10.1021/acs.jafc.3c07536] [PMID: 38284360]

[21] Li J, Zelmat Y, Storck W, *et al.* Drug-induced depressive symptoms: An update through the WHO pharmacovigilance database. J Affect Disord 2024; 350: 452-67.
[http://dx.doi.org/10.1016/j.jad.2024.01.119] [PMID: 38244800]

[22] Sharma R, Longo L, Gonzalez M, *et al.* Nutraceutical and dietary supplement use in the cancer population: The impact of evidence-based education. 2024.

[23] Pandey P, Pal R, Koli M, *et al.* A traditional review: the utilization of nutraceutical as a traditional cure for the modern world at current prospectus for multiple health conditions. J Drug Deliv Ther 2024; 14(3): 154-63.
[http://dx.doi.org/10.22270/jddt.v14i3.6445]

[24] Ahire JJ, Rohilla A, Kumar V, Tiwari A. Quality management of probiotics: Ensuring safety and maximizing health benefits. Curr Microbiol 2024; 81(1): 1.
[http://dx.doi.org/10.1007/s00284-023-03526-3] [PMID: 37935938]

[25] Abdelwahab SI, Elhassan Taha MM, Mariod AA, Al-Foraih M, Al-Asmari H. Exploring nutraceuticals: a comprehensive examination of inception, thematic mapping, evolution, emerging trends, and gaps. Curr Res Nutr Food Sci 2024; 12(1): 41-57.
[http://dx.doi.org/10.12944/CRNFSJ.12.1.04]

[26] Kausar M, Arya RKK, Bisht D, Keservani RK. Current concepts and prospects of herbal nutraceuticals. Herbals as Nutraceuticals 2024; pp. 51-66.
[http://dx.doi.org/10.1201/9781003488392-4]

[27] Kowalska A, Bieniek M, Manning L. Food supplements' non-conformity in Europe – Poland: A case study. Trends Food Sci Technol 2019; 93: 262-70.
[http://dx.doi.org/10.1016/j.tifs.2019.09.022]

[28] Banerjee K, van den Bijgaart H, Holroyd S, Knödlseder M, Konings E. Food safety challenges in the dairy supply chain in India: Controlling risks and developing a structured surveillance system. Int Dairy J 2024; 157: 106004.
[http://dx.doi.org/10.1016/j.idairyj.2024.106004]

[29] Santamarina AB, de Freitas JA, Franco LAM, *et al.* Nutraceutical blends predict enhanced health *via* microbiota reshaping improving cytokines and life quality: a Brazilian double-blind randomized trial. Sci Rep 2024; 14(1): 11127.
[http://dx.doi.org/10.1038/s41598-024-61909-3] [PMID: 38750102]

[30] Dama A, Shpati K, Daliu P, Dumur S, Gorica E, Santini A. Targeting metabolic diseases: the role of nutraceuticals in modulating oxidative stress and inflammation. Nutrients 2024; 16(4): 507.
[http://dx.doi.org/10.3390/nu16040507] [PMID: 38398830]

[31] Katamesh BE, Mickow AA, Huang L, *et al.* Overcoming patient reluctance to statin intolerance. Kardiol Pol 2024; 82(5): 485-91.

[http://dx.doi.org/10.33963/v.phj.100526] [PMID: 38712783]

[32] Agu PC, Afiukwa CA, Orji OU, *et al.* Molecular docking as a tool for the discovery of molecular targets of nutraceuticals in diseases management. Sci Rep 2023; 13(1): 13398. [http://dx.doi.org/10.1038/s41598-023-40160-2] [PMID: 37592012]

[33] Ramli NZ, Yahaya MF, Tooyama I, Damanhuri HA. A mechanistic evaluation of antioxidant nutraceuticals on their potential against age-associated neurodegenerative diseases. Antioxidants 2020; 9(10): 1019. [http://dx.doi.org/10.3390/antiox9101019] [PMID: 33092139]

[34] Wachira SW. Factors to consider in development of nutraceutical and dietary supplements. Pharmacognosy. Elsevier 2024; pp. 757-68. [http://dx.doi.org/10.1016/B978-0-443-18657-8.00032-3]

[35] Parihar N, Naraharisetti T, Patil P, Vathsan S, Deepak BPVP. Future trends in the formulation of nutraceuticals. Formulations, Regulations, and Challenges of Nutraceuticals. Apple Academic Press 2025; pp. 81-104.

[36] A.M. Bhoite, U.P. Patil, H.U. Bagul, S.G. Talele, A. Jadhav, Overview of formulation, challenges, and regulation for the development of nutraceutical, formulations, regulations, and challenges of nutraceuticals. (2025) 3–27.

[37] Colletti A, Procchio C, Pisano M, Martelli A, Pellizzato M, Cravotto G. An evaluation of the effects of pineapple-extract and bromelain-based treatment after mandibular third molar surgery: a randomized three-arm clinical study. Nutrients 2024; 16(6): 784. [http://dx.doi.org/10.3390/nu16060784] [PMID: 38542694]

[38] Vij S, Kumar R, Singh AP, Singh AP, Sharma P. Nutraceuticals: a review. Safety (Basel) 2024; 8: 2.

[39] Ahmad S. India's growing demand of nutraceuticals, asian journal of pharmaceutical research and development 2024.

[40] Yadav VK, Shukla AK, Kumar M, Arya M, Tiwari R. Recent advancements in herbal nutraceuticals. Herbals as Nutraceuticals. Apple Academic Press 2024; pp. 263-87. [http://dx.doi.org/10.1201/9781003488392-16]

[41] Bansal K, Sundram S, Malviya R. Herbal components inspiring current lifestyle disease treatment: role of nutraceuticals. Curr Drug Res Rev 2024; 16(2): 111-27. [http://dx.doi.org/10.2174/2589977515666230512142020] [PMID: 37183457]

[42] Intrasook J, Tsusaka TW, Anal AK. Trends and current food safety regulations and policies for functional foods and beverages containing botanicals. Yao Wu Shi Pin Fen Xi 2024; 32(2): 118-45. [http://dx.doi.org/10.38212/2224-6614.3499] [PMID: 38934687]

[43] Fiebig F. Strategic legal imperatives for directors to consider the context of legalised substance industries: identifying potential future challenges for Psilocybin businesses in South Africa though a comparative study of Cannabis Regulation in the USA. Canada and the Netherlands 2024.

[44] Rao TJM, Kesharwani RK, Keservani RK, Sharma AK. Formulations, regulations, and challenges of nutraceuticals. CRC Press 2024.

[45] Chopra AS, Lordan R, Horbańczuk OK, *et al.* The current use and evolving landscape of nutraceuticals. Pharmacol Res 2022; 175: 106001. [http://dx.doi.org/10.1016/j.phrs.2021.106001] [PMID: 34826602]

[46] Ghosh S, Jung C, Meyer-Rochow VB. Brief account on the history and conceptual evolution of nutrition security: Past, present and future. Emerging Solutions in Sustainable Food and Nutrition Security. Springer 2023; pp. 1-19. [http://dx.doi.org/10.1007/978-3-031-40908-0_1]

[47] Singh A. Herbal-based nutraceuticals in management of lifestyle diseases: experience from indian population, future. Integr Med 2024; 3: 106-15.

[48] Tallon MJ, Kalman DS. The regulatory challenges of placing dietary ingredients on the european and us market, journal of dietary supplements 2024.

[49] Fantasma F, Samukha V, Saviano G, Chini MG, Iorizzi M, Caprari C. Nutraceutical aspects of selected wild edible plants of the italian central apennines. Nutraceuticals 2024; 4(2): 190-231. [http://dx.doi.org/10.3390/nutraceuticals4020013]

[50] Hernández F, Amanpour A, Soltani M, Lipan L. J.M. GARCÍA GARVÍ, Á.A. Carbonell-Barrachina, E. Sendra Nadal, Comparative study on nutraceutical andsensorial characteristics of saffron (Crocussativus L.) cultivated in Iran, Spain, and Türkiye.2024.

[51] Itagi H, Sartagoda KJD, Pratap V, *et al.* Popped rice with distinct nutraceutical properties. Lebensm Wiss Technol 2023; 173: 114346. [http://dx.doi.org/10.1016/j.lwt.2022.114346]

[52] Fernández-García N, Román-García I, Olmos E. The outlook for latin-american crops: challenges and opportunities. Latin-American Seeds 2023; pp. 91-118. [http://dx.doi.org/10.1201/9781003088424-3]

[53] Gautam SS, Talegaonkar S. Nutraceuticals and their applications, anxiety, gut microbiome, and nutraceuticals: recent trends and clinical evidence. 2023; 1.

[54] Singhal P, Kumar A, Singhal RV, Kumar S. Nutraceuticals: the new anti-aging method. Flavonoids as Nutraceuticals. Apple Academic Press 2024; pp. 1-17. [http://dx.doi.org/10.1201/9781003412441-1]

[55] Jadhav HB, Sablani S, Gogate P, *et al.* Factors governing consumers buying behavior concerning nutraceutical product. Food Sci Nutr 2023; 11(9): 4988-5003. [http://dx.doi.org/10.1002/fsn3.3518] [PMID: 37701202]

[56] Ashraf MV, Khan S, Misri S, *et al.* High-altitude medicinal plants as promising source of phytochemical antioxidants to combat lifestyle-associated oxidative stress-induced disorders. Pharmaceuticals (Basel) 2024; 17(8): 975. [http://dx.doi.org/10.3390/ph17080975] [PMID: 39204080]

[57] Alam MS, Kaur G, Zalpouri R. Current trends and techniques in the nutraceutical industry. Fruits and Their Roles in Nutraceuticals and Functional Foods. CRC Press 2023; pp. 29-68. [http://dx.doi.org/10.1201/9781003259213-2]

[58] Oluwole O, Ibidapo O, Arowosola T, *et al.* Sustainable transformation agenda for enhanced global food and nutrition security: a narrative review. Front Nutr 2023; 10: 1226538. [http://dx.doi.org/10.3389/fnut.2023.1226538] [PMID: 37599683]

[59] Dani VV, Ramesh A, Rishi B. PFoods: selecting a segment for a sustainable product. Emerald Emerging Markets Case Studies 2024; 14(2): 1-25. [http://dx.doi.org/10.1108/EEMCS-10-2023-0380]

[60] Kumar M, Pandey SS, Kumar P, Yadav VK, Shukla AK. Nutraceuticals manufacturing challenges in fast growing food segment in india. Formulations, Regulations, and Challenges of Nutraceuticals. Apple Academic Press 2025; pp. 255-84.

[61] Fernandes FA, Carocho M, Prieto MA, Barros L, Ferreira ICFR, Heleno SA. Nutraceuticals and dietary supplements: balancing out the pros and cons. Food Funct 2024; 15(12): 6289-303. [http://dx.doi.org/10.1039/D4FO01113A] [PMID: 38805010]

[62] Saeed A, Zafar SI. Bioactive nutrients as dietary supplements and therapeutic agents: an introduction to nutraceuticals. Cambridge Scholars Publishing 2024.

[63] Apetroaei MM, Adam-dima I, Belc N, *et al.* Integrating nutraceuticals in the one health framework: A path to holistic health solutions. Farmacia 2024; 72(4): 719-29. [http://dx.doi.org/10.31925/farmacia.2024.4.1]

[64] Santini A, Cammarata SM, Capone G, *et al.* Nutraceuticals: opening the debate for a regulatory

framework. Br J Clin Pharmacol 2018; 84(4): 659-72.
[http://dx.doi.org/10.1111/bcp.13496] [PMID: 29433155]

[65] Sharma M, Ojha K, Singh B, Gupta S, Pandey SK. The role of functional foods and nutraceuticals in disease prevention and health promotion. Eur J Nutr Food Saf 2024; 16(2): 61-83.
[http://dx.doi.org/10.9734/ejnfs/2024/v16i21388]

[66] Puzantian T. Nutraceuticals, dietary, and herbal supplements. Age-Adjusted Psychiatric Treatment for the Older Patient. Springer 2024; pp. 321-31.
[http://dx.doi.org/10.1007/978-3-031-53976-3_18]

[67] Coates PM, Bailey RL, Blumberg JB, *et al.* The evolution of science and regulation of dietary supplements: past, present, and future. J Nutr 2024; 154(8): 2335-45.
[http://dx.doi.org/10.1016/j.tjnut.2024.06.017] [PMID: 38971530]

[68] Zovi A, Vitiello A, Sabbatucci M, *et al.* Food supplements marketed worldwide: a comparative analysis between the european and the us regulatory frameworks. J Diet Suppl 2024; 1-16.
[PMID: 39221704]

[69] Fasakin I, von Massow M. Consumer's preferences and willingness to pay for immune enhanced dairy products in canada. Appetite 2024; 196: 107156.
[http://dx.doi.org/10.1016/j.appet.2023.107156] [PMID: 38103791]

[70] Ali H, Singh SK, Iqbal B, Sharma NK, Ali F, Akbar M. Regulations in canada. Global Regulations of Medicinal, Pharmaceutical, and Food Products. CRC Press 2024; pp. 80-101.

[71] Goyal MR, Chauhan A. Holistic approach of nutrients and traditional natural medicines for human health: a review. Future Integrative Medicine 2024; p. 0.

[72] Singh NK, Katiyar R, Kumari R, Mishra B, Mandal SK, Kumar S. Nutraceutical regulation. Asian Countries, in: Formulations, Regulations, and Challenges of Nutraceuticals. Apple Academic Press 2025; pp. 127-52.

[73] Riar CS, Panesar PS. Bioactive compounds and nutraceuticals from dairy, marine, and nonconventional sources: extraction technology, analytical techniques, and potential health prospects. CRC Press 2024.
[http://dx.doi.org/10.1201/9781003452768]

[74] V.A. Tutelyan, B.P. Sukhanov, A.A. Kochetkova, S.A. Sheveleva, E.A. Smirnova, Chapter 18 - Russian regulations on nutraceuticals and functional foods, in: D.B.T.-N. and F.F.R. in the U.S. and A. the W. (Second E. Bagchi (Ed.), Food Science and Technology, Academic Press, San Diego, 2014: pp. 309–326.
[http://dx.doi.org/10.1016/B978-0-12-405870-5.00018-9]

[75] Dhiman N, Habib M, Jan K, Bashir K, Jan S. Proteins as functional foods and nutraceuticals. Functional Foods and Nutraceuticals: Chemistry, Health Benefits and the Way Forward. Springer 2024; pp. 17-35.
[http://dx.doi.org/10.1007/978-3-031-59365-9_2]

[76] Thammisetty N, Yetukuri K. Insights and compliance challenges for nutraceutical regulations in Indian market. Int J Pharm Sci Drug Res 2024; 273-8.
[http://dx.doi.org/10.25004/IJPSDR.2024.160218]

[77] Razzaq A, Ameen H, Aziz R. Commercializing Asian and Australasian Herbal Medicines: Market Potential and Strategies. Australian Herbal Insight, 2023;6(1), 1-11, 21071.

[78] Duran NM. Biological activities from vegetal products in latin america. Food Byproducts Management and Their Utilization. Apple Academic Press 2024; pp. 313-45.

[79] Fogacci F, ALGhasab NS, Di Micoli V, Giovannini M, Cicero AFG. Cholesterol-lowering bioactive foods and nutraceuticals in pediatrics: clinical evidence of efficacy and safety. Nutrients 2024; 16(10): 1526.
[http://dx.doi.org/10.3390/nu16101526] [PMID: 38794764]

[80] Wu H, Wu Y, Cui Z, Hu L. Nutraceutical delivery systems to improve the bioaccessibility and bioavailability of lycopene: a review. Crit Rev Food Sci Nutr 2024; 64(18): 6361-79.
[http://dx.doi.org/10.1080/10408398.2023.2168249] [PMID: 36655428]

[81] Ranjit P, Harikrishna K, Deepu PG, Reddy KV. Acute and chronic effects of contaminants from food crops. Phytoremediation in Food Safety. CRC Press 2025; pp. 125-37.

[82] Saibijaya Rijal , Mandal PK. A study of nutraceutical prescription pattern among patients in an out-patient setting at Birat medical college teaching Hospital. Magna Scientia Advanced Research and Reviews 2024; 10(1): 330-40.
[http://dx.doi.org/10.30574/msarr.2024.10.1.0034]

[83] Zhao M, Ma J, Li M, *et al.* Cytochrome P450 enzymes and drug metabolism in humans. Int J Mol Sci 2021; 22(23): 12808.
[http://dx.doi.org/10.3390/ijms222312808] [PMID: 34884615]

[84] Mrozek W, Socha J, Sidorowicz K, *et al.* Pathogenesis and treatment of depression: Role of diet in prevention and therapy. Nutrition 2023; 115: 112143.
[http://dx.doi.org/10.1016/j.nut.2023.112143] [PMID: 37562078]

[85] Katoch GK, Nain N, Kaur S, Rasane P, Panesar PS. Hyperlipidemia/obesity crisis: healthy food and lifestyle changes to tackle obesity. The Role of Nutrition in Integral Health and Quality of Life. Apple Academic Press 2024; pp. 271-94.

[86] Balahura AM, Moroi ŞI, Scafa-Udrişte A, *et al.* The management of hypertensive emergencies—is there a "magical" prescription for all? J Clin Med 2022; 11(11): 3138.
[http://dx.doi.org/10.3390/jcm11113138] [PMID: 35683521]

[87] F. Tao, Y. Cai, C. Deng, Z. Chen, Y. Shen, H. Sun, A narrative review on traditional Chinese medicine prescriptions and bioactive components in epilepsy treatment, Annals of Translational Medicine; Vol 11, No 2 (January 31, 2023): Annals of Translational Medicine. (2022). Available from: https://atm.amegroups.org/article/view/106373

[88] Kosović E, Sýkora D, Kuchař M. Stability Study of Cannabidiol in the Form of Solid Powder and Sunflower Oil Solution. Pharmaceutics 2021; 13(3): 412.
[http://dx.doi.org/10.3390/pharmaceutics13030412] [PMID: 33808893]

[89] Abu-Sawwa R, Scutt B, Park Y. Emerging use of epidiolex (cannabidiol) in epilepsy. J Pediatr Pharmacol Ther 2020; 25(6): 485-99.
[http://dx.doi.org/10.5863/1551-6776-25.6.485] [PMID: 32839652]

[90] Pant SP, Joshi S, Bisht D, Bisht M. Exploring the historical, botanical, and taxonomical foundations of cannabis: A review. Cannabis and Derivatives 2024; pp. 3-36.
[http://dx.doi.org/10.1016/B978-0-443-15489-8.00001-3]

[91] Melchert D, Schaare F, Winterhalter P, Beuerle T. CBD products: Labeling accuracy of an obscure niche market. Food Control 2024; 160: 110375.
[http://dx.doi.org/10.1016/j.foodcont.2024.110375]

[92] O'Kennedy N, Raederstorff D, Duttaroy AK. Fruitflow®: the first european food safety authority-approved natural cardio-protective functional ingredient. Eur J Nutr 2017; 56(2): 461-82.
[http://dx.doi.org/10.1007/s00394-016-1265-2] [PMID: 27388464]

[93] K. Musa-Veloso, L. Paulionis, T. Pelipyagina, M. Evans, A Randomized, Double-Blind, Placebo-controlled, multicentre trial of the effects of a shrimp protein hydrolysate on blood pressure., international journal of hypertension. 2019 (2019) 2345042.
[http://dx.doi.org/10.1155/2019/2345042]

[94] MegaNatural(®)-BP grape seed extract and maintenance of normal blood pressure: Evaluation of a health claim pursuant to Article 13(5) of Regulation (EC) No 1924/2006., EFSA Journal. European Food Safety Authority 2021; 19: e06776.
[http://dx.doi.org/10.2903/j.efsa.2021.6776]

[95] AlAli M, Alqubaisy M, Aljaafari MN, *et al.* Nutraceuticals: transformation of conventional foods into health promoters/disease preventers and safety considerations. Molecules 2021; 26(9): 2540. [http://dx.doi.org/10.3390/molecules26092540] [PMID: 33925346]

[96] Puri V, Nagpal M, Singh I, *et al.* A comprehensive review on nutraceuticals: therapy support and formulation challenges. Nutrients 2022; 14(21): 4637. [http://dx.doi.org/10.3390/nu14214637] [PMID: 36364899]

[97] Behl T, Kaur G, Sehgal A, *et al.* Elucidating the multi-targeted role of nutraceuticals: a complementary therapy to starve neurodegenerative diseases. Int J Mol Sci 2021; 22(8): 4045. [http://dx.doi.org/10.3390/ijms22084045] [PMID: 33919895]

[98] Andrew R, Izzo AA. Highlights into the pharmacology of nutraceuticals. Br J Pharmacol 2020; 177(6): 1209-11. [http://dx.doi.org/10.1111/bph.15006] [PMID: 32133625]

[99] Surma S, Sahebkar A, Banach M. Nutrition, nutraceuticals and bioactive compounds in the prevention and fight against inflammation. Nutrients 2023; 15(11): 2629. [http://dx.doi.org/10.3390/nu15112629] [PMID: 37299592]

[100] Siddiqui RA, Moghadasian MH. Nutraceuticals and nutrition supplements: challenges and opportunities. Nutrients 2020; 12(6): 1593. [http://dx.doi.org/10.3390/nu12061593] [PMID: 32485839]

[101] Komala MG, Ong SG, Qadri MU, Elshafie LM, Pollock CA, Saad S. Investigating the regulatory process, safety, efficacy and product transparency for nutraceuticals in the usa, europe and australia. Foods 2023; 12(2): 427. [http://dx.doi.org/10.3390/foods12020427] [PMID: 36673519]

[102] Precup G, Marini E, Zakidou P, *et al.* Novel foods, food enzymes, and food additives derived from food by-products of plant or animal origin: principles and overview of the EFSA safety assessment. Front Nutr 2024; 11: 1390734. [http://dx.doi.org/10.3389/fnut.2024.1390734] [PMID: 38863586]

[103] Osadnik T, Goławski M, Lewandowski P, *et al.* A network meta-analysis on the comparative effect of nutraceuticals on lipid profile in adults. Pharmacol Res 2022; 183: 106402. [http://dx.doi.org/10.1016/j.phrs.2022.106402] [PMID: 35988871]

[104] Schilling JM, Hughes CG, Wallace MS, Sexton M, Backonja M, Moeller-Bertram T. Cannabidiol as a treatment for chronic pain: a survey of patients' perspectives and attitudes. J Pain Res 2021; 14: 1241-50. [http://dx.doi.org/10.2147/JPR.S278718] [PMID: 33981161]

[105] Aguilar-Pérez KM, Ruiz-Pulido G, Medina DI, Parra-Saldivar R, Iqbal HMN. Insight of nanotechnological processing for nano-fortified functional foods and nutraceutical—opportunities, challenges, and future scope in food for better health. Crit Rev Food Sci Nutr 2023; 63(20): 4618-35. [http://dx.doi.org/10.1080/10408398.2021.2004994] [PMID: 34817310]

[106] Ambroselli D, Masciulli F, Romano E, *et al.* New advances in metabolic syndrome, from prevention to treatment: the role of diet and food. Nutrients 2023; 15(3): 640. [http://dx.doi.org/10.3390/nu15030640] [PMID: 36771347]

SUBJECT INDEX

A

B

C

D

E

N

O

P

Q

R

S

T

V

X

Z

www.ingramcontent.com/pod-product-compliance
Lightning Source LLC
LaVergne TN
LVHW070945210926
848482LV00002B/100
* 9 7 9 8 8 9 8 8 1 4 0 1 4 *